2008

THE EVALUATION AND MANAGEMENT STEP

An Auditing Tool

CAROL J. BUCK
MS, CPC, CPC-H, CCS-P
Program Director, Retired
Medical Secretary Programs
Northwest Technical College
East Grand Forks, Minnesota

TECHNICAL RESEARCH ASSISTANTS

Judy B. Breuker, CPC, CCS-P, CHCC, CHBME, ACS, CPC-E/M
Medical Educational Services, LLC
Jenison, Michigan

Jacqueline Klitz Grass, MA, CPC
Business Manager/Reimbursement Coding
The Kidney and Hypertension Center
Grand Forks, North Dakota

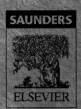

SAUNDERS

ELSEVIER

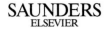

SAUNDERS
ELSEVIER

11830 Westline Industrial Drive
St. Louis, Missouri 63146

THE EVALUATION AND MANAGEMENT STEP:
AN AUDITING TOOL   ISBN: 978-1-4160-3596-1

ISBN: 978-1-4160-3596-1

Publisher: Michael S. Ledbetter
Associate Developmental Editor: Jenna Johnson
Publishing Services Manager: Melissa Lastarria
Project Manager: Mary Pohlman
Senior Designer: Andrea Lutes

Printed in Canada

Last digit is the print number: 9 8 7 6 5 4 3 2 1

Dedication

*To my fellow coders, who endeavor each day to
report services with the greatest precision.
Your dedication
is amazing to behold and is the financial foundation
of our health care system.
Thank you for all you do.*

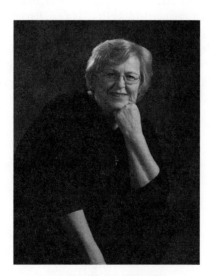

Carol J. Buck

Acknowledgments

There are so many, many people who participated in the development of this text and only through the effort of all the team members has it been possible to publish this text. **Judy Breuker,** who believed in this project from the beginning and was always right there to lend her guidance and knowledge. **Jackie Grass,** who gave unendingly of her technical coding knowledge and provided leadership to this project. **Jody Klitz,** who spent endless hours ensuring that this material was correct. **Joan Wolfgang,** who provided her coding skills and the greatest of determination and who continually demonstrates her caring for students and instructors through collaboration on works such as this text.

   Sally Schrefer, Executive Vice President, Nursing and Health Professions, who possesses great listening skills and the ability to ensure the publication of high-quality educational materials. **Andrew Allen,** Vice President and Publisher, Health Professions, who sees the bigger picture and shares the vision. **Michael Ledbetter,** Publisher, who managed to maintain an excellent sense of humor while jumping into the fray and who is a most valued member of the team. **Josh Rapplean,** Developmental Editor, who has kept us all on track with his exceptional organization skills. **Mary Pohlman,** Project Manager, and **Satyen Vora,** Producer, who both ensured that we all completed our work on time. The employees of Elsevier have participated in the publication of this text and demonstrated the highest levels of professionalism and competence and have my admiration and gratitude for their never-ending patience and desire to produce the highest quality text possible.

Preface

Thank you for purchasing *The Evaluation and Management Step: An Auditing Tool,* the latest resource for evaluation and management coding. This edition has been carefully reviewed and updated with the latest content, making it a current resource. The author and publishers have made every effort to equip you with skills and tools you will need to succeed. To this end, this text presents essential information about the Evaluation and Management codes. No other tool on the market brings together such thorough coverage of the E/M section of the *CPT®* manual in one source.

ORGANIZATION OF THIS TEXTBOOK

Following a basic outline approach, *The Evaluation and Management Step: An Auditing Tool* takes a practical approach to assisting you with your E/M education. The text is divided into three units—E/M, Examinations, and Answers—and there are six appendices for your reference.

Unit I, Evaluation and Management
Provides a review of the categories of the E/M section of the CPT manual.

Unit II, Examinations
Examination 1
Examination 2

Unit III, Answers
Unit I Answers
Examination 1 Answers
Examination 2 Answers

Development of This Edition

This book would not have been possible without a team of educators and professionals, including practicing coders and technical consultants. The combined efforts of the team members have made this text an incredible learning tool.

TEAM LEADER

Jacqueline Klitz Grass, MA, CPC
Business Manager/Reimbursement Coding
The Kidney and Hypertension Center
Grand Forks, North Dakota

TECHNICAL ASSISTANT

Judy B. Breuker, CPC, CCS-P, CHCC, CHBME, ACS, CPC-E/M
Medical Educational Services, LLC
Jenison, Michigan

CODING SPECIALISTS

Jody Klitz, CPC
Coding Reimbursement Specialist
Altru Health System
Grand Forks, North Dakota

Joan E. Wolfgang, BA, CPC, CPC-H
Consultant, Educator, PMCC Certified Instructor
Milwaukee, Wisconsin

Jane A. Tuttle CPC, CCS-P
Owner
Coding Education Endeavors
Westford, Massachusetts

Contents

Unit I   Evaluation and Management, 1

Introduction, 1
E/M Audit Form, 1
E/M Levels, 1
History, 3
Examination, 12
Medical Decision Making (MDM), 13
Counseling, 17
Coordination of Care, 17
Nature of the Presenting Problem, 17
Types of Presenting Problems, 18
Time, 18

E/M Codes, 19
1. Office or Other Outpatient Services (99201-99215), 19
2. Hospital Observation Services (99217-99220), 22
3. Hospital Inpatient Services (99221-99239), 25
4. Consultations (99241-99255), 29
5. Emergency Department Services (99281-99288), 33
6. Pediatric Critical Care Patient Transport (99289-99290), 37
7. Critical Care Services (99291, 99292), 39
8. Inpatient Neonatal and Pediatric Critical Care Services (99293-99300), 43
9. Nursing Facility Services (99304-99318), 45
10. Domiciliary, Rest Home (e.g., Boarding Home), or Custodial Care Services, and Domiciliary, Rest Home (e.g., Assisted Living Facility), or Home Care Plan Oversight Services (99324-99340), 48
11. Home Services (99341-99350), 50
12. Prolonged Services (99354-99360), 53
13. Case Management Services (99363-99368), 58
14. Care Plan Oversight Services (99374-99380), 62
15. Preventive Medicine Services (99381-99429), 64
16. Newborn Care (99431-99440), 67
17. Non-Face-to-Face Physician Services (99441-99444); Special E/M Services (99450-99456); and Other E/M Services (99477-99499), 69

Unit II   Examinations, 71

Examination 1, 71

Examination 2, 85

Unit III   Answers, 99

Unit I Answers, 99

Examination 1 Answers, 125

Examination 2 Answers, 146

Appendix A   **ICD-9-CM Official Guidelines for Coding and Reporting, 169**

Appendix B   **1995 Guidelines for E/M Services, 254**

Appendix C   **1997 Documentation Guidelines for Evaluation and Management Services, 265**

Appendix D   **E/M Audit Form, 296**

Appendix E   **Abbreviations, 303**

Appendix F   **Further Text Resources, 306**

UNIT ■

Evaluation and Management

● INTRODUCTION

E/M AUDIT FORM

Facility may choose to assess E/M services using audit form

Figure 1–1 illustrates an audit form

Designed based on 1995 Guidelines for E/M Services (DG)

    Located in Appendix B of text

Blank audit forms located in Appendix D of this text

You are to complete audit form for cases assigned CPT codes based on key components

Report in Example 1–1 will be used to explain audit form elements

E/M LEVELS

Components that define levels of E/M services

    History (key component)

    Examination (key component)

    Medical decision making (key component)

    Counseling

    Coordination of care

    Nature of presenting problem

    Time

Key components

    History

    Examination

    Medical decision making

HISTORY ELEMENTS	Documented
HISTORY OF PRESENT ILLNESS (HPI)	
1. Location (site on body)	
2. Quality (characteristic: throbbing, sharp)	
3. Severity (1/10 or how intense)	
4. Duration (how long for problem or episode)	
5. Timing (when it occurs)	
6. Context (under what circumstances does it occur)	
7. Modifying factors (what makes it better or worse)	
8. Associated signs and symptoms (what else is happening when it occurs)	
TOTAL	
LEVEL	

REVIEW OF SYSTEMS (ROS)	Documented
1. Constitutional (e.g., weight loss, fever)	
2. Ophthalmologic (eyes)	
3. Otolaryngologic (ears, nose, mouth, throat)	
4. Cardiovascular	
5. Respiratory	
6. Gastrointestinal	
7. Genitourinary	
8. Musculoskeletal	
9. Integumentary (skin and/or breasts)	
10. Neurologic	
11. Psychiatric	
12. Endocrine	
13. Hematologic/Lymphatic	
14. Allergic/Immunologic	
TOTAL	
LEVEL	

PAST, FAMILY, AND/OR SOCIAL HISTORY (PFSH)	Documented
1. Past illness, operations, injuries, treatments, and current medications	
2. Family medical history for heredity and risk	
3. Social activities, both past and present	
TOTAL	
LEVEL	

History Level	1	2	3	4
	Problem Focused	Expanded Problem Focused	Detailed	Comprehensive
HPI	Brief 1-3	Brief 1-3	Extended 4+	Extended 4+
ROS	None	Problem Pertinent	Extended 2-9	Complete 10+
PFSH	None	None	Pertinent 1	Complete 2-3
			HISTORY LEVEL	

EXAMINATION ELEMENTS	Documented
CONSTITUTIONAL	
1. Blood pressure, sitting	
2. Blood pressure, lying	
3. Pulse	
4. Respirations	
5. Temperature	
6. Height	
7. Weight	
8. General appearance	
NUMBER	

BODY AREAS (BA)	Documented
1. Head (including face)	
2. Neck	
3. Chest (including breasts and axillae)	
4. Abdomen	
5. Genitalia, groin, buttocks	
6. Back (including spine)	
7. Each extremity	
NUMBER	

ORGAN SYSTEMS (OS)	Documented
1. Ophthalmologic (eyes)	
2. Otolaryngologic (ears, nose, mouth, throat)	
3. Cardiovascular	
4. Respiratory	
5. Gastrointestinal	
6. Genitourinary	
7. Musculoskeletal	
8. Integumentary	
9. Neurologic	
10. Psychiatric	
11. Hematologic/Lymphatic/Immunologic	
NUMBER	
TOTAL BA/OS	

Exam Level	1	2	3	4
	Problem Focused	Expanded Problem Focused	Detailed	Comprehensive
	Limited to affected BA/OS	Limited to affected BA/OS & other related OSs	Extended of affected BA & other related OSs	General multi-system or complete single OS
# of OS or BA	1	2-7 limited	2-7 extended	8+
		EXAMINATION LEVEL		

MDM ELEMENTS	Documented
# OF DIAGNOSIS/MANAGEMENT OPTIONS	
1. Minimal	
2. Limited	
3. Multiple	
4. Extensive	
LEVEL	

AMOUNT OR COMPLEXITY OF DATA TO REVIEW	Documented
1. Minimal/None	
2. Limited	
3. Moderate	
4. Extensive	
LEVEL	

RISK OF COMPLICATION OR DEATH IF NOT TREATED	Documented
1. Minimal	
2. Low	
3. Moderate	
4. High	
LEVEL	

MDM*	1	2	3	4
	Straightforward	Low	Moderate	High
Number of DX or management options	Minimal	Limited	Multiple	Extensive
Amount or complexity of data	Minimal/None	Limited	Moderate	Extensive
Risks	Minimal	Low	Moderate	High
			MDM LEVEL	

*To qualify for a given type of MDM complexity, 2 of 3 elements in the table must be met or exceeded.

History:

Examination:

MDM:

Number of Key Components:

Code:

Figure **1-1.** E/M audit form based on 1995 Guidelines for E/M Services.

EXAMPLE 1-1

SURGICAL CONSULTATION
(Note: The patient had a gastrointestinal operation four weeks ago, but the report does not clearly indicate that the current obstruction is due to the surgical procedure, therefore, a "complication of surgery" code would not be appropriate in this case.)

LOCATION: Inpatient Hospital
PATIENT: Martin Newwell
PHYSICIAN: Alma Naraquist, M.D.
CONSULTANT: Daniel Olanka, M.D.

HISTORY OF PRESENT ILLNESS: This patient was operated on by Dr. Sanchez approximately 4 weeks ago for a misdiagnosis of appendicitis. He underwent ileocecal resection. He has had a variety of problems in the postoperative period, including renal failure, respiratory failure, tracheostomy, etc. He is currently under the care of Dr. Naraquist and is off the ventilator and breathing through the tracheostomy. He has been intermittently fed through small bowel Cor-Flo tube, but this has the appearance of a bowel obstruction. Dr. Naraquist has asked me to evaluate the patient, and the family has requested that another surgeon get involved in his care, and so I have been tagged to review his case.

PHYSICAL EXAMINATION: On examination, the patient is resting comfortably in bed. He does have a tracheostomy in place. He is alert and does respond. The chest is clear to auscultation. There is a catheter in place for dialysis, although the patient is not currently on dialysis. The abdomen is markedly distended. It is tympanitic. Tinkling bowel sounds are heard. There are no rushes. The midline scar is well healed. There is no particular focal tenderness, and no hernias are appreciated.

Review of the patient's films shows marked dilatation of the small bowel. Review of the CT scan shows marked dilatation of the small bowel with what appears to be a transition zone in the distal ileum. The colon is deflated.

DISCUSSION: By physical examination, this patient has chronic bowel obstruction, at least partial in nature. Certainly his x-rays support that there is a major problem intra-abdominally. My recommendation would be that the patient should be considered for re-exploration for bowel obstruction. I do not know whether the problem is at the anastomosis or near the anastomosis. I think patient would benefit from some total parenteral nutrition (TPN) and aggressive hydration over the next few days, and then we will plan to take him to the operating room next week.

HISTORY

Complete history has four components

Chief Complaint (CC)

Brief summary describing reason for encounter

   Usually in patient's own words

   Required at all E/M levels

Includes

    Symptom

    Problem

    Condition

    Diagnosis

    Physician's recommendations

    Any other significant factors

In Example 1–1

    CC is obstruction of intestine

History of the Present Illness (HPI)

Description of current problem

Described in order in which symptoms

    Occurred

    Have occurred since the previous encounter

Must be documented in medical record by physician

HPI elements

    Location

        Site on body (e.g., arm, leg, neck)

    Quality

        Patient's description of problem (e.g., dull, constant, throbbing)

    Severity

        Patient's description concerning pain caliber (1-10 scale or how intense)

    Duration

        Length of time patient has experienced symptom or episode

    Timing

        When problem is experienced (e.g., morning, noon, when lying down) or when started

    Context

        Under what circumstances does it occur (e.g., bending, standing)

    Modifying factors

        Actions patient used to treat symptoms (e.g., aspirin, antacids, heat)

    Associated signs and symptoms

        What else is happening when it occurs (e.g., stress or incontinence)

Two levels of HPI

    Brief, 1-3 elements

        Problem focused and extended problem focused

    Extended, 4+ elements

        Detailed and comprehensive

In Example 1–1, the HPI elements **(Figure 1–2)** are:
Location (abdomen)
Duration (4 weeks)
Associated signs and symptoms (renal failure, respiratory failure)
Modifying factors (tracheostomy, feeding tube)
Level: 4 elements = extended (detailed level)

The level is the same whether using either the 1995 or 1997 Documentation Guidelines

HISTORY ELEMENTS	Documented
HISTORY OF PRESENT ILLNESS (HPI)	
1. Location (site on body)	✗
2. Quality (characteristic: throbbing, sharp)	
3. Severity (1/10 or how intense)	
4. Duration (how long for problem or episode)	✗
5. Timing (when it occurs)	
6. Context (under what circumstances does it occur)	
7. Modifying factors (what makes it better or worse)	✗
8. Associated signs and symptoms (what else is happening when it occurs)	✗
TOTAL	4
LEVEL	4

Figure **1–2.** HPI Elements.

Review of Systems (ROS)

Used to identify subjective symptoms that the patient

Deemed unimportant

Neglected to mention

May be obtained from

Questionnaire completed by patient or ancillary staff

To qualify, physician must evaluate and document in medical record

ROS aids in

Defining problem(s)

Clarifying differential diagnoses

Identifying tests useful for diagnosis

Providing physician broader knowledge of patient

Assisting physician in decision regarding management options

Three types of ROS

Problem Pertinent

Inquiry about system directly identified in HPI

Patient's positive/negative responses must be documented in medical record

Extended

Inquiry about system directly related to problems identified in HPI, 2-9 related body systems

Patient's positive/negative responses must be documented in medical record

Complete

Inquiry about the system identified in HPI and all other systems

CPT recognizes the following for an ROS

Constitutional factors

Blood pressure (lying)

Blood pressure (sitting)

Pulse

Respiration

Temperature

Height

Weight

General appearance

Organ systems (OSs)

Ophthalmologic (eyes)

Otolaryngologic (ears, nose, mouth, throat)

Cardiovascular

Respiratory

Gastrointestinal

Genitourinary

Musculoskeletal

Integumentary (skin and/or breast)

Neurological

Psychiatric

Endocrine

Hematologic/Lymphatic

Allergic/Immunologic

In Example 1-1, there were no ROS elements
 With no elements, this is a problem focused ROS
 See **Figure 1-3** for completed ROS portion of audit form

Note: The level of ROS is the same whether using the 1995 or 1997 DGs

REVIEW OF SYSTEMS (ROS)	Documented
1. Constitutional (e.g., weight loss, fever)	
2. Ophthalmologic (eyes)	
3. Otolaryngologic (ears, nose, mouth, throat)	
4. Cardiovascular	
5. Respiratory	
6. Gastrointestinal	
7. Genitourinary	
8. Musculoskeletal	
9. Integumentary (skin and/or breasts)	
10. Neurologic	
11. Psychiatric	
12. Endocrine	
13. Hematologic/Lymphatic	
14. Allergic/Immunologic	
TOTAL	0
LEVEL	I

Figure **1–3.** ROS Elements.

Past, Family, and/or Social History (PFSH)

Past History

Catalogues patient's medical history

All-inclusive record of

Past illnesses

Operations

Injuries

Treatments

Specific information

Prior

Major illnesses

Injuries

Operations

Hospitalizations

Current medication(s)

Allergies (e.g., related to drug or food)

Age-appropriate

Immunization

Feeding

Dietary status

Family History

Identifies medical events within patient's family

Focuses on health issues of

Parents

Siblings

Children

Specific information

    Causes of death

        Parents

        Siblings

        Children

    Specific diseases shared by family members pertaining to

        CC

        HPI

        System review

    Potential risk factors for the patient

        Commonly identified with hereditary diseases

Social History

    Focuses on vital age-appropriate relevant information

    Specific information

        Marital status

        Current living arrangements

        Current employment and occupational history

        Use of drugs, alcohol, tobacco

        Sexual history

        Any other socially relevant factors

In Example 1–1, there were no PFSH elements
   No elements assigned: This is an expanded problem focused PFSH
   See **Figure 1–4** for the audit form with the PFSH portion completed

Note: The level of PFSH is the same whether using the 1995 or 1997 Documentation Guidelines

---

Four History Levels

Based on amount of data gathered

Clinical judgment of physician determines extent of history

PAST, FAMILY, AND/OR SOCIAL HISTORY (PFSH)		Documented
1. Past illness, operations, injuries, treatments, and current medications		
2. Family medical history for heredity and risk		
3. Social activities, both past and present		
	TOTAL	0
	LEVEL	2

Figure **1-4.** PFSH Elements.

Problem Focused

Centers on CC

Brief history of present illness/problem (1-3 elements)

Reviews pertinent information of CC in terms of

Severity

Duration

Symptoms

Does not include a PFSH or ROS

Expanded Problem Focused

Focused on CC

Brief history of present illness/problem (1-3 elements)

Review of organ system associated with CC

Detailed

CC

Extended HPI

Pertinent system review (4+ elements)

Related systems reviewed

Documentation shows positive and negative responses regarding multiple organ systems (total of 2-9 systems reviewed)

Pertinent PFSH

Related to CC

Comprehensive

CC

Extended HPI (4+ elements)

Review of all body systems (at least 10)

Complete PFSH

In Example 1–1, the following elements were present:
HPI:	Detailed
ROS:	Problem focused
PFSH:	Expanded problem focused
Level:	Problem focused

See **Figure 1–5** for the audit form with the History level assigned

---

History Level	1	2	3	4
	Problem Focused	Expanded Problem Focused	Detailed	Comprehensive
HPI	Brief 1-3	Brief 1-3	Extended 4+	Extended 4+
ROS	None	Problem Pertinent	Extended 2-9	Complete 10+
PFSH	None	None	Pertinent 1	Complete 2-3
			HISTORY LEVEL	1

Figure **1–5.** History level assigned.

Requirements for History Levels

Problem-Focused History

1-3 HPI elements

No ROS

No PFSH

Expanded Problem-Focused History

1-3 HPI elements

Problem-pertinent ROS (1 system)

No PFSH

Detailed History

4+ HPI elements

   Status of each condition must be reported by patient

Extended ROS

   2-9 ROS systems

Problem-pertinent PFSH

   1-2 history elements

Comprehensive History

4+ HPI elements

   Status of each condition must be reported by patient

Comprehensive ROS (10+ systems)

Complete PFSH

To qualify for a given level of history, all elements must be met

---

Additional Guidelines for Documenting History

CC, ROS, and PFSH may be listed separately or included in HPI

If during a previous encounter a ROS and/or PFSH has been recorded

   The ROS and/or PFSH does not need to be re-recorded

   Physician must indicate review of ROS and/or PFSH and any updates

Questionnaire completed by ancillary staff or patient considered valid for ROS and/or PFSH if

   Physician review is documented in medical record

If patient or other source is unable to provide history

   Medical record must describe patient's condition or circumstance

   Document the reason for patient/other source not providing HPI

Another Example of History Level

CC: Right elbow pain

HPI: The patient is a 44-year-old female who states she has had worsening pain in her right elbow (location) for 2 weeks (duration). The pain is described as stabbing (quality) and is worse after knitting (context). She experiences some relief with ice and acetaminophen (modifying factors).

ROS: Constitutional: No fevers or weight change within the past 3 months

   Musculoskeletal: Negative for muscle or joint pain

   Skin: No rashes, complains of mild dryness

PFSH: Positive for hyperthyroidism (past history) which is controlled with Synthroid (medication)

History Level

HPI elements: 5 equal an extended HPI

   Location (right elbow)

   Duration (2 weeks)

   Quality (stabbing)

   Context (knitting)

   Modifying factors (ice, acetaminophen)

ROS: 3 meets the requirements of a detailed ROS

   Constitutional

   Musculoskeletal

   Skin (integumentary)

PFSH: 1 meets pertinent PFSH

   Past history revealed a thyroid condition controlled with medication

   No mention of a family or social history

Detailed history includes

   Extended HPI

      4 or more elements

      Or status of 3 or more chronic and/or inactive conditions

   Extended ROS

      2-9 systems

   Pertinent PFSH

      1 element

Case report meets requirements of a detailed history with

   Extended HPI

   Extended ROS

   Pertinent PFSH

Note: The level of History level is the same whether using the 1995 or 1997 Documentation Guidelines

---

EXAMINATION

Objective portion of the encounter

Performed by the medical provider

Level of examination based on clinical judgment and nature of the presenting problem(s)

Examination Levels

Problem Focused

Limited to affected body area (BA)/organ system (OS) identified by CC

1 BA/OS

Expanded Problem Focused

Limited examination of BA(s) or OS(s) identified by CC and other related BA(s)/OS(s)

2-7 BA/OS

Detailed

Extended examination of affected BA(s) or OS(s) and other symptomatic or related OS(s)

2-7 BA/OS

Comprehensive

General multisystem examination OR complete examination of single organ system

8+ OS

FROM EXAMPLE 1–1

PHYSICAL EXAMINATION:
On examination, the patient is resting comfortably in bed. He does have a tracheostomy in place. He is alert and does respond. The chest is clear to auscultation. There is a catheter in place for dialysis, although the patient is not currently on dialysis. The abdomen is markedly distended. It is tympanitic. Tinkling bowel sounds are heard. There are no rushes. The midline scar is well healed. There is no particular focal tenderness, and no hernias are appreciated.

Review of the patient's films shows marked dilatation of the small bowel. Review of the CT scan shows marked dilatation of the small bowel with what appears to be a transition zone in the distal ileum. The colon is deflated.

In Example 1–1, using the 1995 Documentation Guidelines, the physical examination includes 1 constitutional element (general appearance, resting comfortably, tracheostomy in place, alert, does respond), for 1 OS. There was 1 BA: abdomen (marked distention). There are 4 OSs examined: respiratory (clear to auscultation), genitourinary (catheter in place), gastrointestinal (tympanitic, tinkling bowel sounds), integumentary (midline scar is well-healed), for a total of 6 BAs/OSs. This is a level 2 expanded problem-focused examination. See **Figure 1–6** for completed audit form for the examination portion of the audit form.

EXAMINATION ELEMENTS				Documented
CONSTITUTIONAL				
1. Blood pressure, sitting				
2. Blood pressure, lying				
3. Pulse				
4. Respirations				
5. Temperature				
6. Height				
7. Weight				
8. General appearance				✗
			NUMBER	I
BODY AREAS (BA)				Documented
1. Head (including face)				
2. Neck				
3. Chest (including breasts and axillae)				
4. Abdomen				✗
5. Genitalia, groin, buttocks				
6. Back (including spine)				
7. Each extremity				
			NUMBER	I
ORGAN SYSTEMS (OS)				Documented
1. Ophthalmologic (eyes)				
2. Otolaryngologic (ears, nose, mouth, throat)				
3. Cardiovascular				
4. Respiratory				✗
5. Gastrointestinal				✗
6. Genitourinary				✗
7. Musculoskeletal				
8. Integumentary				✗
9. Neurologic				
10. Psychiatric				
11. Hematologic/Lymphatic/Immunologic				
			NUMBER	4
			TOTAL BA/OS	6

Exam Level	1	2	3	4
	Problem Focused	Expanded Problem Focused	Detailed	Comprehensive
	Limited to affected BA/OS	Limited to affected BA/OS & other related OSs	Extended of affected BA & other related OSs	General multi-system or complete single OS
# of OS or BA	1	2-7 limited	2-7 extended	8+
			EXAMINATION LEVEL	2

Figure **1-6.** Examination portion of audit form.

MEDICAL DECISION MAKING (MDM)

Complexity of MDM addresses the complications involved in

Establishing a diagnosis and/or

Selecting a management option(s)

Factors in MDM Process

Number of possible diagnoses and/or management options

Information from medical records, diagnostic tests, and other relevant information must be

Obtained

Reviewed

Analyzed

Factors associated with patient's presenting problem, the diagnostic procedures, and the possible management options

Risk of significant complications

Morbidity

Mortality

Comorbidities

Four Types of MDM

2 of 3 elements must be met or exceeded to assign the level

Straightforward decision making involves

Minimal number of diagnoses or management options

Data and/or complexity of data is minimal or nonexistent

The complications and risk of morbidity are minimal

Low-complexity decision making involves

Limited management options

Data limited in scope and complexity

Low risk of morbidity

Moderate-complexity decision making involves

Multiple diagnoses and management options available

Moderate amount of data and complexities

Moderate risk of complications and/or morbidity

High-complexity decision making involves

Extensive management options and diagnoses

Extensive amount and complexity of data

High risk of complications and/or morbidity

Guidelines used to document management options

Each encounter requires documentation that is explicitly stated or implied, and describes an assessment, clinical impression, or diagnoses

For a presenting problem **WITH** an established diagnoses, the documentation must indicate the problem is either

Improved, well controlled, resolving, or resolved

OR

Inadequately controlled, worsening or failing to change

For a presenting problem **WITHOUT** an established diagnosis, the assessment is recorded in the context of a differential diagnosis

Commonly used terms are

Possible

Probable

Rule out

Any initiation of or change in a treatment must be documented

Changes in management options include those in

Either patient or nursing care instructions

Any therapies

Medication usage changes

MDM ELEMENTS				Documented
# OF DIAGNOSIS/MANAGEMENT OPTIONS				
1. Minimal				
2. Limited				
3. Multiple				
4. Extensive				✗
			LEVEL	4
AMOUNT OR COMPLEXITY OF DATA TO REVIEW				Documented
1. Minimal/None				✗
2. Limited				
3. Moderate				
4. Extensive				
			LEVEL	I
RISK OF COMPLICATION OR DEATH IF NOT TREATED				Documented
1. Minimal				
2. Low				
3. Moderate				
4. High				✗
			LEVEL	4
MDM*	I	2	3	4
	Straightforward	Low	Moderate	High
Number of DX or management options	Minimal	Limited	Multiple	Extensive
Amount or complexity of data	Minimal/None	Limited	Moderate	Extensive
Risks	Minimal	Low	Moderate	High
			MDM LEVEL	4

*To qualify for a given type of MDM complexity, 2 of 3 elements in the table must be met or exceeded.

Figure **1–7.** Medical decision making portion of audit form.

When a referral is made, documentation must show the following

Consultation(s) requested or advice that has been sought

To whom or where the request has been made

The origination of the request

In Example 1–1, using the 1995 Documentation Guidelines, the MDM includes extensive diagnosis and management options, minimal data, and high risk to the patient. The patient does have a chronic condition (chronic bowel obstruction), is breathing through a tracheostomy, and is going to have another major surgery at a time when he is not yet recovered from his prior surgery. This would indicate a high risk.

See **Figure 1–7** with the audit form completed and with the Medical Decision Making portion of the form completed.

When considering all levels on this case, when using the 1995 Documentation Guidelines, (See **Figure 1–8** for completed form), the level on this code is 99251 based on that history element.

HISTORY ELEMENTS				Documented
HISTORY OF PRESENT ILLNESS (HPI)				
1. Location (site on body)				✗
2. Quality (characteristic: throbbing, sharp)				
3. Severity (1/10 or how intense)				
4. Duration (how long for problem or episode)				✗
5. Timing (when it occurs)				
6. Context (under what circumstances does it occur)				
7. Modifying factors (what makes it better or worse)				✗
8. Associated signs and symptoms (what else is happening when it occurs)				✗
			TOTAL	4
			LEVEL	4

REVIEW OF SYSTEMS (ROS)				Documented
1. Constitutional (e.g., weight loss, fever)				
2. Ophthalmologic (eyes)				
3. Otolaryngologic (ears, nose, mouth, throat)				
4. Cardiovascular				
5. Respiratory				
6. Gastrointestinal				
7. Genitourinary				
8. Musculoskeletal				
9. Integumentary (skin and/or breasts)				
10. Neurologic				
11. Psychiatric				
12. Endocrine				
13. Hematologic/Lymphatic				
14. Allergic/Immunologic				
			TOTAL	0
			LEVEL	1

PAST, FAMILY, AND/OR SOCIAL HISTORY (PFSH)				Documented
1. Past illness, operations, injuries, treatments, and current medications				
2. Family medical history for heredity and risk				
3. Social activities, both past and present				
			TOTAL	0
			LEVEL	2

History Level	1	2	3	4
	Problem Focused	Expanded Problem Focused	Detailed	Comprehensive
HPI	Brief 1-3	Brief 1-3	Extended 4+	Extended 4+
ROS	None	Problem Pertinent	Extended 2-9	Complete 10+
PFSH	None	None	Pertinent 1	Complete 2-3
			HISTORY LEVEL	1

EXAMINATION ELEMENTS	Documented
CONSTITUTIONAL	
1. Blood pressure, sitting	
2. Blood pressure, lying	
3. Pulse	
4. Respirations	
5. Temperature	
6. Height	
7. Weight	
8. General appearance	✗
NUMBER	1

BODY AREAS (BA)	Documented
1. Head (including face)	
2. Neck	
3. Chest (including breasts and axillae)	
4. Abdomen	
5. Genitalia, groin, buttocks	
6. Back (including spine)	
7. Each extremity	
NUMBER	0

ORGAN SYSTEMS (OS)	Documented
1. Ophthalmologic (eyes)	
2. Otolaryngologic (ears, nose, mouth, throat)	
3. Cardiovascular	
4. Respiratory	✗
5. Gastrointestinal	✗
6. Genitourinary	✗
7. Musculoskeletal	
8. Integumentary	✗
9. Neurologic	
10. Psychiatric	
11. Hematologic/Lymphatic/Immunologic	
NUMBER	4
TOTAL BA/OS	6

Exam Level	1	2	3	4
	Problem Focused	Expanded Problem Focused	Detailed	Comprehensive
	Limited to affected BA/OS	Limited to affected BA/OS & other related OSs	Extended of affected BA & other related OSs	General multi-system or complete single OS
# of OS or BA	1	2-7 limited	2-7 extended	8+
			EXAMINATION LEVEL	2

MDM ELEMENTS				Documented
# OF DIAGNOSIS/MANAGEMENT OPTIONS				
1. Minimal				
2. Limited				
3. Multiple				
4. Extensive				✗
			LEVEL	4
AMOUNT OR COMPLEXITY OF DATA TO REVIEW				Documented
1. Minimal/None				✗
2. Limited				
3. Moderate				
4. Extensive				
			LEVEL	1
RISK OF COMPLICATION OR DEATH IF NOT TREATED				Documented
1. Minimal				
2. Low				
3. Moderate				
4. High				✗
			LEVEL	4

MDM*	1	2	3	4
	Straightforward	Low	Moderate	High
Number of DX or management options	Minimal	Limited	Multiple	Extensive
Amount or complexity of data	Minimal/None	Limited	Moderate	Extensive
Risks	Minimal	Low	Moderate	High
			MDM LEVEL	4

*To qualify for a given type of MDM complexity, 2 of 3 elements in the table must be met or exceeded.

History: Problem Focused
Examination: Expanded Problem Focused
MDM: High

Number of Key Components: 3 of 3

99251

Figure **1–8.** Completed audit form for Example 1–1.

COUNSELING

Some aspect of counseling will usually take place during physician-patient encounters

One or more of following items are present in discussion with patient, family members, and/or caregivers

Diagnostic results, impressions, and/or recommended diagnostic studies

Prognosis of CC

Management options presented with

Potential risks and/or benefits

Instructions given for

Treatment of the CC

Follow-up directions

Communication explaining importance of patient following through with management/treatment option(s)

Discussion of risk factor reduction

Education (patient and/or family) regarding the physician's clinical judgment(s)

COORDINATION OF CARE

Physician makes arrangements to provide the patient with additional services from other agencies or healthcare providers

NATURE OF THE PRESENTING PROBLEM

Actual CC/situation for which physician makes a clinical judgment concerning appropriate level of care to diagnose and treat patient

Medical record should include physician's observations regarding the level of care determined necessary to diagnose and treat patient

CPT describes the present problem by using the following terms

Disease

Condition

Illness

Injury

Symptom

Sign

Findings

Complaints

A diagnosis need not be made during the physician-patient encounter for these terms to be used

TYPES OF PRESENTING PROBLEMS

Minimal

May/may not require the presence of physician

Service provided must be done under the physician's supervision

    Example: Blood pressure readings, dressing changes

Self-Limited

Also known as minor presenting problem

Problem

    Follows normal course

    Is transient, and

    Does not permanently alter patient's health status

Good prognosis possible with proper management and compliance

Low Severity

Risk of morbidity without treatment is minimal

Full recovery is likely

No indication of future health impairment

Moderate Severity

Risk of morbidity without treatment exists

Prognosis uncertain

Possibility of future impairment exists

High Severity

Risk of morbidity without treatment is very high/extremely likely

Moderate to high risk/morbidity

Presenting problem in which severe, prolonged, and functional impairment is highly probable

TIME

"Time" in E/M code description is not meant to be precise measurement tool

Estimated amount of time based on the average physician-patient encounter

Used to aid in determining level of service

Three Measures of Time

Direct Face-to-Face Time

Describes office visits, outpatient visits, and office consultations

Refers to the time the physician actually spends in the presence of patient and/or family and/or other caregivers

Typical face-to-face time includes obtaining history and performing examination of patient and counseling

Non Face-to-Face Time

Time spent by physician before/after encounter

While this information is not specifically addressed with E/M codes, it is factored in calculations of time based upon physician's surveys

Face-to-face time stated in E/M codes reflects the physician's work before, during, and after physician-patient encounter

Unit/Floor Time

Time spent by physician at the hospital unit

Time the physician provides direct bedside services to patient

Further Time

Intra-service time is face-to-face time during which the physician

Reviews the patient chart

Conducts the examination

Engages in discussion with other professionals concerning patient

Communicating with patient's family and/or caregivers

Time is not a descriptive element to be used when evaluating emergency department services due to the difficulties involving the physician's multiple encounters with a variety of patients. Time is not considered in the selection of E/M codes unless it specifically addresses counseling/coordinating care.

Most important question to answer with time in E/M codes:

Did the counseling or coordination of care comprise more than 50% of the visit?

If counseling or coordination of care did not comprise 50% or more of the visit, then the level of service selected would be based on the level of history, examination, and MDM

● E/M CODES

1. OFFICE OR OTHER OUTPATIENT SERVICES (99201-99215)

Two subcategories of problem-focused patients

New patient is one who has

Never had health care services provided by the physician or anyone in the same group or specialty

Not sought care from either the physician or someone in the same group or specialty for at least 3 years

Established patient is one who has

Received services within the last 3 years from the physician or from another physician of the same specialty in the same group

Criteria that must be documented in the medical record as having been met or exceeded

New patient

3 of 3 key components must be met or exceeded

Established patient

2 of 3 key components must be met or exceeded

Note: These codes should never be used to report "annual physicals" or "well-child" visits

Patients receiving care are considered to be outpatients unless admitted to a health care facility

If directly admitted to a health care facility during the course of physician/patient encounter

Services performed by physician are considered part of initial hospital care service when all records have same date

Initial office visit would not be reported

Bundled into initial hospital care code

Admitting physician must record all services related to admission

Including those that occurred prior to admission when services were same date as the admission

PRACTICE 1, OFFICE OR OTHER OUTPATIENT SERVICES

Now it is time to put this information to practice by coding two reports. The first report is multiple choice and you are to select the correct choice to report the services provided and diagnosis(es) documented in the report.

The second report is fill-in-the-blank in which you assign the CPT service and ICD-9-CM diagnosis codes. Be certain to complete an audit form for each of the fill-in-the-blank reports in which the code selection is based on key components.

Once you have coded the two cases, check your answers in Unit III of this text, where you will locate the answers and rationales.

Practice 1, Report A

LOCATION: Outpatient Clinic

Brooke is a 7-year-old established patient who presents to the clinic today with a cough that she has had for more than a week. It is definitely worse at night; however, it is there all the time. It is quite harsh and she is having productive green sputum. She has had a low-grade temperature and has not really felt very well.

PHYSICAL EXAMINATION reveals both tympanic membranes are normal. Her nose is clear. Throat is clear. Lungs are really coarse in both bases. There is an occasional wheeze. Heart has a normal sinus rhythm without murmur.

IMPRESSION: Bronchitis.
We gave her a prescription for Zithromax Z-Pak liquid 200 mg/5 cc two teaspoons today and then one teaspoon daily for the following four days. We will see how she does. If she has difficulty next week, we will recheck her.

A. 99212, 490

B. 99213, 490, 786.2

C. 99213, 490

D. 99202, 490

Practice 1, Report B

LOCATION: Outpatient, Clinic

NOTE: Start Augmentin. Stat CT of abd/pelvis.
This is a woman well known to me 4 months status post open cholecystectomy for gallstone pancreatitis. She had some fevers and gastrointestinal pain. CT scan of the abdomen shows a persistent pseudocyst. No hydronephrosis gross abscess. She looks better today. Her abdomen is soft.

ASSESSMENT AND PLAN: A 44-year-old woman with gallstone pancreatitis and abdominal pain. CT scan showing pseudocysts, but no frank abscess. I will have her continue her Augmentin and I would like to see her again in one week.

Codes:_____

2. HOSPITAL OBSERVATION SERVICES (99217-99220)

Purpose of patient observation is to determine the severity of patient's condition

Patient's illness does not meet acute inpatient criteria

Codes apply to either new or established patients

All codes are based on level of services provided

All codes require 3 of 3 key components be met

When patient status changes from observation status to inpatient status on the same date, the observation is not reported separately

Rather bundled into initial hospital admission service

Codes do not apply to post-surgery care (RPPR = Routine post procedure recovery)

That care is part of surgical package and not reported separately

Two subcategories of codes

Observation Care Discharge Services

Initial Observation Care

PRACTICE 2, HOSPITAL OBSERVATION SERVICES

Once you have coded the two cases, check your answers in Unit III of this text, where you will locate the answers and rationales.

Practice 2, Report A

LOCATION: Outpatient, Hospital

REASON FOR ADMISSION: Hyperglycemia.

HISTORY OF PRESENT ILLNESS: The patient is well-known to me. He has end-stage renal disease and is on CAPD. I was called by his daughter last night informing me that a couple of days ago he was driving in bad weather and he went in the ditch. There have been lots of problems at his home with his wife and the daughter was worried about him and was wondering if he needs to be committed. I was called by the emergency room staff for guidance. His son-in-law brought him to the emergency room. At that time, the patient was seen by the emergency physician and myself. He seemed to have been oriented x 3 without any focal neurological deficits and vital signs were stable. He had some edema in the lower extremities but he was walking and talking. His STATs were maintained. His PO2 was 65. His chest x-ray showed bilateral infiltrates which seemed to be getting better. His blood sugar was 895 and a couple of hours later went up to 1,468. Magnesium was 1.3 and phosphorus was 6.2.

His white count was only 11,000. Hemoglobin was 9.5. He had some metamyelocytes and myelocytes in his differential with eosinophilia.

After long discussions with the patient and his son-in-law, we convinced him to be admitted for observation to control his sugar at least and be discharged the next morning. I also found out yesterday that he had an M-spike on serum protein electrophoresis suggestive of a multiple myeloma. This was ordered because of elevated protein and low albumin in addition to an episode of hypercalcemia.

He has not been compliant with his medications and probably more ignorant of how to manage insulin rather than compliance issues. He had some personality changes over the past 2 months.

The patient expressed sorrow and he was depressed and cried a couple of times in the emergency room and was concerned about the situation at home. He was not suicidal at the time I saw him in the emergency room. Obviously, his sugar was elevated because he did not take his insulin all day and was eating cookies and candy all the day, in addition to his peritoneal dialysis fluid.

Finally, the patient agreed to be admitted for observation. His sugar will be controlled with 20 units of regular insulin IV and insulin drip and he will be discharged in the morning.

Because of chronic cough and the infiltrates, he is scheduled to have CT scan next week. I will have to also schedule him to see our hematologist/oncologist to do a bone marrow aspiration and biopsy.

A. 99220, 250.82, 585.6, 786.2, 793.1, 790.99

B. 99218, 99354, 99355 ×3, 250.82, 585.6, 786.2, 793.1, 790.99

C. 99218, 250.82, 585.6, 790.99

D. 99218, 250.82, 585.6, 786.2, 793.1, 790.99

Practice 2, Report B

LOCATION: Outpatient, Hospital (Observation status)

DIAGNOSES:
1. Chronic renal failure secondary to renovascular disease.
2. Renovascular disease.
3. Right-sided renal artery stent re-stenosis post angioplasty and placement of new stent by interventional radiology.
4. Anemia secondary to peri-procedure bleeding without evidence of hematomas.
5. Longstanding hypertension.
6. Hypotension secondary to angioplasty and stent placement of the right renal artery and peri-procedure bleeding.

HOSPITAL COURSE: The patient is an 87-year-old female known to have chronic renal failure and renovascular disease with right-sided renal artery stenosis with previous in-stent restenosis. She had her procedure done on the day of admission. She had blood pressure of 70 systolic afterwards with some peri-procedure bleeding at the site in the right inguinal area but she did not seem to have any hematoma. She was asymptomatic with her low blood pressure. Her antihypertensive medications were held. The patient was given IV fluids. Her hemoglobin was monitored. She was around 8.8 to 9.3 grams.

On the day of discharge her hemoglobin was 8.8. Her creatinine has come down to 1.4 with a BUN of 31, sodium of 143, chloride of 117, bicarb of 21.1, and glucose of 94.

The patient was asymptomatic on the day of discharge and she was discharged in good general condition.

Code Level I.

DISCHARGE PLAN:
1. The patient will not be on any antihypertensive medications at least until I see her again next week. Altace and Toprol both will be on hold.
2. Return to clinic next week with basic panel and CBC before her appointment.
3. I have advised her to contact me immediately if she has dizzy spells or if she has any questions or any problems. She knows how to contact me.

Codes:_____

3. HOSPITAL INPATIENT SERVICES (99221-99239)

Attending physician is one who is

Qualified on the basis of education and training and has staff membership/appointment and is therefore

Qualified to oversee patient care

Authorized to order/perform therapeutic/diagnostic procedures

Codes apply to patients officially admitted into the hospital

Key components of history, examination, and MDM determine code assignment

Subcategories

Initial Hospital Care

Codes only used by admitting physician

Any service performed by physician in a setting other than the hospital on the day the patient was admitted is considered when assigning admission code

Requires 3 of 3 key components be met

Subsequent Hospital Care

Codes apply to services rendered to patient after admission date

Requires 2 of 3 key components be met

History component in this subcategory reflects any new information that has been recorded in interval since most recent physician/patient encounter

Three levels of service are recognized

When the patient demonstrates improvement

When the patient has experienced a relatively minor complication or is not responding to current therapy as desired

When patient is significantly unstable or has developed either serious complications or new problem(s)

These codes can be used by physicians other than admitting physicians when physician provides a different services from the admitting physician on the same day

Hospital Discharge Services

Apply to time spent by attending physician when discharging the patient

Time based codes

Two levels

30 minutes or less, and more than 30 minutes

Include following services when applicable

Final patient examination

Discussion about patient's hospital stay

Discussion with the family and/or caregiver regarding continuing care

Paperwork for discharge records

Prescriptions

Referral forms

Patient is deceased and the above mentioned services were provided

PRACTICE 3, HOSPITAL INPATIENT SERVICES

Once you have coded the two cases, check your answers in Unit III of this text.
The answers, written rationales, and completed audit forms are located in Unit III.

Practice 3, Report A

LOCATION: Inpatient, Hospital

CHIEF COMPLAINT: Extreme shortness of breath for the last 8-10 days.

HISTORY OF PRESENT ILLNESS: Lewis is a 33-year-old white male, well known to me, who came to the office this morning and was sent directly to the hospital with a complaint of progressively worsening shortness of breath for the last 10 days. It has gotten to the point he cannot even walk from the house to the mailbox without having to stop to catch his breath. He even gets short of breath while changing his clothes or during routine activities inside the house. He even gets short of breath while just sitting and talking. He denies any productive cough, fever, chest pains, or any other problems. His symptoms are mainly located in the chest, all the time. He describes it as tightness around his chest and he has difficultly breathing. Exertion makes it worse, rest makes it feel better. He rates it as a 8-9/10. It has been going on for the last 10 days and the only associated signs and symptoms are decreased exercise tolerance and some dry cough.

REVIEW OF SYSTEMS: CONSTITUTIONAL: As noted above, no fever. Also denies change of weight. HEENT: He denies any blurry vision or discharge. He denies any earaches, runny nose, or sore throat. HEMATOLOGY: He denies any bleeding from any site. Denies unusual bruising. CARDIAC: he denies any chest pain or palpitations. RESPIRATORY: He is complaining of severe shortness of breath and dry cough. GI: He denies any abdominal pain, nausea, vomiting, diarrhea, constipation, melena, hematochezia. GENITOURNINARY: He denies any burning micturition. DERMATOLOGICAL: He denies any jaundice or rash. NEUROLOGICAL: He denies any loss of consciousness, light-headedness, dizziness or any weakness on any one side. PSYCHIATRIC: He denies feeling depressed or anxious.

PAST MEDICAL HISTORY:
1. Nodular sclerosing Hodgkin's disease, abdomen only, diagnosed in 08/1991, status post Adriamycin, bleomycin, viblastine and decarbazine therapy.
2. Post radiation hypothyroidism.
3. Gastroesophageal reflux disease, hiatal hernia with subsequent stricture formation requiring repeated balloon dilation of the esophagus.
4. Possible Gilbert's syndrome.
5. Relative lymphocytosis persistent since chemotherapy.
6. Hemorrhoids.

PAST SURGICAL HISTORY:
1. Neck/groin lymph node biopsy.
2. Exploratory laparotomy with splenectomy in 1983.
3. Right subclavian Port-A-Cath insertion and removal.
4. Multiple esophagogastroduodenoscopies with esophageal balloon dilations. The last esophagogastroduodenoscopy was in 2002.

CURRENT MEDICATIONS: Synthroid 75 mcg qam, Prilosec 20 mg qam, Anusol HC cream prn.

ALLERGIES: No known drug allergies.

SOCIAL HISTORY: He denies any history of smoking, alcohol, or drug abuse. He is single and has no children.

FAMILY HISTORY: His mother had hypertension, hyperlipidemia, and multiple ventral hernias.

LABORATORY STUDIES: White blood count 10, hemoglobin 15.9, hematocrit 48.7, platelets 701, glucose 118, BUN 9, creatinine 1.1, calcium 10.1, albumin 4.7, alkaline phosphatase 142, sodium 137, potassium 4.5, CO2 30, PT 13.6, INR 1.14, PTT 26.8.

RADIOLOGY STUDIES: Chest x-ray shows complete whitening of the left lung field. CT Scan of the chest shows complete fluid accumulation on the left side with complete collapse of the left lung. It also shows some lymphadenopathy.

PHYSICAL EXAMINATION:
VITAL SIGNS: blood pressure 120/88, pulse 104 regular, respirations 18, temperature 97.7, weight 168.4 pounds, oxygen saturation 98% on room air. GENERAL: He is alert, awake, in mild to moderate respiratory distress at this time. EYES: Pink conjunctiva, anicteric sclera. Pupils are equal, round, and reactive to light. Extraocular movements are intact. NECK/LYMPH: Neck is supple. No jugular venous distention or cervical lymphadenopathy. LUNGS: He has absent breath sounds on the left side. Good air entry on the right side. No wheeze or rhonchi. HEART: Regular rate and rhythm. Tachycardia. Normal S1 and S2. No murmurs. ABDOMEN: Soft, non-tender, nondistended. No hepatosplenomegaly. Normoactive bowel sounds. MUSCULOSKELETAL: No CVA tenderness. EXTREMITIES: No cyanosis, clubbing or edema. Good distal pulses. NEUROLOGICALLY: There is no evidence of any focal neurological deficits. PSYCHOLOGICALLY: Alert and oriented times three.

ASSESSMENT:
1. Huge left sided pleural effusion with shortness of breath.
2. History of nodular sclerosing Hodgkin's disease, status post Adriamycin, bleomycin, viblastine, and decarbazine therapy and status post nodo irradiation and splenectomy.
3. Gastroesophageal reflux disease.
4. Post radiation hypothyroidism.
5. Hemorrhoids.

PLAN: The patient was sent directly from the office to radiology to get a chest x-ray. I reviewed the chest x-ray showing there is a complete opacification of the left lung, subsequently we immediately got a CT scan of the chest which showed complete collapse of the left lung and the left side is full of fluid. It also showed some lymphadenopathy. At that time, the decision was made to admit the patient as a direct admit. He was sent to the third floor. We will start oxygen 2 liters nasal cannula. We will have Dr. Green on consult for a left sided thoracocentesis. We will give him a regular diet. IV Heplock. Synthroid 75 mcg qam, Prilosec 20 mg qam. We will repeat a complete blood count and basic metabolic profile tomorrow morning. All of the above findings and plan were discussed with the patient. He seems to understand and agree. The patient has a guarded prognosis.

A. 99205

B. 99223

C. 99215

D. 99221

Practice 3, Report B

LOCATION: Inpatient, Hospital
Discharge Summary

FINAL DIAGNOSIS:
1. Acute gastrointestinal bleed with anemia, stable.
2. Coronary artery disease/stents.
3. Severe peripheral vascular disease.
4. Moderate to severe chronic obstructive pulmonary disease.

HOSPITAL COURSE: He is a 63-year-old white male with a known history of coronary artery disease, status post stents, peripheral vascular disease, chronic obstructive pulmonary disease who was admitted to the general medical floor on the 5th of August as a direct admit because of persistently low hemoglobin level and persistent melena. An esophagogastroduodenoscopy was performed yesterday, which did not show any source of active bleeding. He was transfused two units of packed red blood cells and his hemoglobin has been stable around 11.4. He denies any complaints and wishes to go home.

DISCHARGE MEDICATIONS: He has been instructed to resume all his home medications as before.

PLAN: He is scheduled for a colonoscopy as an outpatient with Dr. Blue on the 9th of August at 6:30 a.m. All instructions and the preparatory material have been given to the patient. If his colonoscopy does not show any source of bleeding we will get a capsule endoscopy done. We will get a hemoglobin level one day prior to his visit. He is scheduled for a follow-up visit with me in the office in one week.

Codes:_____

4. CONSULTATIONS (99241-99255)

Requesting physician or other appropriate source is the one asking for opinion/advice of another physician

Physician who gives the opinion/advice is consultant

Consultation codes reflect inquiries between physicians or other qualified personnel

Written or verbal request for consultation must be documented in medical record

Consulting physician must provide requesting physician documentation of

- Examination
- Clinical judgment(s)
- Treatment(s) prescribed

Consulting physician is authorized to order all medically necessary tests/services

According to CPT and CMS, only one consultation should be reported per inpatient stay

Same physician may be consulted more than once regarding same patient provided there is documentation in the medical record indicating a change in patient's status to support another consultation or a new condition in office setting

- This varies by payer
- Medicare states no consultation if same condition has been treated by same physician in the past

Requires 3 of 3 key components be met

Types of consultations

- Office or other outpatient consultations
  - Applies to both new and established patients
  - Reflects consultations occurring in one of the following sites
    - Physician's office
    - Hospital's observation services
    - Home services
    - Rest home or custodial care
    - Emergency department
    - Any other ambulatory facility
- Inpatient consultation
  - Reported for both new and established patients
  - Documentation on all three key components must either be met or exceeded
  - Limited to one initial inpatient consultation per patient/hospitalization by a consultant

PRACTICE 4, CONSULTATIONS

Once you have coded the two cases, check your answers in Unit III of this text, where you will locate the answers and rationales.

Practice 4, Report A

LOCATION: Outpatient, Office

Dear Dr. Green:

Thank you for asking me to evaluate Ms. N., a 50-year-old female. She is referred for fever, rash, and mouth sores occurring after a trip.

The patient and her husband tell me that they traveled to Hawaii in November. They flew into San Diego and took a bus to the ship in Ensenada, Mexico. The cruise ship then went to the islands of Hawaii. While in Hawaii, they took tours by bus to volcanoes. She did shopping in the towns they stopped in. The patient did no swimming while there and had no fresh water exposure. She was not around any animals. There were no ill contacts on the cruise ship. She did not eat any food while in Mexico, but did drink bottled water.

The patient and her husband returned to town on December 6. The patient notes that two weeks ago she began feeling fatigued and "not good". Twelve days ago she developed a fever to 103.8, as well as "sores" along the side of her tongue and her throat. Since then, she notes that she has developed both gingival and buccal lesions. She did have severe odynophagia and reports trouble drinking water. She denies any lesions on her lips.

Eight days ago, due to ongoing oral pain as well as pain that had developed in the neck and on the right side of her face and ear, she was seen as an outpatient. She tells me that she was given Prednisone because of oral swelling. She does not know the dosage of her Prednisone, but states that it was given for five days.

Six to seven days ago, the patient developed a cough. She tells me that this was nonproductive until this morning, when she began having "phlegmy, yucky stuff". She had a chest x-ray done three days ago and tells me that it was "free of pneumonia".

Three to four days ago, the patient began developing lesions on her neck and scalp. They are non pruritic, but are associated with sharp "nerve pain" which the patient describes as "intense".

The patient's fevers have decreased since her initial illness. She tells me that she is still having maximum temperatures of 101, and is taking Advil and Tylenol around the clock.

Past medical history is well known to you, and will not be reiterated here. Social history includes that the patient is married. She has three dogs and three cats, all of which are full grown. The cats are declawed on all four paws. She has had no nips or bites. The patient does not work outside the home. She was taking care of her 18-month-old granddaughter two days per week, up until the time that the patient became ill. The patient notes that the granddaughter has not been ill throughout this time.

On physical examination in my clinic, temperature was 99.0. Her pulse was 78 and her blood pressure was 118/86. Her weight was 168 pounds (decreased 15 pounds from October). The exam was significant only for skin, head, and neck exam. The mouth had multiple small punctate ulcers, all of which were on a white base. These were all between 1 and 3 mm and were on the buccal mucosa and in the oropharynx. There were labial lesions and no palatal lesions. There was mild anterior cervical lymphadenopathy, which was mildly to moderately tender. This all measured less than 2 cm and there was no associated erythema or fluctuance. Skin exam revealed several small pustular lesions located on the scalp and neck.

I suspect that the patient has a Coxsackie virus infection with predominance of oral lesions. With no exposure to animals or fresh water while in Hawaii, more unusual infections such as Leptospirosis would be exceedingly unusual. Additionally, her symptom complex (and particularly her oral ulcers) is not suggestive of either Typhus or Leptospirosis. Also in the differential diagnosis would be an adverse drug reaction to her chronic Augmentin. The patient was due to complete this in one week with a planned total duration of Augmentin of six months. I recommended that the patient stop her Augmentin one week early. I think that it would safe to re-challenge her with Augmentin into the future, if she required antibiotics. However, if she redeveloped oral ulcers with re-challenge of Augmentin, she would then need to be labeled as allergic to Augmentin.

Follow up will be on an as-needed basis in our clinic.

A. 99243

B. 99244

C. 99203

D. 99215

Practice 4, Report B

LOCATION: Inpatient, Hospital

REASON FOR CONSULTATION: Nausea, vomiting, and abdominal pain.

HISTORY OF PRESENT ILLNESS: The patient is a 33-year-old woman with a past medical history of diabetes, diabetic gastroparesis, status post J-tube placement in 2004, who now presents with an approximately two-day history of nausea and vomiting. According to old records, the patient had been made n.p.o. with strict J-tube feedings; however, the patient has been noncompliant with this therapy and admits to taking moderate p.o. intake. The patient also complains of diffuse abdominal pain that does not radiate. The patient states that she has had this pain in the past. It is not specific and is not localized to any one point. The patient denies any chest pain, shortness of breath, fevers, or chills. She denies any change in her bowel movements. She states that she has been somewhat more constipated lately with her last formed bowel movement approximately one day prior. The patient states that she had diarrhea this morning. She denies any hematochezia or melena. She denies any dysuria or symptoms related to gastroesophageal reflux disease.

PAST MEDICAL HISTORY:
1. Diabetes.
2. Hypertension.
3. Diabetic gastroparesis.

PAST SURGICAL HISTORY:
1. Cholecystectomy.
2. Tubal ligation.
3. J-tube placement.

MEDICATIONS: Duragesic patch, Diflucan, insulin, Prevacid, Phenergan, Reglan, lisinopril, Lexapro, methadone.

ALLERGIES: No known medical allergies.

SOCIAL/FAMILY HISTORY: The patient does not smoke or drink alcohol. No family history of GI problems.

REVIEW OF SYSTEMS: The patient has an extensive review of systems and as per history and physical examination of three days prior to admission to hospital.

PHYSICAL EXAMINATION:
GENERAL: The patient is a 33-year-old woman who appears older than her stated age. She is in no acute distress. She closes her eyes easily during questioning and responds only to repeated questions. VITAL SIGNS: Temperature 97.4 degrees, heart rate 91, blood pressure 106/57, oxygen saturation 97% on room air. HEENT: Pupils equal, round, reactive to light and accommodation and extraocular motions intact. Sclerae are anicteric. Oropharynx is benign. Mucous membranes are dry. NECK: Soft, supple, and nontender. No masses were felt.

LUNGS: Clear to auscultation, bilaterally. There are no rhonchi, rales, or wheezes. The patient is not in respiratory distress. HEART: Regular rate and rhythm, normal S1 and S2, no S3, murmurs, or rubs heard. ABDOMEN: Shows a well-healing midline scar, as well a J-tube. Abdomen is soft and slightly distended. There is no focal tenderness. There are hypoactive bowel sounds. There is no guarding, hepatosplenomegaly, or masses felt. The patient does not have any growing hernias. EXTREMETIES: Non-tender without edema.

NEUROLOGIC: The patient is intact.

LABORATORY STUDIES: Electrolytes are within normal limits. Alkaline phosphatase is 119, ALT 583, AST 679, bilirubin 0.4, albumin 2.8, white blood count 6.6, and hemoglobin 12.1.

RADIOLOGY STUDIES: Upright abdominal x-ray showed minimal distention of the small bowel. There were some small associated air fluid levels. There is a small amount of gas and stool in the colon. There are no signs of free air or free fluid. CT scan of abdomen and pelvis is pending at this time.

IMPRESSION/RECOMMENDATIONS: The patient is a 33-year-old woman with a history of diabetic gastroparesis who presents now with nausea, vomiting, and abdominal pain.

1. These symptoms could represent diabetic gastroparesis. The patient will need a nasogastric tube placed. We will keep the patient n.p.o., as well as hold her J-tube feeding for now. We will review the CT scan findings with the radiologist. Otherwise, we will continue to treat this conservatively with intravenous fluids. In addition to her past medical history, the patient is on methadone, as well as Duragesic patch, which could cause significant ileus. The patient may need further small bowel imaging if the CT scan is inconclusive and her symptoms persist. However, the CT scan is a good modality for evaluating partial small-bowel obstructions.

2. Elevated transaminase. The patient was admitted with normal ALT and AST; however, on admission the patient developed AST and ALT elevations. This could be due to multiple causes; however, drug induced is likely given that the patient was started on Diflucan and Zosyn, both with known hepatic toxicity profiles. We will defer changing these antibiotics per the primary service. Bilirubin is within normal limits and the patient is not clinically jaundice or complaining of any upper quadrant pain suggestive of biliary obstruction. We will discuss this case with the general surgeon who is on call for general surgery today.

Codes:_____

5. EMERGENCY DEPARTMENT SERVICES (99281-99288)

Limited to use by ED (Emergency Department) staff physicians

No distinction is made between new and established patients

Requires 3 of 3 key components be met

ED services may be billed by physicians who are not assigned to the ED

Any physician who provides services in the ED may use these codes to report the service

If the physician asks the patient to meet him/her in ED as an alternative to the physician's office and the patient is not registered as an ED patient

Report the service with appropriate office/outpatient visit codes

Facilities qualifying as EDs must be

Available 24 hours a day

Located in organized hospital-based facility

Exist to provide immediate medical attention to persons without the constraints of prior scheduled appointments

Code assignment determined by severity of patient's condition as reported by physician in medical record

Facilities may use acuity sheet, such as that in **Figure 1–9** to assign level of ED service

Level 1—99281	Level 2—99282	Level 3—99283
1. Initial (triage) assessment 2. Suture removal 3. Wound recheck 4. Note for work or school 5. Simple discharge information	Interventions from previous level plus any of the following: 1. OTC med administration 2. Tetanus booster 3. Bedside diagnostic tests (stool hemoccult, glucometer) 4. Visual acuity 5. Orthostatic vital signs 6. Simple trauma not requiring x-ray 7. Simple discharge information	Interventions from previous level plus any of the following: 1. Heparin/saline lock 2. Crystalloid IV therapy 3. X-ray, one area 4. RX med administration 5. Fluorescein stain 6. Quick cath 7. Foley cath 8. Receipt of ambulance patient 9. Mental health emergencies (mild) not requiring parenteral medications or admission 10. Moderate complexity discharge instructions 11. Intermediate layered and complex laceration repair
Level 4—99284	**Level 5—99285**	**Critical Care 99291, 99292**
Interventions from previous level plus any of the following: 1. X-ray, multiple areas 2. Special imaging studies (CT, MRI, ultrasound) 3. Cardiac monitoring 4. Multiple reassessments of patient 5. Parenteral[1] medications (including insulin) 6. Nebulizer treatment (1 or 2) 7. NG placement 8. Pelvic exam 9. Mental health emergencies (moderate). May require parenteral medications but not admission 10. Administration of IV medications *[1]not through the alimentary canal but rather by injection through some other route, such as subcutaneous, intramuscular, intraorbital, intracapsular, intraspinal, intrasternal, or intravenous*	Interventions from previous level plus any of the following: 1. Monitor/stabilize patient during in hospital transport and/or testing (CT, MRI, ultrasound) 2. Vasoactive medication 3. Administration (dopamine, dobutamine, multiple) nebulizer treatments (3 or more) 4. Conscious sedation 5. Lumbar puncture 6. Thoracentesis 7. Sexual assault exam 8. Admission to hospital 9. Mental health emergency (severe) psychotic and/or agitated/combative 10. Requires admission 11. Fracture/dislocation reduction 12. Suicide precautions 13. Gastric lavage 14. Complex discharge instructions	Interventions from any previous level plus any of the following: 1. Multiple parenteral medications 2. Continuous monitoring 3. Major trauma care 4. Chest tube insertion 5. CPR 6. Defibrillation/cardioversion 7. Delivery of baby 8. Control of major hemorrhage 9. Administration of blood or blood products

Figure **1-9.** Example of an acuity sheet used to determine level of emergency department services.

PRACTICE 5, EMERGENCY DEPARTMENT SERVICES

*Using the acuity sheet (**Figure 1–9**), code the following two cases and then check your answers in Unit III of this text, where you will locate the answer and written rationales.*

Practice 5, Report A

CHIEF COMPLAINT: Abdominal pain.

HISTORY OF PRESENT ILLNESS
This is a 34-year-old female who presents to the ED and has had upper abdominal pain, nausea, and diarrhea today not associated with fevers, pain with urination, urgency, or frequency. The patient had similar problems about a month ago, and that workup was negative. It is not associated with food, melena, hematochezia, fever, pain with urination, urgency, frequency, and no sick contacts that she is aware of.

PAST MEDICAL HISTORY: Asthma, hypertension, depression, migraines, esophageal reflux, and arthritis.

MEDICATIONS/ALLERGIES: (Reviewed. See nursing notes.)

PAST SURGICAL HISTORY: She has had a tubal ligation.

FAMILY HISTORY: Unremarkable.

SOCIAL HISTORY: Denies alcohol, drug, or tobacco use.

REVIEW OF SYSTEMS: Positive for abdominal pain, nausea, and diarrhea. Remainder of ten-point review of system performed is negative.

PHYSICAL EXAMINATION
General—the patient is a 34-year-old female who does not appear toxic or in distress. Vital signs—she has stable vitals and afebrile. HEENT—nonicteric sclerae. Oropharynx does not appear significantly dry. Neck—supple. Lungs—clear. Heart—regular rate and rhythm without murmur. Abdomen—she has some diffuse abdominal tenderness, possibly some right upper quadrant discomfort, but no peritoneal signs nor flank discomfort. Skin—exam is unremarkable. Neurological—she is awake, alert, appropriate, and ambulates normally.

EMERGENCY DEPARTMENT COURSE
The patient was given pain medication and IV fluids. She had an ultrasound performed 1 month ago and was essentially negative. All her lab work was normal. Her pain was controlled. I felt she probably was coming down with some type of viral syndrome.

PROVISIONAL DIAGNOSIS/DIAGNOSES: Evaluation of abdominal pain, etiology undetermined.

PLAN(S)
1. The patient was given abdominal pain instruction sheet.
2. Sent home with a prescription for Bentyl.
3. I recommend that she follow up with her primary care physician if she has persistent problems.
   Condition at discharge was stable.

A. 99284, 789.09, 787.02, 787.91

B. 99285, 789.00, 079.9

C. 99283, 789.00

D. 99284, 789.09, 079.99

Practice 5, Report B

CHIEF COMPLAINT: Ankle injury.

HISTORY OF PRESENT ILLNESS
The patient is a 16-year-old male who was skateboarding today and had an inversion injury of his left ankle. He is ambulatory but complains of pain and swelling. No other complaints or injuries at this time. See nurse's notes for medications and allergies.

ROS
Patient states no dizziness prior to or after the fall. No recent muscle or joint problems. No broken skin.

HISTORY
No past surgeries. The patient is a junior in school and does play sports.

PHYSICAL EXAMINATION
Height 68″, weight 185, BP 120/58. He is an alert and pleasant male in no acute distress. Examination of the left lower extremity shows a soft tissue swelling of the lateral malleolus. He has no base of the 5th metatarsal tenderness. He has no proximal tibial tenderness. Neurovascularly intact distally.

EMERGENCY DEPARTMENT COURSE
Plain films were performed and showed no evidence of acute fracture or malalignment and told this represented sprain. I recommend symptomatic care, air cast, ice, crutches, and Motrin. Follow up with primary care physician. Return for any problems. He is agreeable to this plan. He was discharged home in stable condition.

PROVISIONAL DIAGNOSIS/DIAGNOSES: Left ankle sprain.

Codes:_____

6. PEDIATRIC CRITICAL CARE PATIENT TRANSPORT (99289-99290)

Time is a factor in choosing the correct code

Face-to-face care as reported by the physician is limited to time physician has assumed primary responsibility for patient care

All services provided during patient transport by physician in charge of critical care that pertain to routine monitoring of a patient's condition during transport are not reported with these codes

Examples of services that may not be reported separately during transport include

Monitoring

Heart rates

Respiratory rates

Blood pressure monitoring

Pulse monitoring

Interpretation of cardiac output measurements

Blood gas information

Any data from computers

PRACTICE 6, PEDIATRIC CRITICAL CARE PATIENT TRANSPORT

These are time-based codes, so no audit form is required. Once you have coded the two cases, check your answers in Unit III of this text, where you will locate the answers and written rationales.

Practice 6, Report A

The physician accompanies a 13-month-old critical-care patient during transport from one hospital to another. The documented time spent was 1 ½ hours with the patient in the first hospital, two hours transporting the patient to the second hospital.

A. 99291, 99292, 99299, 99290 ×2

B. 99289, 99290 ×4

C. 99291, 99289, 99290 ×2

D. 99289, 99290 ×5

Practice 6, Report B

Total of 2 hours, 40 minutes spent with 18-month-old burn patient that went into shock. Patient was be transported to The Children's Burn Center by air flight.

Codes:_____

7. CRITICAL CARE SERVICES (99291, 99292)

Critical care is provided when

Used for patients age over 2 years

29 days-24 months is pediatric critical care, not critical care

One or more of the vital organ(s) is in/has high probability for being in a life-threatening state

A high complexity of MDM is required for treating vital organ(s) failure and/or prevention of further deterioration in the patient's condition

Examples of vital organ failure

Central nervous system

Circulatory failure

Presence of shock

Renal failure

Hepatic failure

Metabolic failure

Respiratory failure

Threats to vital organs are not limited to the above list

Most (but not all) critical care involves an interpretation of either advanced technology and/or multiple interpretations with physiologic parameters

Codes may also be assigned for critical care services for

Postoperative patient

Patient with a deteriorating condition

Type of physician time and location is an important key in assigning these codes

Time spent on critical care may include time

On medical unit reviewing patient care with or without other medical staff

Spent documenting patient's status into medical record

Spent with the patient's family or caregivers compiling a history and/or discussing medical management if patient is clinically incompetent

Time spent in a face-to-face encounter may be accumulated over course of day

Example: Three 30-minute encounters result in 90 minutes of time

Time spent must be documented in the medical record

PRACTICE 7, CRITICAL CARE SERVICES

These are time-based codes, so no audit form is required. Once you have coded the two cases, check your answers in Unit III of this text, where you will locate the answers and rationales.

Practice 7, Report A

CHIEF COMPLAINT: Syncope.

HISTORY OF PRESENT ILLNESS
An 88-year-old male who presents to the ED after he apparently had a syncopal episode at home. Unfortunately, the patient does not remember the episode. He was found by his wife, he was able to stand on his own. He complained of some neck pain and was placed on a backboard and transported via EMS. The patient does not remember walking around the house this morning and does not know what he was feeling, does not remember if he had any symptoms prior to the collapse. Vital signs documented per supplemental sheet. I do not believe the patient is a reliable historian.
Per the family, he has had a history of cancer, COPD, atrial fibrillation.

PSH: Left carotid endarterectomy and a Nissen. The patient quit smoking 40 years ago.

FH: Positive for coronary disease.

MEDICATIONS/ALLERGIES: A full 10-point review of systems is otherwise negative.

PHYSICAL EXAMINATION
The patient was afebrile, vital signs notable for a pulse of 116, otherwise normal. In general, a pleasant male on a backboard, wearing a C-collar, in no acute distress. HEENT: Pupils equal, round and reactive, extraocular movements intact. There are no signs of trauma about the face or scalp. Neck is examined with in-line stabilization, in a C-collar. The patient had some tenderness over the upper cervical spine and was kept in a C-collar. CV tachy and irregular but no murmur. Lungs are clear. Abdomen is soft, nontender. Extremities unremarkable with no rash, no focal tenderness. Back exam revealed no tenderness. Neurologically the patient was oriented to person and place.

EMERGENCY DEPARTMENT COURSE
The patient was carefully log-rolled off the backboard. Did have an EKG which showed atrial fibrillation with some lateral ST depression consistent with digitalis effect. Patient did have a metabolic panel which showed the glucose of 114, otherwise normal. CBC showed a white count of 10.9, hemoglobin 12.1. Troponin 0.04, myoglobin 611, thought to be elevated secondary to his syncope. Urinalysis was negative. CT of the head was unremarkable except for possible left basal ganglia lacunar infarct. CT of the C-spine did show fracture of the C4 left pedicle and left transverse foramina. With this finding, the patient was kept in a C-collar, was seen by orthopedics. Discussed with primary care physician. The patient will be admitted in guarded condition.

PROVISIONAL DIAGNOSIS/DIAGNOSES
1. C4 fracture.
2. Syncope of uncertain cause.

The patient is neurologically intact. Total critical care time did exceed 30 minutes.

A. 99291, 806.00, 780.09, E888.8

B. 99221, 805.04, 780.2, E888.8

C. 99291, 805.04, 780.2

D. 99221, 806.00, 780.2

Practice 7, Report B

CHIEF COMPLAINT: Altered level of consciousness.

HISTORY OF PRESENT ILLNESS

This is an 84-year-old male who was found by his son to be somewhat unresponsive and seeming to have difficulty with gasping for air. This was at his nursing home where he is in assisted living. The son had the staff check an oxygen level and it was 70%, so EMS was called and the patient was brought here. The patient has responded to verbal stimuli, but has not indicated any pain. The son is not aware of any fever or vomiting, although the patient has not been eating well for the last week or so. PAST MEDICAL HISTORY: There is a history of bladder cancer. There is also a history of pulmonary embolism and deep venous thrombosis and the patient is on Coumadin. He has also had a history of stroke. SOCIAL HISTORY: The patient is here with his son. There is a "do not resuscitate order" within his advance directive that indicates he does not want intubation or CPR according to the son. The son does want to see the patient get necessary medication or fluids. As noted above, he lives in assisted living. ROS: I was not able to do a review of systems on the patient because of his lethargy. The son stated he did not know of any recent fever or cough. He did not know of any vomiting or urinary difficulties.

PHYSICAL EXAMINATION

Vital signs show a low blood pressure of 89/48 with a normal pulse of 90 and regular. Increased respiratory rate of 28, but not labored. Now that the patient is on oxygen he is not using accessory muscles respiration or gasping. The pharynx shows no inflammation or exudate, but is very dry. There is no cervical adenopathy and his neck is supple. Pupils equal, round, and reactive to light.

Cranial nerves II-XII are intact. The patient is able to cooperate enough to squeeze my fingers or to lift his arms and legs, and he does this in a symmetrical way in all 4 extremities. The heart has normal S1-S2 without murmur. Lungs are clear to auscultation and percussion. The abdomen is soft and nontender throughout without mass, guarding or rebound tenderness. Lower extremities show no swelling, tenderness, or cords. Skin is clear of significant rashes.

DIAGNOSTIC STUDIES

LABORATORY/PATHOLOGY: Pulse oximetry is adequate at 96% on an oxygen mask by nonrebreather. CBC shows low hemoglobin of 11.1 and elevated white count of 14,300. Electrolytes shows high potassium of 5.1, high chloride of 114 and low CO2 of 19. BUN is high at 50 and creatinine high at 3.3. These are significant elevations since a previous level done 8 days ago when he had a BUN of 17 and creatinine of 1.3. Glucose is high at 154, albumin is low at 2.7. Liver studies are basically normal. Urinalysis is positive for probable infection with 11 white cells and small leukocyte esterase.
Troponin I is normal at less than 0.03.

IMAGING: Chest x-ray shows no active infiltrate.

EKG: A 12-lead electrocardiogram was done for the indication of lethargy and hypotension, and the computer interpretation was reviewed. The tracing shows normal sinus rhythm with frequent premature atrial contractions. There is nonspecific T-wave flattening present in the inferior and lateral leads. There are Q waves in leads III and aVF consistent with old inferior MI. There are no acute ischemic changes.

EMERGENCY DEPARTMENT COURSE

I gave the patient a liter of IV fluids in the emergency department over a couple of hours and this with the oxygen resulted in definite improvement of his mental status. He was alert and easily responsive after the first 700 mL of saline. I ordered Levaquin 250 mg IV. I spoke with his primary physician and he is going to come over to the emergency department and admit the patient.

PROVISIONAL DIAGNOSIS/DIAGNOSES

1. Upper respiratory infection with urosepsis.
2. Transient hypotension, which has now improved.
3. History of bladder cancer.
4. History of anticoagulation for pulmonary embolism and deep venous thrombosis.

DISPOSITION

He was admitted as noted. Condition on discharge from the emergency department is improved. Critical care time was 30 minutes on this patient.

Codes:_____

8. INPATIENT NEONATAL AND PEDIATRIC CRITICAL CARE SERVICES (99293-99300)

Same definition used to describe critical care for adults is used to describe critical care for children/neonates

Care includes care given by a physician when providing services of

Management

Monitoring

Treatment

Codes apply to patient services rendered to neonate in intensive care unit that include patient management monitoring and treatment

Inpatient Pediatric Critical Care (99293, 99294)

Initial or subsequent care

Per day

Critically ill

29 days through 24 months of age

Inpatient Neonatal Critical Care (99295, 99296)

Initial or subsequent care

Per day

Critically ill

Require cardiac and/or respiratory support

Includes life-threatening surgical/cardiac conditions

28 days of age or less

Continuing Intensive Care Services (99298-99300)

Subsequent care

Per day

Based on body weight

LBW (low birth weight), less than 1500 grams (3.31 pounds) assign 99298

VLBW (very low birth weight), 1500-2500 grams (3.31 to 5.51 pounds) assign 99299

Normal weight, 2501-5000 grams (5.51 to 11.02 pounds) assign 99300

PRACTICE 8, INPATIENT NEONATAL AND PEDIATRIC CRITICAL CARE SERVICES

These are time-based codes, so no audit form is required. Once you have coded the two cases, check your answers in Unit III of this text, where you will locate the answers and rationales.

Practice 8, Report A

NICU INPATIENT PROGRESS NOTE

S: No event overnight, brief bradycardia, sleep study overnight

O: Resp: Rate: 32-76   Exam: Upper airway congestion
         CV: Rate: 94-154   Map: 50-69
                    Exam: RRR, good perfusion
         FEN/GI: I: 630   TF: 134   Wt: 4696 grams
         O: 345
                    Exam: Soft NT ND with +BS
         HEME: none
         GU: Within normal limits.
         ID: Temp Max: 36.7
         Cultures: none
         NEURO:
                    Exam: warm, no edema. Alert and appropriate, good tone

A/P: 2 month 1 wk old male was admitted for require of unilateral, incarcerated inguinal hernia and subsequently developed acute lung congestion. Sleep study done yesterday. Continue to monitor perfusion. Continue with 22 kcal feedings.

A. No code; post-operative global period

B. 99231, 764.09, V45.89, 550.10

C. 99300, 550.10, 486, 427.89

D. 99300, 550.10, 486, V45.89

Practice 8, Report B

NICU INPATIENT

S: Quiet night

O: Resp: Rate: 26-73   Exam: Lungs clear
         CV: Rate: 131-174   Map: 44-51
                  Exam:
         FEN/GI: I: 250   TF: Wt: 2100 grams
                  O: 138
                  Exam: Abd soft with +BS
         HEME:
         ID: Temp Max: 37
         Cultures: 0
         NEURO:
                  Exam: AF soft, ext: good tone

A/P: 55 day old, 27 week premature, resp stable, PE benign. Occ desats monitor. Follow up echo this week to look at coronary arteries. Monitor weight.

Codes:_____

9. NURSING FACILITY SERVICES (99304-99318)

These codes are used for patients in

Nursing facilities

Intermediate care facilities

Long-term care facilities

Psychiatric residential treatment centers

Psychiatric residential treatment centers are those that

Provide a 24-hour therapeutically planned living and/or learning environment with professionally trained staff

Medical psychotherapy is not included in codes

There are four subcategories of codes in nursing facility codes

Dependent on assessment instruments used by the nursing facility to assess a resident's functional capacity

Initial Nursing Facility Care

Subsequent Nursing Facility Care

Nursing Facility Discharge Services

Other Nursing Facility Services (Annual Assessments)

Two forms are used to determine the patient's status

Resident Assessment Protocols (RAP)

Residential Assessment Instrument (RAT) with uniform Minimum Data Set requirements (MDS)

Uniform minimum data (MDS) for nursing facilities must include or exceed following information

Medically defined conditions and prior medical history

Medical status measurement

Physical and mental functional status

Discharge potential

Dental condition

Activities potential

Rehabilitation potential

Cognitive status

Drug therapy

MDS must contain input from physician for evaluation and formulation of multidisciplinary care

When an MDS appears incomplete or signals a need for supplementary information, Resident Assessment Protocols (RAPs) are used

RAP must be used by nursing facility in following situations

At time of patient admittance to facility

When 12 months have lapsed since previous assessment

When a major permanent change in patient's status is observed

RAP is helpful in assessing potential problems and provide useful information for follow-up procedures

When a patient is admitted to nursing care facility from another medical service site, such as physician office or an emergency department, all services performed on date of admission are evaluated (considered) as part of initial facility care codes

Codes are not used when either a discharge from a hospital or observation status in a hospital occurs on same date as admission to nursing facility

Note: When a physician discharges a patient from a nursing facility, the appropriate axle is based on the time spent with the patient and/or family and/or caregiver discussing both the facility stay and management options, which the physician bases on his/her final examination

PRACTICE 9, NURSING FACILITY SERVICES

Once you have coded the two cases, check your answers in Unit III of this text.

Practice 9, Report A

LOCATION: Light Hills Nursing Home
Emily is seen for a review of chronic controlled conditions listed below. The chart is reviewed along with the nursing notes. Advanced directives are in place.

S: No fevers or chills. No chest pain or shortness of breath.

O: This well-developed, well-nourished lady is sitting without distress. HEENT is normal, normocephalic, and atraumatic. Neck is supple. Lungs clear to auscultation.

A: 1. Chronic headaches
2. Bipolar disorder
3. Hypertension
4. Tardive dyskinesia secondary to antidepressants
5. Urinary incontinence

P: 1. The patient has chronic headaches for which she has been taking Fioricet as needed, but I will go ahead and start her on Topamax for preventative measures, 25 mg one p.o. H.S. for 10 days and then one p.o. bid for 10 days and then one in the A.M. and two at H.S. for 10 days. Then we will start 50 mg p.o. bid.
2. Reassess in four weeks.
3. In the meantime, the case was discussed with the charge nurse and I advised that the Topamax may cause a little increased fatigue and hypersomnolence but if it is clinically significant, we might have to decrease the doses.

A. 99309, 784.0, 296.90, 401.9, 333.82, 788.30, E939.3

B. 99308, 784.0, 296.80, 401.1, 333.82, 788.30, E939.3

C. 99336, 784.0, 296.90, 401.9, 969.3, 788.30, E939.3

D. 99309, 784.0, 296.80, 401.9, 333.82, 788.30, E939.3

Practice 9, Report B

LOCATION:
Nursing Facility
This patient is seen for a routine visit. No code in place. The chart is reviewed along with the nursing notes. Advanced directives are in place. The graphic chart is also reviewed.

S: No fevers or chills. No chest pain or shortness of breath. Nurse states patient continues to be frequently delusional.

O: This well-developed, well-nourished gentleman is sitting without distress. HEENT—normocephalic and atraumatic. Neck is supple. Lungs—clear to auscultation.

A: 1. Alzheimer dementia
2. Atypical psychosis with delusions

P: 1. As the patient is otherwise clinically stable; the rest of the treatment is without change.

Codes:_____

10. DOMICILIARY, REST HOME (E.G., BOARDING HOME), OR CUSTODIAL CARE SERVICES, AND DOMICILIARY, REST HOME (E.G., ASSISTED LIVING FACILITY), OR HOME CARE PLAN OVERSIGHT SERVICES (99324-99340)

Domiciliary, Rest Home (e.g., Boarding Home), or Custodial Care Services (99324-99337)

These codes are used to report services in two settings

- Facility providing room, board, and other personal assistance services on a long-term basis
- Assisted living facility

Code choice based on whether patient is new or established patient

- For a new patient all 3 key components must be met or exceeded
- For an established patient, 2 of 3 key components must be met or exceeded

Time spent by a physician is considered a contributing factor when assigning a code for service

Domiciliary, Rest Home (e.g., Assisted Living Facility), or Home Care Plan Oversight Services (99339-99340)

Reports physician supervision of patient, when patient is not present

Patient resides in

- Own home
- Rest home or domiciliary
  - Includes assisted living facility

Codes based on time spent during calendar month

Not for patients receiving

- Home health care (99374-99375)
- Hospice care (99376-99377)
- Nursing facility services (99379-99380)

Physician provides the following types of services

- Review subsequent reports, laboratory studies, or other studies
- Integrates new data into patients' care plan
- Adjust medical therapy
- Develops or revises care plans
- Communicate with other health care professionals

PRACTICE 10, DOMICILIARY, REST HOME (E.G., BOARDING HOME), OR CUSTODIAL CARE SERVICES, AND DOMICILIARY, REST HOME (E.G., ASSISTED LIVING FACILITY), OR HOME CARE PLAN OVERSIGHT SERVICES (99324-99340)

Once you have coded the two cases, check your answers in Unit III of this text, where you will locate the answers and rationales.

Practice 10, Report A

LOCATION: Custodial Care Center

Patient evaluated today for a rash on her arms for the last 3 days. Nursing staff reports that lotion has been applied with no relief. Examined the patient and rash is contained to her arms. Staff also noticed that the patient has been sleeping a lot during the day. When I questioned the patient on her sleeping, she let me know that she has not been sleeping at night. Other than the rash and her sleeping habits, the patient is overall healthy.

Benadryl cream will be given prn for the patient's rash. Watch to make sure it doesn't spread. There is no change in her care plan at this time.

A. 99335, 782.1

B. 99307, 782.1

C. 99347, 782.1

D. 99325, 782.1, 780.52

Practice 10, Report B

LOCATION: Shady Lane Rest Home

This is an 80-year-old man, who resides in a rest home, complaining of painful urination. The pain is 5 out of 10. He has a suprapubic catheter due to urinary retention. He has been treated for urinary tract infections in the past with Cipro. He is having acute abdominal pain and fever. He has been eating fair.

EXAMINATION: When I visit with him today, he denies any weight loss, SOB, or palpitations. He is mildly confused. He answers yes and no, but there is very little conversation. His color is pink. His HEART is regular without murmur. His CHEST is diminished breath sounds with mild crackles at both bases. ABDOMEN is soft and nontender with active bowel sounds. His EXTREMITIES show no edema.

PLAN: Medications and treatments have been reviewed. I will place the patient on Cipro to treat UTI. No other changes to care plan at this time.

Codes:_____

11. HOME SERVICES (99341-99350)

Reports interaction between a physician and either new/established patient within the patient's residence

"Homebound" status required by many payers

New patient visit

   3 key components must be met or exceeded

Established patient visit

   2 of 3 key components must be met or exceeded

PRACTICE 11, HOME SERVICES

Once you have coded the two cases, check your answers in Unit III of this text.

Practice 11, Report A

LOCATION: Patient's Home

CHIEF COMPLAINT: Cough.

HISTORY OF PRESENT ILLNESS: This 89-year-old male, who is well known to me, has been coughing somewhat more as reported by the nurse and his wife but he seems to be sleeping rather well, without having to be propped up for any possible paroxysmal nocturnal dyspnea. He does not awaken through the night with difficulty breathing. His appetite appears to be normal. He is otherwise not complaining of any other discomforts.

EXAMINATION:
General: The patient is seen in his home. Vital signs are stable. He has some coughing and has more swelling of his right leg than the left. He is mostly bed-bound but does get up in the wheelchair and eat his meals and gets out sometimes with help. HEENT: Head is normocephalic. Ears are clear bilaterally. Throat is slightly dry. Neck is supple. LUNGS: Lungs demonstrate rhonchi bilaterally. No wheezes are noted. HEART: Heart demonstrates a regular rate and rhythm with no murmur, click, or rub. ABDOMEN: Abdomen is protuberant. Benign with no masses or tenderness. GENITALIA: Normal, no swelling. RECTAL: Deferred. EXTREMITIES: Pitting edema bilaterally, the right a little more than the left. He does have several decubiti which are currently being treated and appear to be healing and not getting worse.

IMPRESSION:
1. Bronchitis.
2. Severe osteoarthritis.
3. Multiple decubiti.
4. Pitting edema.

RECOMMENDATION:
He will be started on Zithromax Z-pak as directed.
    He will continue his cough syrup, Robitussin AC 1 tsp 4 times a day.
    Continue Lasix 40 mg a day.
    Decrease salt intake. His wife is instructed to not add any salt at the table and to make sure that he does not eat any potato chips or obviously salty foods.

A. 99343, 491.0, 715.90, 782.3, 707.00

B. 99343, 490, 715.90, 782.3, 707.00

C. 99349, 490, 715.90, 707.00, 782.3

D. 99349, 491.0, 715.90, 707.00, 782.3

Practice 11, Report B

LOCATION: Patient's Home

PATIENT: 91-year-old male

CC: Cough with underlying CHF

The 91-year-old gentleman is seen at home in bed. He has had more of a productive cough since Monday with no swelling of his ankles. He has been continuing on his usual medication including Tequin 400 mg once a day and Robitussin AC one teaspoon 4 times a day, with some relief. I have asked for his head to be elevated 30 degrees while he is in this respiratory condition. Today he is doing much better. He awakens every now and then. I believe he still recognizes me.

ROS is not obtained due to the patient's condition. The patient does suffer from CHF and Parkinsons.

Vital signs: BP 130/62, R 16, T 37. Head is normocephalic, atraumatic. Lungs: few basilar rales; otherwise clear. Heart: RRR. Abdomen: benign with no mass or tenderness. He certainly does not grimace when palpating his abdomen. Extremities: 1+ edema bilaterally. Pulses are 2+ bilaterally in the lower extremities.

IMPRESSION:
1. CHF
2. Cough
3. Bronchitis
4. Osteoarthritis
5. Parkinson's

RECOMMENDATIONS
Finish the antibiotics.
Continue to monitor.

Codes:_____

12. PROLONGED SERVICES (99354-99360)

Under the Prolonged Services subsection there are three categories of

Prolonged Physician Service With Direct (Face-to-Face) Patient Contact (99354-99357)

Prolonged Physician Service Without Direct (Face-to-Face) Patient Contact (99358, 99359)

Physician Standby Services (99360)

Prolonged Physician Service With or Without (Face-to-Face) Patient Contact

Codes 99354-99359 are all add-on codes

Only assigned when estimated service exceeds the time listed by more than 30 minutes

First 30 minutes of prolonged services are not reported but are considered part of initial service

Used in addition to codes reported for other E/M services

Used in addition to other codes to show an extension of the service

Unusual length of service may be in inpatient or outpatient setting

Codes available for services with or without face-to-face provider and patient contact

PRACTICE 12A, PROLONGED SERVICES WITH OR WITHOUT DIRECT PATIENT CONTACT (99354-99359)

These are time based codes, so no audit form is required. Once you have coded the two cases, check your answers in Unit III of this text.

Practice 12A, Report A

LOCATION: Outpatient Clinic

Chief Complaint:	Chronic Renal Failure and Hypertension
Hx of Present Illness:	The patient presents to the clinic today for a follow-up appointment for hypertension and chronic kidney disease. At her last visit the Norvasc was increased to 5 mg PO QD. She has been seeing a cardiologist and pulmonologist for breathing problems. The Labetalol was discontinued and she was started on Toprol XL 50 mg PO QD. She was also started on an Advair inhaler b.i.d. by the pulmonologist. Her breathing has been much better. Her BP has been higher running 150's systolic at home. She has been feeling relatively well. She does have a history of renal artery stenosis with right renal artery stent placement. Labs today include: BUN 26, sodium 140, creatinine is better at 1.2 mg/dL, CO2 28.6, K+ 4.5.
Urinary Symptoms:	Patient has no urinary symptoms.
Uremic Symptoms:	Patient has no uremic symptoms.
Cardiovascular Symptoms:	Patient has no cardiovascular symptoms.
PAST MEDICAL HISTORY:	Hypertension Proteinuria Atrial Fibrillation Osteoarthritis in lt knee Coronary Artery Disease Cataract surgery Open cholecystecomy
CURRENT MEDICATIONS:	1. Insulin 70/30 2. Insulin 3. Aspirin 4. Pravachol 5. Labetolol 6. Bumex 7. Tylenol 8. Multivitamin/Iron 9. Norvasc 10. Toprol XL 11. Advair inhaler
SOCIAL HISTORY:	Marital Status: Current Occupation: Past Occupation: Current Alcohol use: No Current Smoker: No Ex-Smoker: No Residence:

REVIEW OF SYSTEMS:	
Constitutional:	Negative
Eyes:	Wear glasses
ENT:	Negative
Cardiovascular:	Mentioned in HPI
Respiratory:	Dry cough
Gastrointestinal:	Negative
Genitourinary:	Mentioned in HPI
Musculoskeletal:	Arthritis
Skin:	Negative
Neurological:	Negative
Psychological:	Negative
Endocrine:	Diabetes Mellitus
Hematology:	Negative
PHYSICAL EXAMINATION:	
	Patient does not appear in any respiratory, cardiac, or neurological distress. No pallor, jaundice, or cynosis.
	Temperature: 97.9° F, Respiration 28/min, Pulse 72/min and regular
	Height: Weight: 155 lbs.
Blood Pressure:	Left (sitting): 166/72 mmHg Left (standing): 162/73 mmHg
Eyes:	Pupils are equal and reactive to light and accommodation. No evidence of conjunctivitis.
Fundoscopy:	Not done
ENT:	No hearing loss. Normal oropharyngeal and nasal mucosa.
Neck:	Normal jugular venous pressure. No carotid bruits.
Lungs:	Good air entry bilaterally. No wheezes or crackles.
Heart:	Regular S1, S2.
Abdomen:	Not done.
Extremities:	No edema.
Neurologic:	Patient was awake, alert and oriented x 3. Cranial nerves II through XII were intact. Motor power was 5/5 bilaterally. Normal gait.
Skin:	No lesions or rashes.
Other:	None
Diagnosis:	Hypertension, Chronic kidney disease, Renal Artery Stenosis. Direct face-to face time spent with patient was 80 minutes.
Plan:	1. Increase the Toprol XL to 100 mg PO QD. Script written. 2. She will continue to monitor her BP at home. 3. She knows to call with any questions or concerns. 4. Return to clinic in 3-4 week with a basic metabolic panel. 5. Continue other medications for now.

A. 99215, 99354, 403.90, 585.9, V45.89
B. 99214, 403.90, V45.89
C. 99214, 99358, 401.9, 585.9, 440.1
D. 99215, 99354, 401.9, 585.9, V45.89

Practice 12A, Report B

HOSPITAL-PROGRESS NOTE

CC: Worsening Acute Renal Failure

The patient was seen and examined multiple times today. His BUN was down to 40, sodium 135. His hiccups are better. He is getting them intermittently. His potassium was 3.9. He had no shortness of breath, no chest pain. Ultrasound was done. I evaluated him later in the evening. The patient was found to have right-sided hydronephrosis and right-sided hydroureter. I had a a long discussion with him and his family and I discussed the case with the consulting physicians. We proceeded with right-sided percutaneous nephrostomy and nephrostomy tube placement. The patient had bloody urine. He tolerated that procedure well. He was evaluated afterwards again. The patient also had a PD catheter placed, without difficulty and uneventfully.

EXAMINATION: The patient had no edema and felt well. His LUNGS are clear. His VITALS remain stable, BP 138/82, Pulse 126. He is afebrile.

I spent quite a bit of time with this patient today and with his family at bedside. Had lots of discussions on the different procedures that were done. His family asked a lot of questions. They were all answered. We discussed hemodialysis and peritoneal dialysis. We discussed nephrostomy tube and distal ureteric obstruction could be related to his surgery. We have addressed all of the concerns and issues. We discussed the fact that we might end up placing a stent, either cystoscopically or antegrade. I discussed this with his surgeon and we decided to proceed again tomorrow with antegrade stent placement.

IMPRESSION:

1. Acute renal failure.
2. Obstructive uropathy.
3. Right-sided hydronephrosis.
4. Chronic renal failure.
5. Hyponatremia from fluid overload state.

PLAN:

1. Hold dialysis for now.
2. Repeat laboratories in the morning.
3. High protein boost t.i.d.
4. Will keep him n.p.o. after midnight.
5. We will proceed with antegrade stent placement.
6. Consult urologist.
7. The patient is code level 1.

    Total time spent on this patient today was 2 hours and 25 minutes.

Codes:_____

Standby Services (99360)

Used when a physician, at request of attending physician, is standing by in case his/her services are needed

Standby physician cannot be rendering services to another patient during standby time

Reported in increments of 30 minutes

Only reported when no service is performed and there is no face-to-face contact with the patient

> Not used when a standby status ends, and the physician is providing a service to a patient

> The service the physician provides is reported as any other service would be, even though it began as a physician standby service

PRACTICE 12B, STANDBY SERVICES

These are time-based codes, so no audit form is required. Once you have coded the two cases, check your answers in Unit III of this text, where you will locate the answers and rationales.

Practice 12B, Report A

LOCATION: Outpatient Hospital

Surgeon is called in to be on standby for a female patient with proteinuria that has ungone a biopsy of her right kidney. Specimen was sent for frozen section. Patient remains in surgery suite prepped for a procedure if diagnosis comes back malignant. Surgeon had been on standby for approximately 15 minutes when he received a call regarding another patient. Surgeon spent 6 minutes on the phone. Within 10 minutes of ending his call he was notified that his services would not be needed as the biopsy came back negative for malignancy.

A. Not reportable/billable service

B. 99360

C. 50205-80

D. 99360-52

Practice 12B, Report B

LOCATION: Inpatient, Hospital

OB/GYN physician on call has asked me to standby due to 19-year-old patient in labor with fetal monitoring showing increased fetal distress. Patient is at 32-weeks gestation. Possible neonatal resuscitation may be required. After 1 hour and 40 minutes of constant standby, patient delivered without my assistance to newborn.

Codes:_____

13. CASE MANAGEMENT SERVICES (99363-99368)

Anticoagulant Management (99363, 99364)

Codes used to report anticoagulant (warfarin) therapy management

Require physician review and interpretation

Reported based initial or subsequent services

Outpatient management only

Assessments taken based on International Normalized Ratio (INR)

A system developed to report blood coagulation (clotting)

Reported for each 90 days

Initial service must include a minimum of 8 assessments

Subsequent service must include at least 3 assessments

Any period less than 60 days is not reported

Medical Team Conferences (99366-99368)

Management of complex cases involving individuals, such as

Hospice patient

Patient who is homebound and receives majority of health care from visiting nurse

Reported when a team of at least 3 different specialists meet to discuss

Revising care plan

Coordinating treatment plan with other professionals

Adjusting therapies

Medical Team Conferences codes

Face-to-face with patient and/or family—**99366**

Participation by nonphysician qualified health professional

30 minutes or more

Without patient and/or family—**99367**

Participation by physician

30 minutes or more

Without patient and/or family—**99368**

Participation by nonphysician qualified health professional

30 minutes or more

PRACTICE 13A, CASE MANAGEMENT SERVICES (99363-99368)

These are time- and complexity-based codes, so no audit form is required. Once you have coded the two cases, check your answers in Unit III of this text, where you will locate the answers and rationales.

Practice 13A, Report A

PHONE CALL

I spoke to the family today in conference. Present were 2 sons, 1 daughter and the patient's husband. The interdisciplinary team of 5 was present for the conference. We spoke in great detail the prognosis of the patient and that the ongoing chemotherapy is not working and that decisions had to be made on behalf of the patient as far a code status. Besides the patient's stomach cancer with mets to the lungs, she is also deteriorating in regards to chronic pneumonia along with CHF. We explained to the family that the patient should be put on comfort measures, maybe bringing in hospice.

We will meet in my office next week to discuss this further.

The patient's prognosis is very grim, but we have left the decision to family to decide the care of their mother/wife. The conference lasted 45 minutes.

A. 99366, V66.7, 151.9, 197.0, 428.0, 515

B. 99367, V65.49, 151.9, 197.0, 428.5, 515

C. 99368, V66.7, 151.9, 197.0, 428.0, 515

D. 99366, V65.49, 151.9, 197.0, 428.0, 515

Practice 13A, Report B

TEAM CONFERENCE

This is an 87-year-old female that was discharged from the Rehabilitation Center to the Lilly Basic Care Facility. She was admitted with the diagnosis of nephritis and previous right below-the-knee amputation. An interdisciplinary team of 4 met to discuss the best plan for this patient. No family was in attendance during the conference.

The patient's goal was to improve with her strength and overall health status. The patient has shown improvement with both her health status cares and mobility. At this time, she is ambulatory with the wheeled walker and her prosthesis modified independent. She is managing well enough at this time with mobility, transfers, and toileting to be a candidate for transition to a basic care facility. The basic care facility will provide assistance with bathing, meals, housekeeping, and medication monitoring. A physical therapy exercise program is planned. The patient does receive renal dialysis three days a week for her ESRD and will continue dialysis on Tuesday, Thursday, and Saturdays. She will receive her IV antibiotic dosing during her dialysis treatments under the direction of pharmacy. Dial-A-Ride has been arranged for transport for her Tuesday and Thursday appointments at dialysis and family will assist with transport for Saturday dialysis appointments. A referral has been made through County Social Service to assess eligibility for vouchers for the Saturday Dial-A-Ride. Referral information was faxed to the basic care facility on the day of discharge as requested. Family did provide transport at discharge. Time spent on conference was approximately 60 minutes.

Codes:_____

Anticoagulant Management (99363, 99364)

Codes used to report anticoagulant (warfarin) therapy management

  Require physician review and interpretation

Reported based initial or subsequent services

Outpatient management only

Assessments taken based on International Normalized Ratio (INR)

  A system developed to report blood coagulation (clotting)

Reported for each 90 days

  Initial service must include a minimum of 8 assessments

  Subsequent service must include at least 3 assessments

Any period less than 60 days is not reported

PRACTICE 13B, ANTICOAGULANT MANAGEMENT

These are time- and complexity-based codes, so no audit form is required. Once you have coded the two cases, check your answers in Unit III of this text.

Practice 13B, Report A

LOCATION: Outpatient

Patient was initially seen in the office to establish an anticoagulant regiment. The patient had some high risk of clot formation, so the initial INR needed to be higher and he was started at 3.3. The tests and instruction were discussed with the patient. He returned for INR measurements and adjustment of his medications 9 times during the initial three months of therapy.

A. 99363

B. 99363, 99364

C. 99364

D. 99364, 99363

Practice 13B, Report B

LOCATION: Outpatient

The patient has been responding well to the initial 3 months of therapy and his dosage of warifin was reduced significantly to 2.5 at the end of the initial 3-month treatment period. He was then seen once a month for the next three months for INR measurements. He responded well to treatment and his coagulation rates were within normal limits.

Codes:_____

The patient presented for warifin therapy due to deep vein thrombosis of the lower legs.

14. CARE PLAN OVERSIGHT SERVICES (99374-99380)

Codes are divided according to whether physician is supervising a patient being cared for by

Home health agency

Hospice

Nursing facility

Time-based codes

15-29 minutes

30 minutes or more

Reporting is by time over a month

One physician may report the code per month

Reports physician supervision of patient, when patient is not present over a 30-day period

Patient resides in

Own home

Rest home or domiciliary

Includes assisted living facility or hospice

For patients under

Home health care (99374-99375)

Hospice (99376-99377)

Nursing facility services (99379-99380)

Physician provides the following types of services

Review subsequent reports, laboratory studies, or other studies

Integrates new data into patients' care plan

Adjust medical therapy

Develops or revises care plans

Communicate with other health care professionals

PRACTICE 14, CARE PLAN OVERSIGHT SERVICES (99374-99380)

Once you have coded the two cases, check your answers in Unit III of this text, where you will locate the answers and rationales.

Practice 14, Report A

Care plan review of 77-year-old female in the local nursing facility. Patient suffers from advanced ovarian cancer and is currently receiving chemotherapy. Spoke with gynecologist and patient seems to be doing well with current treatments, although has increased pain. Per nurse's remarks in chart, patient seems to have increased edema in the lower extremities. Plan includes continuing with current dose of chemotherapy per gynecologist, IV morphine infusion for pain, and IV diuretics for edema. After reviewing her labs, I have ordered Aranesp 100 mcg if her hemoglobin drops below 12, currently it is 12.4. Documentation includes review of chart, nurse's remarks noted and medication adjustments of patient's care plan. Total time spent this month formulating care plan was 40 minutes.

A. 99367, 99380, 183.0, 338.3, 782.3

B. 99380, 183.0, 338.3, 782.3

C. 99308, V58.11, 183.0, 338.3, 782.3

D. 99380, V58.11, 183.0

Practice 14, Report B

CARE PLAN OVERSIGHT

Care plan oversight for terminal care of a 78-year-old male hospice patient with advanced lower lobe lung cancer. Plan includes continuous oxygen and pain control management involving IV morphine infusion. Have had contact with nurses, family members, and patient's social worker. Phone conference with patient's family to discuss concerns of continuing supportive care, from which patient wishes to withdraw. Documentation includes review and modification of patient's care plan and orders to pharmacy. Total time spent this month formulating care plan was 45 minutes.

Codes:_____

15. PREVENTIVE MEDICINE SERVICES (99381-99429)

There are two categories under Preventive Medicine Services

Preventive Medicine Services (99381-99397)

Counseling and/or Risk Factor Reduction Intervention (99401-99429)

Preventive Medicine Services (99381-99397)

Reports routine E/M for patient who is healthy and has no complaint

Used to identify comprehensive services, not a single-system examination

Such as an annual gynecologic examination

Codes based on age and if new or established patient

If physician encounters a problem or abnormality that requires significant additional service during preventative service

Report appropriate level office visit code with −25

Code descriptions indicate terms "comprehensive history" and "comprehensive examination" are used

Not same definition as in 99201-99350

Comprehensive means a complete history and a complete examination appropriate for age/gender

Examination is a multisystem examination

Extent of examination is determined by age of patient and risk factors for patient

Counseling and/or Risk Factor Reduction and Behavior Change Intervention (99401-99429)

Both new and established healthy patients

Based on whether individual or group counseling is provided and time spent in service

Used to report a physician's services to a patient for risk factor interventional counseling

Codes used to report services focused on promoting health and preventing illness/injury

Patient does NOT have symptoms or an established illness

If patient does have symptoms or an established illness, report service with appropriate E/M code

Examples

Diet and exercise program

Smoking cessation

Contraceptive management

PRACTICE 15, PREVENTIVE MEDICINE SERVICES

These are age-based codes, so no audit form is required. Once you have coded the two cases, check your answers in Unit III of this text.

Practice 15, Report A

SUBJECTIVE: This is an established 43-year-old white female, four previous pregnancies, two children, in today for a GYN exam and Pap smear. Her only physical complaint is weight gain over the last couple of years. She had tried switching her antidepressant medicine from Zoloft to Wellbutrin and reacted very severely to the Wellbutrin. She is now back on Zoloft which she is aware can increase appetite. She has never tried portion control and increased exercise. She has generalized body aches.

CURRENT BIRTH CONTROL METHOD: She had a hysterectomy.

OTHER MEDICATIONS: 1. Protonix. 2. Lipitor. 3. Zoloft

ALLERGIES: Poppy seeds.

IMMUNIZATIONS: Tetanus and flu shot are up to date.

MENSTRUAL HISTORY: Hysterectomy for a bicornuate uterus. The cervix was adhesed on to the bladder so the cervical stub was left. Last Pap smear was August 2 years ago. Pap smears are being done every two to four years.

MEDICAL HISTORY, SOCIAL HISTORY, AND FAMILY HISTORY are unchanged since her last appointment. Please refer to consultation.

REVIEW OF SYSTEMS: No current HEENT, respiratory, cardiovascular, or breast problems. Irritable bowel symptoms are relieved by diet and Protonix. Multiple musculoskeletal problems related to bursitis and hip and back pain. No neurological, endocrine, or integumentary problems. Depression symptoms are well controlled by Zoloft.

PHYSICAL EXAMINATION: Declines the presence of a chaperone in the room today. Blood pressure: 106/66. Weight: 189. Height: 5 feet 5 inches. Thyroid is normal to palpation without enlargement. Cervical nodes are negative. Lungs are clear to auscultation without rates or wheezes. Heart: Regular rate and rhythm without murmurs. Breasts are normal to inspection and bilaterally symmetrical. Normal to palpation. No nipple discharge. Negative axillary nodes. Negative CVAT. Abdomen is soft without organomegaly or hernia. Vulva is normal to inspection. Normal hair distribution. Negative BUS. Negative inguinal nodes. Vagina has a scant amount of creamy discharge. Cervix is normal. A Pap smear was obtained. Bimanual exam shows no masses. Skin is warm and dry. Distal pulses are equal. No edema of the extremities.

ASSESSMENT:
1. Gynecologic examination with Pap.
2. Health maintenance issues.

PLAN:
1. We will notify her of her Pap within two weeks.
2. She will schedule a mammogram in the near future. Fasting lab work has all been done within the last two years.
3. Return to the clinic p.r.n. and for GYN care.

A. 99396, V70.0, V72.31

B. 99213, V70.0, 783.1

C. 99386, 783.1, 311

D. 99395, V70.0

Practice 15, Report B

Patient is a 44-year-old white female who comes to our office this afternoon for a yearly physical. She denies any active complaints. She is established with our clinic.

PMH: None.

PSH: Tubal ligation in 1982.

MEDICATIONS: None.

ALLERGIES: NKA.

SOCIAL HISTORY: She smokes one pack per day for the last twenty years. She denies any history of alcohol or drug abuse. She is married and has three adult children. Her husband is currently in the service. She lives alone at home.

FAMILY HISTORY: Her father died at age 62 from unknown reasons. Her mother died at age 35 from unknown reasons. She has three brothers and one sister who are in good health.

PE: Declines the presence of a chaperone in the room today. Blood pressure: 108/78. Weight: 228 pounds. Height: 5 feet 5 inches. Thyroid is normal to palpation without enlargement. Cervical nodes are negative. Lungs are clear to auscultation without rates or wheezes. Heart: Regular rate and rhythm without murmurs. Breasts are normal to inspection and bilaterally symmetrical. Normal to palpation.

No nipple discharge. Negative axillary nodes. Abdomen is soft without organomegaly or hernia. Vulva is normal to inspection. Normal hair distribution. Negative BUS. Negative inguinal nodes. Vagina is clean with a scant amount of creamy discharge. On opening of the speculum to visualize the cervix, the patient complains of some discomfort and there is a slight amount of oozing at the posterior aspect of the cervical apex under the cervical stump. A Pap smear was obtained. Bimanual exam shows tenderness with deep penetration into the vagina and tenderness with cervical stump movement anteriorly. No masses palpated in the cut-de-sac or with bimanual exam. Skin is warm and dry. Distal pulses are equal. No edema of the extremities.

ASSESSMENT/PLAN:
1. Yearly physical done today.
2. Smoking cessation.

I talked to the patient about quitting smoking and she told me she has been thinking about it and will try. We will get a CBC, fasting CMP, fasting lipid panel, TSH, UA, EKG, chest x-ray, mammogram and stool occult cards x 3. We will do a Pap smear with her next visit. The patient is scheduled for a follow-up visit in one month.

Codes:_____

16. NEWBORN CARE (99431-99440)

Report services provided to newborns provided in several settings

    Such as hospital or birthing room

Usually used for normal, healthy newborns

Hospital care codes would be used if the newborn were ill

Apgar assessment at 1 minute and 5 minutes after delivery

    Physician assesses

        Muscle tone (activity)

        Heart rate (pulse)

        Reflex response (grimace)

        Color (appearance)

        Breathing (respiration)

    Each assessment area is assigned a rating of 0 to 2

    Recorded on the newborn's medical record

Includes codes for attendance at delivery and newborn resuscitation.

PRACTICE 16, NEWBORN CARE

Once you have coded the two cases, check your answers in Unit III of this text, where you will locate the answers and rationales.

Practice 16, Report A

36-week male born at 1:27 AM by vaginal delivery. APGAR 8/9. Disorganized suck, but once eating, takes 10-20 cc per feeding. Patient has (+) urine and stool output. Patient is discharged from the hospital the same day at 7:30 PM.

A. 99435, V30.1, 779.3

B. 99234, V30.1

C. 99234, V30.00, 779.3

D. 99435, V30.00

Practice 16, Report B

	Normal	Abnormal	**NEWBORN EXAM RECORD** ADMISSION EXAM Comments Date: 07/28/XX	Normal	Abnormal	DISCHARGE EXAM Comments Date:
Head/Fontanels		✓	Scalp bruised			
Eyes	✓					
Ears/Nose/Throat	✓					
Heart	✓					
Lungs	✓					
Abdomen	✓					
Trunk/Spine	✓					
Anus	✓					
Genitalia	✓					
Negative Barlow Test	✓					
Negative Ortolani Test	✓					
Extremities/Clavicles	✓					
Skin	✓					
Neurological/Tone	✓					

PROGRESS NOTES: 07/29/XX

Day two: Vitals stable, afebrile. Exam is unchanged.	
(+) urine and stool. Weight is up 2.3%.	
Continue normal newborn care.	

Codes:_____

17. NON-FACE-TO-FACE PHYSICIAN SERVICES (99441-99444); SPECIAL E/M SERVICES (99450-99456); AND OTHER E/M SERVICES (99477-99499)

Non-Face-to-Face Physician Services (99441–99444)

Report physician E/M services using the telephone or internet

99441-99443 used to report telephone E/M services

> Provided to an established patient, family member of the patient, or a guardian

> Cannot originate from an E/M service within the previous seven days

> Cannot lead to an E/M service within the next 24 hours or the next available appointment

> Reported based on the time documented in the medical record

99444 used to report online E/M services

> Provided to an established patient, family member of the patient, or a guardian

> Cannot originate from an E/M service within the previous seven days

> Cannot lead to an E/M service within the next 24 hours or the next available appointment

Special E/M Services (99450-99456)

Reports examination for life, work, or disability insurance

Establishes patient health baseline information

Provided in office or other setting

Reported for both new and established patients

If other E/M services provided the same day

> Report additional service with appropriate E/M code(s)

99455 reports examination by treating physician

99456 reports examination by other than treating physician

Other E/M Services (99477–99499)

99477 reports an initial hospital E/M service for a neonate

> 28 days of age or less

> Requires intensive observation, interventions, and intensive care services

99499 reports unlisted E/M services

> Accompanied by a special report

PRACTICE 17, NON-FACE-TO-FACE PHYSICIAN SERVICES; SPECIAL E/M SERVICES; AND OTHER E/M SERVICES

No audit form is required for these codes. Once you have coded the two cases, check your answers in Unit III of this text.

Practice 17, Report A

DISABILITY ASSESSMENT

This patient has suffered neck and low back injuries from an automobile accident. We determined from her Spinal Disability Evaluation that she has a Spinal Disability Rating of 50%.

Lost Pre-Injury Capacity: Disability precluding heavy lifting, repeated bending, stooping, and crawling. This individual has also lost approximately HALF of her pre-injury capacity of lifting, bending, stooping, and crawling.

Patient will continue with the prescribed chronic pain management regimen and ongoing physical therapy 3 times a week.

A. 99455, 723.1, 724.2, 846.8, E819.9

B. 99456, 723.1, 724.2, 905.7, E920.0

C. 99456, 723.1, 724.2, 846.8, E819.9

D. 99455, 723.1, 724.2, 338.21, 905.7, E929.0

Practice 17, Report B

DISABILITY ASSESSMENT

This is a 42-year-old man who has been disabled due to work-related injury for about 6 months now. He is unable to use his hands or arms in any type of lifting due to carpal tunnel syndrome status post surgery with no relief and chronic pain.

The patient's pain level today is 7 out of 10. He will continue with his prescribed medication at the current dosage. I will also consult physical therapy to strengthen his arms. I will see this patient back after his first treatment in therapy.

Completion of performance examination has been completed.

Codes:_____

UNIT ▌▌

Examinations

● EXAMINATION 1

EXAMINATION 1, REPORT 1

LOCATION: Shady Lane Nursing Facility
Nursing Facility Admission

HISTORY
Chief Complaint: Dementia, Parkinson's disease, and inability to care for self.

HISTORY OF CHIEF COMPLAINT: (Obtained mostly from the patient's guardian and wife of 27 years, Margaret.) The patient's wife relates that the patient was diagnosed in 2001 at Community General with Alzheimer's dementia that has progressively worsened. In addition, he has also had a 10-year history of Parkinson's disease. He is very unsteady on his feet and has recurrent falls. He is also an insulin requiring diabetic.

The wife, until recently, had been having an aide come in twice a week to assist with showering and activities of daily living of the patient. An RN was also coming in twice a week to check on his medications and diabetic status. Unfortunately, the falls have progressively worsened and the wife is becoming overwhelmed by the need now for 24 hr care. He has also become more assaultive and is exhibiting inappropriate behaviors. It should be noted he was placed on Prozac and the wife indicates he responded well in terms of his inappropriate behaviors. In addition to his other signs and symptoms, he has now developed some sundowning. All of these have culminated in the need for admission to this nursing facility.

CURRENT MEDICATIONS: Bumex .5 mg daily, Celexa 20 mg daily, Sinemet 25-100 mg tid, Humulin 70/30 insulin 30 units in AM.

MEDICAL HISTORY: Surgeries—myocardial infarction six years ago with stenting at Community General.

ILLNESSES: Myocardial infarction six years ago, diabetes mellitus type II—approximately 15 years, Parkinson's disease—approximately 15 years.

ALLERGIES: NO KNOWN DRUG ALLERGIES.

FAMILY HISTORY: Mother and father both died in their 70's. The remainder of the family history is not really known by the patient or the wife.

SOCIAL HISTORY: He has a 10th grade education. He served in the US Navy in World War II. A previous marriage ended in divorce. His current marriage, as noted, has been for 27 years. There are no biologic children from either of the marriages.

REVIEW OF SYSTEMS
Gastrointestinal: Good appetite; no reported nausea, vomiting, melena, fecal incontinence, or hematochezia. Genitourinary: He had long-standing incontinence but no reported dysuria or gross hematuria. Cardiovascular: As noted above; sleeps on 1 pillow. No paroxysmal nocturnal dyspnea. He has intermittent dependent edema. Neuromuscular: As noted above; he has severely impaired balance and has had frequent falls. No fractures. Respiratory: As noted above. Habits: Cigarettes—20 to 30 pack-a-year history of nicotine abuse; stopped about 20 years ago. Alcohol—history of abuse that he also stopped about 20 years ago.

PHYSICAL EXAMINATION
General: This is a very pleasant, well-nourished, well-developed Caucasian male who appears his stated age. He's reasonably alert. His speech is clear and fairly fluent. He knows the year, but doesn't know his exact birth date. He's a somewhat inconsistent historian. He recalls remote events more easily than any short-term memories.

HEENT: Head—normocephalic with male pattern baldness. Eyes—pupils are slightly myotic but reactive. Extraocular movements are intact. Sclerae are non-icteric. Conjunctivae are non-injected. Fundi suggest arteriolar narrowing without any obvious hemorrhages or exudates. No papilledema. Ears—otic canals are cerumen filled bilaterally. Face is symmetrical. There's evidence of some actinic keratoses. Mouth/Throat—lips, tongue, and mucous membranes are moist. Tongue is in the midline. He has multiple indigenous teeth, but there are many absent teeth. There's a suggestion of halitosis. Neck: Supple; thyroid gland is not palpable. Carotid upstrokes are satisfactory. No overt delays or bruits noted. Lymphadenopathy is not evident in the neck and supraclavicular region. Cervical neck veins are non-distended. Chest/Lung: Symmetrical and moves symmetrically with inspiration and expiration. No thrills or heaves. Rate and rhythm are regular. There's a faint grade 2/6 aortic ejection murmur radiating along the left sternal border without any concomitant 53 or 54 gallops. Lungs reveal some dry crackles in the right lower lobe. Abdomen: Round, non-distended, and non-tender. No scars visible. No inguinal hernias noted. Liver, spleen, kidneys, and urinary bladder are not palpably enlarged. Normal bowel sounds. No abdominal or flank bruits. Genitalia: External- penis is uncircumcised with normal scrotal contents. Rectal: Digital exam—anal sphincter is tonic. The prostate gland is slightly atrophic and smooth. There's a moderate amount of semi-solid, light brown stool in the rectal vault. Hemoccult is obtained. Extremities: There is +1/+4 bilateral pitting pretibial and ankle edema. Dorsalis pedis and posterior tibial pulses are not palpable. Popliteals are trace/+4 on the right and +1/+4 on the left. Neurologic: Deep tendon reflexes are hypoactive but symmetrical. He's not exhibiting any drooling or tremor at this time. He has positive cogwheel rigidity.

MINI-MENTAL STATE: He can only recall 2 out of 3 objects within one minute. He is unable to spell the word "world" backwards. He cannot do any simple arithmetic problems. It is obvious that this gentleman is not capable of making decisions regarding his personal, medical, or financial affairs.

IMPRESSIONS:
1. Alzheimer's dementia.
2. Parkinson's disease.
3. Diabetes mellitus type II.
4. Arteriosclerotic heart disease.
   a. History of myocardial infarction—stented seven years ago at Community General.
5. Urinary incontinence.
6. Seborrhea.
7. Actinic keratoses.
8. Peripheral vascular disease.
   a. Bilateral tibial artery occlusive disease.

He is now being admitted to this nursing facility.

PLAN: The patient is to have a Do Not Resuscitate code status. The patient will be assessed by the doctor in the Musculoskeletal Clinic for PT/OT evaluation. Glucoscan monitors will be instituted. We'll monitor renal function and serum electrolytes in light of the diuretic therapy. It certainly appears he's, possibly, exhibiting increased signs of left ventricular failure and we'll certainly increase the Bumex dosage.

The goals for this gentleman are to provide a reasonably safe and secure environment and maximize his comfort in life. He's functioning at a fairly high level for a dementia individual and may very well integrate pretty well into the unit and facility with participation in those activities for which he's capable of appreciating and enjoying, as well as interacting with his peers and members of the staff. General medical status is fair at this time. Unfortunately, the overall prognosis in this gentleman with irreversible neurologic disorders superimposed on significant comorbidities, certainly, doesn't portend well for long-term life expectancy.

Codes:_____

EXAMINATION 1, REPORT 2

LOCATION: Outpatient, Hospital
Patient is admitted to observation for left heart catheterization.

INDICATION: Abnormal stress test with exercise intolerance.

HISTORY OF PRESENT ILLNESS: The patient is a very pleasant 79-year-old gentleman, past medical history significant for unstable angina, multivessel coronary disease. After identifying multivessel coronary disease at cardiac catheterization, the patient went on to 5-vessel coronary artery bypass grafting surgery. Surgery performed in June included LIMA to LAD, saphenous vein graft to OM-1, reverse saphenous vein graft to PDA at junction of PDA and PLV with extension to the main body of the right coronary artery. Utilization of PADCAB (perfusion assisted direct coronary artery bypass) for infusion of graft during the off pump coronary bypass grafting surgery and utilization of VasoView for harvesting leg vein for saphenous vein graft was performed.

Shortly thereafter the patient underwent exercise treadmill stress testing with complaints of exercise intolerance. The patient underwent exercise treadmill stress testing in August where he was found to have functional capacity class II/III under modified Bruce protocol.

Double product (this is the systolic blood pressure times the heart rate) was 26,280, disproportionately elevated from a minimal amount of physical exertion and provocation, challenged the patient by modified Bruce protocol stress test.

The patient did exercise 9 minutes at 1.7 miles per hour, 10% grade maximum, METs 4. Initial heart rate 74 beats per minute, reached a maximum of 147 beats per minute, 98% maximum predicted heart rate for age with initial blood pressure of 150/86 and a maximum of 180/82. There was appropriate heart rate and blood pressure response to exercise and the treadmill stress test was discontinued once maximum heart rate achieved. There was clear evidence of disproportionate amount of fatigue, exercise intolerance to the minimal amount of stress challenge given patient. There was no chest pain. No significant electrocardiogram changes were found.

He went on to imaging which showed ejection fraction of 54%, no significant regional wall motion abnormalities, mixed largely reversible perfusion defect at the lateral wall involving the base and reversible perfusion defect, apex extending to the inferior wall and a mild anterior wall perfusion defect.

The patient now comes for left heart catheterization.

REVIEW OF SYSTEMS: The patient has had intermittent chest pain and some dyspnea on exertion.

PHYSICAL EXAMINATION: Well-developed, well-nourished gentleman, alert and oriented to time, place, and person. Mood congruent, affect appropriate, goal oriented speech, lying on stretcher in holding area in the cardiac catheterization laboratory. VITAL SIGNS: Reveal BLOOD PRESSURE of 140/80, HEART RATE 80, RESPIRATIONS 14 per minute. The patient is afebrile. HEAD, EYES, EARS, NOSE, AND THROAT: Unremarkable. HEART: Reveals regular rate and rhythm. LUNGS: Clear. ABDOMEN: Benign.

LABORATORY STUDIES: CBC shows a white count of 4.3, hemoglobin of 9.6, chronically anemic. Hematocrit is 31.1, platelets 198,000. The patient has microcytic, hypochromic anemia with an MCV of 76, MCH of 23, MCHC of 31. Basic metabolic profile shows sodium of 138, potassium of 4.1, chloride of 105, bicarb 26, BUN 13, creatinine 1.2, glucose 133, calcium 8.4, GFR greater than 60. PT, INR is 10.4, 1.0 respectively. PTT is 23.1 baseline. Normal differential and CBC.

IMPRESSION: 87-year-old gentleman status post multivessel coronary artery bypass grafting surgery after coronary disease identified, now with exercise intolerance on cardiolite stress testing, comes for left heart catheterization.

Codes:_____

EXAMINATION 1, REPORT 3

LOCATION: Outpatient, Office

Thank you for referring Mr. W. to me for consultation and care. The following is a summary of my findings and recommendations.

SUBJECTIVE: The patient is a seventy-one-year-old white male who presents complaining of right knee pain. This has been ongoing for a few months. When he goes to pivot on his knee he is having buckling and giving way. He was coming out of his pickup truck a couple of weeks ago his knee did give way. He is not having any swelling to speak of, but he has the same problems stair climbing and he does feel unstable. He denies any paresthesias.

PAST MEDICAL HISTORY: Significant for coronary artery disease, cardiac arrhythmia, hypercholesterolemia, hypertension, reflux, right inguinal hernia, Dupuytren's disease.

His current medications are:
1. Atenolol 50mg three tablets daily
2. Coumadin 2mg daily

3. Cozaar 50mg daily
4. Prilosec 20mg daily
5. Aspirin 81mg daily
6. Pravachol 80mg daily
7. Lopid 600mg bid
8. IMDUR daily, dose unknown
9. Nitro sublingual on a prn basis

PAST SURGICAL HISTORY: Significant for coronary artery bypass grafting ×2, coronary stenting ×3, right inguinal herniorrhaphy repair, and bilaterally Dupuytren's contracture release.

REVIEW OF SYSTEMS: The history form was reviewed. Neurologic: denies any history of seizure disorder, tinnitus, and vertigo. Cardiovascular: positive for coronary disease, occasional chest pain, positive for essential hypertension, controlled. No lower extremity edema. GI: positive for gastroesophageal reflux disease, but no change in bowel habits, weight loss or gain. GU: no frequency, dysuria, hematuria, but does complain of nocturia ×2. Constitutional, ophthalmologic, otolaryngologic, respiratory, musculoskeletal, integumentary, psychiatric, endocrine, hematologic, and immunologic were negative.

PHYSICAL EXAM: Well developed, well nourished white male 5' 8" in height and 200 pounds. BP: 176/86, pulse: 60, respiratory rate: 24, temperature: 97.3. He has a genu varus deformity of the right knee with atrophy of his right quadriceps, which is mild. He has a positive McMurray's medially, equivocal anterior drawer, negative posterior drawer, medial joint line tenderness, no lateral joint line tenderness is noted. The left knee has 5/5 quadriceps strength, very minimal Grade I valgus instability, no varus instability. Negative McMurray's medially or laterally.

X-RAYS: Standing AP, as well as sunrise, notch, and lateral views of the right knee. There is a mild genu varus deformity of the right knee of about 5 to 10 degrees with total loss of joint space in the medial femoral compartment. Lateral view shows spurring on the superior and inferior poles of the patella with decreased joint space in the patellofemoral compartment. The notch view shows chondromalacia and varus deformity of the right knee, chondromalacia in the lateral femoral compartment.

Review of the MRI, which is accompanying the patient, reveals a very large tear of the posterior horn of the medial meniscus as well as chondromalacia in the patellofemoral compartment, large medial plica, and cysts noted in the anterior and posterior horns of the lateral meniscus.

ASSESSMENT:
1. Degenerative joint disease with meniscal tears bilateral medial and lateral femoral compartments with associated genu varus deformity.
2. Coronary artery disease.
3. Hypercholesterolemia.

PLAN: The patient will need arthroscopy intervention in the hopes of saving the knee. I did explain to him that we would not be able to give him 100% relief, probably because of the chronicity of the problem and the medial femoral compartment is pretty much at this point Grade IV chondromalacia in several spots with bare bone "kissing lesions" noted. He will need medical clearance/consultation by Dr. G prior to any surgical intervention and will probably have to get a preoperative INR level and stop the Coumadin one to two days prior to surgical intervention and repeat the PT INR the day of surgery. This will be under general anesthetic and he will be placed back on Cournadin postoperatively. We also gave him Celebrex samples 200mg once daily, which he can take while taking Coumadin. He can take his Tylenol with this. Continue his regular medication.

Thank you for allowing me to participate in the care of your patient. If you have any questions don't hesitate to call.

Codes:_____

EXAMINATION 1, REPORT 4

LOCATION: Emergency Department

CHIEF COMPLAINT: Sore throat.

HISTORY OF PRESENT ILLNESS
This is a 53-year-old female with history of bipolar disorder who has had 5-7 days of sore throat, constitutional symptoms, generalized aches and some fatigue. She has had no fever. Some slight cough but no shortness of breath. No abdominal pain. No other complaints at this time. She comes for evaluation today.

Please see nursing notes for medications and allergies.

ROS
The patient has had no fever or weight loss. Has had some fullness of the ears. No SOB. No rashes.

SOCIAL HISTORY
The patient does not smoke and only consumes occasional alcohol.

PHYSICAL EXAMINATION
Blood pressure 128/68, respirations 20, afebrile. She is an alert, pleasant female in no apparent distress. HEENT—clear tympanic membranes bilaterally. Oropharynx has some slight posterior oropharyngeal erythema. There is no exudate. There is no mass or asymmetry. She has nasopharynx and oropharynx cobblestoning with postnasal drip. Neck supple. Cervical lymphadenopathy. Heart regular. Lungs clear to auscultation bilaterally.

EMERGENCY DEPARTMENT COURSE
It was felt that this represented a viral pharyngitis. Recommended continued symptomatic care. Motrin, warm salt water gargles. Administered 800 mg oral Motrin. Return for any problems. Follow up with primary care physician. She is agreeable with this plan. Discharged home in stable condition.

PROVISIONAL DIAGNOSIS/DIAGNOSES: Pharyngitis.

Codes:_____

EXAMINATION 1, REPORT 5

LOCATION: ED (Critical Care Service)

CHIEF COMPLAINT: Weakness, fever, mental status changes.

HISTORY OF PRESENT ILLNESS
The patient is an 83-year-old male with multiple medical problems who presents to the ED accompanied by his wife. Apparently has had increased lethargy and decreased level of consciousness for the last 3 days. Wife states it has been progressively worse, especially over the last 24 hours. She did notice several days ago that he would occasionally choke and cough on some food. He has had very little food over the last 24 hours. States he has been trying to

up his fluid intake. She denies any recent trauma, other than falling and hitting his buttocks up against the countertop. Denies chest pain. Has had no cough or abdominal pain or vomiting. He was brought to the ED for further evaluation and treatment.

ROS/SH/FH/PMH: Not able to obtain due to patient status. Please see supplemental sheet from what I could get from the chart.

MEDICATIONS/ALLERGIES: Please see nursing notes.

PHYSICAL EXAMINATION
Oral temperature 38.2 degrees, vitals as charted. General—this is an elderly male, ill-appearing. HEENT—mucous membranes appear dry. Neck is supple. Cardiac exam is regular. Chest—there is apparent asymmetry of the rales, best heard in the right base. No extra accessory muscle use. Chest wall is nontender. Pacemaker in place. Abdomen is soft, flat, and nontender. Neurologic—the patient does move all 4 extremities spontaneously. Appears somewhat fatigued. He is able to answer a few questions and converse. Integumentary—skin warm and dry. He has abrasions by the left lower extremity as well as the right buttock from a recent fall. Please see supplemental sheet for exam findings.

EMERGENCY DEPARTMENT COURSE
The patient was seen and evaluated by myself. IV access was established. He was given supplemental oxygen to keep his saturations in the mid-90 percents. He was placed on continuous cardiac monitor. A 12-lead EKG was obtained. This revealed a ventricularly paced rhythm. His CMP reveals BUN 76, creatinine 3.1, total bilirubin 2.1, AST 43, and ALT 39. WBC 6.8, hemoglobin 10.0 (previous hemoglobins were in the 9 to 10 range), and he has had previous renal insufficiency. His INR is 3.2. Troponin is 7.64. BNP 1457. Digoxin level 2.0. Urinalysis does not reveal any white blood cells, negative leukocyte esterase and nitrite. He was given IV fluids. CT scan of the head was obtained and pending at time of this dictation. Blood and urine cultures were sent. Single-view chest radiograph has an apparent right-sided infiltrate. Administered IV Claforan and clindamycin, given his history of possible aspiration. Discussed the findings with the patient as well as his family members present, including his wife. Reviewed his labs and condition here. They did re-affirm he is a DNR/DNI (do not resuscitate/do not intubate). They understand that he has multiple organs that are failing at this point and that he is very sick, and that his condition very well could be terminal. He was admitted to monitored bed in guarded condition.

PROVISIONAL DIAGNOSIS/DIAGNOSES
1. Acute febrile illness/acute mental status changes.
2. Pneumonia.
3. Acute renal failure.
4. Elevated troponin/myocardial infarction.
5. Elevated BNP (elevated in cardiac disease).
6. Evaluation of dyspnea/hypoxemia.
   Critical care time 90 minutes.

Codes:_____

EXAMINATION 1, REPORT 6

LOCATION: Patient's Home

PATIENT: 89-year-old male

SUBJECTIVE: The patient is an 89-year-old gentleman who is cared for at home by his wife and attendant along with home health nurses. He has COPD and Parkinson's and has gotten over an episode of pneumonia. He has occasional anxiety episodes for which he takes Xanax with good relief. He sits up in a chair several times a week and is doing relatively well. He has minimal edema and his appetite is good. He has occasional coughing spells for which he uses a nebulizer with good results.

OBJECTIVE: He is afebrile. Pulse is 68 per minute and regular, respiratory rate is 18 per minute and unlabored. He is in no acute distress. He is somewhat lethargic today. Lungs are clear with no wheezes, rales or rhonchi. Heart demonstrates a regular rate and rhythm. Abdomen is soft, benign with no masses or tenderness. Extremities demonstrate no edema.

ASSESSMENT:
1. COPD.
2. Parkinson's.
3. Osteoarthritis, severe, bilateral knees.

PLAN:
He will continue his current therapy. He has had excellent care with no breakdown or pressure sores at this point.
   He will be seen again in one month.

Codes:_____

EXAMINATION 1, REPORT 7

LOCATION: Hospital, Inpatient

NEPHROLOGY/PROLONGED SERVICE PROGRESS NOTE:
CC: Pericardial Effusion
   The patient was seen, examined, and evaluated multiple times. Discussions were held with him and his wife.
   The patient did well overnight. He was making adequate amounts of urine. His blood pressure was maintained in the 130 range. Saturations were maintained in the high 90s on 3 liters per nasal cannula. I gave him 6 units of fresh frozen plasma and it brought his INR down to 1.7 this morning.

PHYSICAL EXAMINATION: He feels tired and weak. He has some chest pressure but no chest pain. He does not seem to be in any distress. He has good air entry bilaterally. He has a few crackles, if any, in the bases. ABDOMEN: Nontender. He has right IJ tunneled dialysis catheter. He does have slight generalized edema all over.

LABS TODAY: Phosphorus is 3.7, ionized calcium 4.2, INR 1.7. White count is 18.9, hemoglobin 8.9 grams and platelets 361,000. His BUN is 58, creatinine down to 1.5, sodium 131, potassium 4.1, chloride 97, glucose 151, albumin 3, alkaline phosphatase up to 190, total bilirubin 2.2, AST 279, ALT 350, bicarb 21.

IMPRESSION:
1. Pericardial effusion without tamponade yet.
2. Acute renal failure, improved.
3. Hyponatremia, improving.
4. Hypocalcemia secondary to blood transfusion.
5. Leukocytosis, improving.
6. Urinary tract infection.
7. Anemia secondary to subcutaneous bleeding and multiple blood draws in addition to the pericardial effusion.
8. Elevated liver function tests secondary to pericardial effusion most likely.

PLAN:
1. I attempted to contact his cardiologist twice this morning but I have been unsuccessful. I have talked to his nurse practitioner; she informed me that Cardiothoracic Surgery probably should be involved in the case. I have discussed the case with the patient's surgeon, and he indicated to me that the procedure could be done in our facility without any problems and the patient could be drained percutaneously.
2. I will have 2 units packed red blood cells ready to be transfused on-call to the cardiac catheterization laboratory.
3. Repeat labs in the morning.
4. Will hold on any IV fluids unless his blood pressure drops.
5. Replace his calcium with calcium gluconate 2 grams IV q.2.h. for 3 doses.
6. Expect liver function tests to improve once his pericardial effusion is drained.
7. Hold Coumadin for the time being.
8. Continue with Cipro.
9. Will keep NPO.

I discussed the case with cardiology and I appreciate his help on the case. We will await the patient's cardiologist recommendations.

I discussed the case with the patient and his family. They were in agreement with our approach and they were satisfied with the service today. All their questions were answered. I discussed the case with the patient's primary care physician, who was here this morning, as well. I have discussed my entire plan with the nursing staff.

Total time spent on this patient this morning was 1 hour and 55 minutes.

Codes:_____

EXAMINATION 1, REPORT 8

LOCATION: Hospital

Surgery operator paged me to be on standby for Neurosurgery. The patient is a 67-year-old male who was having a hemilaminectomy due to stenosis of the lumbar region. I arrived to the operative suite at 8:45 AM. I stayed in the suite until I was notified by one of the surgical team members that I was not needed at 9:25 AM.

Codes:_____

EXAMINATION 1, REPORT 9

CASE MANAGEMENT SERVICES

LOCATION: Office

I called Mrs. Johnson at home regarding the results of her chest x-ray that she had at our facility this morning for a chronic cough. I met with the radiologist in conference for 35 minutes to discuss the case. I discussed with her that there was a very small shadow in the lower lobe of the left lung. I told her that there wasn't anything to be concerned about and that we are going to follow-up in 3 months with another chest x-ray. I called in a prescription to her pharmacy for Robitussin with codeine to help her with her cough at nighttime. I notified her that if she worsens or has any questions to call our office immediately. Will follow-up with her in 3 months.

Codes:_____

EXAMINATION 1, REPORT 10

LOCATION: Office

ANNUAL PHYSICAL EXAM

SUBJECTIVE: This patient is a 39-year-old white female, four previous pregnancies, two children, in today for a GYN exam and Pap smear. She has some concerns about some occasional right lower quadrant pain and some vaginal bleeding that she has had off and on for the last couple of weeks. She did have a urinalysis done that showed no blood in the urine. She states the discharge is very minimal and she has not found any contributing factors.

CURRENT HORMONE THERAPY: Nothing.

MENSTRUAL HISTORY: She had a hysterectomy for a bicornuate uterus and menorrhagia. The cervix was adhered to the bladder so a cervical stump has been left. She has no hot flashes or steep disturbances. Last Pap was March 30. She has never had a previous abnormal pap.

MEDICAL HISTORY: Chronic illnesses include gastroesophageal reflux disease, high cholesterol, anxiety, history of one kidney, and history of irritable bowel.

SURGERIES:
1. Hysterectomy.
2. Two cesarean sections.

HOSPITALIZATIONS: For surgery only.

SOCIAL HISTORY: She is married and has no concerns of STD risks or abuse in this 23-year relationship. She works in an office. She feels that her diet has been fairly healthy. She is down over 15 pounds with healthy eating over the last few months and hoping to lose a lot more. She has two to three servings of calcium a day and no caffeine. She does continue to smoke rarely and has minimal secondhand smoke exposure. She has no alcohol intake. She is trying to walk consistently for exercise. She does wear a seatbelt, does use a sunscreen, and does do a breast exam.

FAMILY HISTORY: Father has high blood pressure, high cholesterol, coronary artery disease. Maternal grandmother had breast cancer. No ovarian or colon cancer history. Father is diabetic. No family history of thyroid disorders or osteoporosis. No depression or mental health issues.

REVIEW OF SYSTEMS: No current HEENT, respiratory, cardiovascular, breast, or GI problems. Lower abdominal pain and vaginal bleeding as noted above on a couple of instances. No pain during intercourse. No neurological, endocrine, or integumentary problems. No further depression symptoms.

PHYSICAL EXAMINATION: Declines the presence of a chaperone in the room today. Blood pressure 108/78. Weight 168 pounds. Height: 5 feet 4 inches. Thyroid is normal to palpation without enlargement. Cervical nodes are negative. Lungs are clear to auscultation without rales or wheezes. Heart: Regular rate and rhythm without murmurs. Breasts are normal to inspection and bilaterally symmetrical. Normal to palpation.

No nipple discharge. Negative axillary nodes. Negative CVAT. Abdomen is soft without organomegally or hernia. Vulva is normal to inspection. Normal hair distribution. Negative BUS. Negative inguinal nodes. Vagina is clean with a scant amount of creamy discharge. On opening of the speculum to visualize the cervix, the patient complains of some discomfort and there is a slight amount of oozing at the posterior aspect of the cervical apex under the cervical stump. A Pap smear was obtained. Bimanual exam shows tenderness with deep penetration into the vagina and tenderness with cervical stump movement anteriorly. No masses palpated in the cul-de-sac or with bimanual exam. Skin is warm and dry. Distal pulses are equal. No edema of the extremities.

ASSESSMENT:
1. Gynecologic examination with Pap.
2. Vaginal tenderness and slight vaginal bleeding, post hysterectomy.
3. Health maintenance issues.

PLAN:
1. We will notify her of her Pap results within two weeks.
2. I did give the patient two samples of vaginal Premarin cream and advised that she apply weekly to thicken the vaginal skin to decrease vaginal bleeding.
3. Mammogram will be scheduled in the near future.
4. Reinforced that she does a monthly breast exam, maintain an adequate calcium intake, and encouraged her efforts towards resuming a Weight Watcher's food plan and consistent exercise regimen.
5. Return to the clinic p.r.n. and for gynecologic care.

Codes:_____

EXAMINATION 1, REPORT 11

LOCATION: Office

This 58-year-old woman comes in for a life insurance examination. She currently has no complaints.

EXAM: Ht: 5′ 4″, Wt: 171, BP: 130/72. The patient's lungs are clear, heart regular with no murmur present. Abdomen is soft with bowel sounds. Extremities show no edema.

The patient is a healthy 58-year-old female with no complaints. I will send her to the lab for a basic metabolic panel and UA. I will contact her with the results. At that time I will complete the insurance form and forward a copy to the insurance company as well as the patient.

Codes:_____

EXAMINATION 1, REPORT 12

LOCATION: NICU INPATIENT

S: No events overnight

O: Resp: Rate: 38-73   Exam: upper airway congestion
CV: Rate: 110-150   Map: 50-63
Exam: RRR and well perfused
FEN/GI: I: 710   TF: 150   Wt: 4725
          O: 490
          Exam: Soft NT ND with +BS
HEME: none
GU: Right side of scrotal sac enlarged and unable to reduce, nontender.
ID: Temp Max: 36
Cultures:
NEURO:
          Exam: Alert, no edema.

A/P: 2 month 1 wk old male status post incarcerated hernia repair and status post supraglottoplasty now working on increasing weight. Continues to PO well, formula had mistakenly been formulated to 18 kcal vs. 22 kcal, mistake fixed and subsequently we should see much better weight gain.

Codes:_____

EXAMINATION 1, REPORT 13

LOCATION: Office

CARE PLAN OVERSIGHT

Six-month care plan for a 90-year-old Alzheimer patient on hospice. Patient also has COPD and stage IV renal failure, currently on peritoneal dialysis. Plan includes current medications, oxygen prn and to continue dialysis daily. Patient is to see nephrologist in dialysis center for monthly service and labs next Monday. Documentation includes review, nurse's remarks noted and modification of patient's care plan. Total time spent this month formulating care plan was 20 minutes.

Codes:_____

EXAMINATION 1, REPORT 14

LOCATION: Office

Home Care Plan Oversight

Gladys is a 92-year-old woman that I have had the pleasure of seeing in the past. She now resides in a rest home about 30 miles from here. The purpose of this note is to go over her monthly care plan. Gladys has severe arthritis in her knees and uses a walker. She also has emphysema from years of smoking, for which she is on oxygen prn. I have gone over her latest labs, which show hemoglobin of 9.2. I have a standing order of Aranesp 60 mcg if her hemoglobin drops below 11, in which case she will receive in the clinic. This will be increased to 100 mcg every two weeks. Per conversations with family members, Gladys seems in good spirits when they visit. The order for Aranesp 100 mcg will be sent to clinic. She will continue with her current dose of medication and current dose of oxygen prn. Total time spent this month formulating care plan was 45 minutes, plus 38 minutes conversing with family via telephone.

Codes:_____

EXAMINATION 1, REPORT 15

LOCATION: Outpatient, Clinic

SUBJECTIVE: This is a 42-year-old Caucasian female who presents to the clinic today to establish with me as her primary care provider. At this particular service she is complaining of right hip pain and would also like to be weaned off her Zoloft because she is thinking that this is contributing to her increase in weight. She also complains of a nagging dry cough and would like to find out what might possibly be causing that. Her right hip pain has been going on for about three months now, which is constant and is aggravated by standing up from sitting. She does not feel the pain as much when walking and she says that this pain sometimes radiates to the buttocks and all the way down to her heel area. She occasionally feels a tingling sensation at the lateral aspect of the thigh, particularly at night. She has been treating this with over-the-counter pain medication but that is not found to be helpful. In terms of her cough, she noticed that she usually gets this whenever she has heartburn. She also thought that it might be related to her smoking as well.

PAST MEDICAL HISTORY is remarkable for:
1. Gastroesophageal reflux disease and has been taking medication for this but she cannot recall the name of that medication right now.
2. She also was found to have only one kidney and this was thought to be congenital.
3. Obesity, BMI, 34.

PAST SURGICAL HISTORY is remarkable for a hysterectomy due to a bicornuate uterus.

PSYCHIATRIC HISTORY: She suffered from a major depressive disorder and anxiety.

SCREENINGS: She gets a Pap smear and mammogram every year. Last time was last year, which were normal.

CURRENT MEDICATIONS:
1. Aspirin 81 mg daily.
2. Tums as needed.
3. Zoloft 100 mg daily.

ALLERGIES: She otherwise has no known drug allergies.

FAMILY MEDICAL HISTORY: Her father died at the age of 70 from a myocardial infarction. Mother is presently having high blood pressure and is taking medication for her heart. She also has high blood cholesterol. She is presently 67 years old. There is one brother who has ankylosing spondylitis and she has a total of three sisters. One sister has a benign breast tumor.

PERSONAL AND SOCIAL HISTORY: She is married. She has been doing her job for about 11 years now. She smokes and currently one pack will last her about two weeks. She denies alcohol use. I have established a quitting date of smoking with her and that would be May 1, 2007. She has a total of two children. One is 18 years old and one is 6 years old. She had a miscarriage and one stillbirth. She does not particularly exercise but has been watching her diet, drinking Slim-Fast once a day, and following Weight Watchers.

REVIEW OF SYSTEMS: Constitutional, eyes, head, mouth, chest and lungs, cardiovascular, gastrointestinal, genitourinary, and extremities are otherwise negative other than what is already mentioned above.

OBJECTIVE FINDINGS: Vital signs: Blood pressure is 110/70. Pulse rate of 88. Weight is 201 pounds. General survey: She is an obese middle-aged lady who is pleasant, in no acute distress. Head and neck: Normocephalic and atraumatic. Pink conjunctivae and anicteric sclerae. Pupils are equal, round, and reactive to light and accommodation. Extraocular movements are intact. Neck is supple. No jugular venous distention. No carotid bruit. No thyromegaly. No cervical lymphadenopathy. Chest and lungs: Symmetrical expansion. Clear breath sounds. No rales or wheezes. Cardiovascular: Normal rate and regular rhythm. No murmur and no gallop. Abdomen is obese, soft; normoactive bowel sounds; non-tender. No organomegaly. Extremities: She has no edema, cyanosis, or clubbing. Palpable distal pulses. Straight-leg testing on both lower extremities is essentially negative. She has pain on internal rotation of the right hip joint. No pain on external rotation. On the left side internal and external rotation of the hip joints are negative.

ASSESSMENT/PLAN:

1. Hip pain, exact etiology is uncertain but this could be most likely secondary to degenerative joint disease of the hip versus mild bursitis. Superficial femoral nerve syndrome is also a consideration but not very likely. Discussed management with patient and we will just continue to observe for now. I advised her to give us a call when she develops progression of symptoms and referral to orthopedics might be appropriate if that happens.

2. Cough, dry, probably related to heartburn symptoms. Advised her to elevate her bed at night and continue to take a proton pump inhibitor for heartburn and also to quit smoking at the established quitting day.

3. Major depressive disorder, presently stable. She wants to be weaned off Zoloft and we are therefore decreasing her dose to 50 mg in the next two weeks and 25 mg after that. Then we will just discontinue it after one month. She agrees to this plan. She does not need to come to the clinic unless there is a new concern.

Codes:_____

EXAMINATION 1, REPORT 16

LOCATION: Hospital Inpatient

PROGRESS NOTE

SUBJECTIVE: Patient feels better. He was up and around yesterday and he felt very much better. Shortness of breath has improved. He has no orthopnea but some apparent dyspnea.

REVIEW OF SYSTEMS: Constitutional, ophthalmologic, otolaryngologic, cardiovascular, respiratory, GI, GU, musculoskeletal, integumentary, neurologic, psychiatric, endocrine, hematologic, immunologic negative other than what I have mentioned.

OBJECTIVE: He looks okay, in no acute distress. VITALS are stable. He is afebrile. HEAD, EYES, EARS, NOSE, and THROAT unremarkable. NECK supple, no JVD. The ABDOMEN is benign. EXTREMITIES: The swelling has gone down but he still has some swelling on the feet. NEUROLOGIC examination is grossly intact and nonfocal. His WEIGHT today is 194 pounds.

LABORATORY: Basic metabolic panel: BUN 43, creatinine 1.8, glucose 122. During the day his glucose has come up to around 200. Platelet count today is 128.

ASSESSMENT:

1. Congestive heart failure.
2. Aortic stenosis.
3. Chronic renal failure, currently on hemodialysis.
4. Fluid overload state, improving.

RECOMMENDATIONS:

1. We will resume Amaryt 2mg p.o. qd, watch his Accu-Cheks.
2. Follow up kidney function.
3. Increase activity and discharge.

Codes:_____

EXAMINATION 1, REPORT 17

LOCATION: Hospital

Ten-month-old male is admitted straight to NICU after going into cardiac arrest due to electrical shock when he chewed on an electrical cord. Patient also has second degree burns to lower face, lips and oral cavity (9% body surface). Patient was prepped for transport to The Children's Hospital and stabilized for air flight. During the air flight I personally spoke to the transport team, via two-way radio, instructing them on pulmonary and cardiac resuscitation when the patient again went into cardiac arrest. Total direct face-to-face time spent trying to stabilize the patient for air flight was 70 minutes.

Codes:_____

EXAMINATION 1, REPORT 18

LOCATION: Domiciliary Facility

I am evaluating the patient today, in the domiciliary care setting, for complaints of cough and wheezing. The nursing staff reports that the patient started coughing yesterday afternoon. He denies feeling short of breath. There is no peripheral edema and his weight has been stable.

Today, he is alert and oriented. He denies any complaints other than he feels he has a sore throat. He says his glands in his neck have also been swollen. He is very pleasant. His vitals are stable.

EXAMINATION: BLOOD PRESSURE is 105/61. PULSE is 73. RESPIRATIONS are 20. TEMPERATURE is 97.4 degrees. He is lying flat in his bed and gets very upset when I attempt to elevate his head. His LUNGS have wheezes throughout, more accentuated in the upper airway. His abdomen is soft and nontender. EXTREMITIES show no edema.

PLAN: He does have some DuoNebs ordered p.r.n. and I am going to schedule them for a few days and see how he does. I know that he does not like using these nebutizers, but I think it will help his breathing. We will also have the patient go to the clinic for a chest x-ray because he does have a history of pneumonia.

Codes:_____

● EXAMINATION 2

EXAMINATION 2, REPORT 1

LOCATION: Office

CHIEF COMPLAINT: Complete physical exam of new patient.

SUBJECTIVE:
The patient is a 55-year-old Caucasian male who is here for complete physical exam. His health history form was reviewed. His last exam was in 1997. The patient was recently in the emergency room for a bladder infection and tachycardia. He had heart evaluation done. Stress test was normal. He was discharged on antibiotics. He finished the course and he is feeling fine. Previous medical history is negative, and he never had any surgery. He is not allergic to any medication. The patient does not have any previous medical problem

diagnosed. His family history does include some arthritis. Mother had throat cancer. There is also coronary artery disease with mother. Father had COPD.

SOCIAL HISTORY: He is married. He does not smoke. He does not drink alcohol. He is fairly active. The patient is self-employed as a carpenter.

REVIEW OF SYSTEM is very stable. He denied any skin changes. He sees a dentist. The patient denied any chest pain. He does have some costochondritis type symptoms. He had chest x-ray during this recent sickness, which was reported normal. The patient denies frequent heartburn. He has some spasms of the right hand. He has minimal arthritic changes. The patient denied any urinary symptoms or urgency. He may have some weak urinary stream. The patient denies any tingling or numbness in the lower extremity, joint swelling, or any pedal edema.

OBJECTIVE:
VITAL SIGNS: Reviewed. GENERAL: Awake, alert, and in no apparent distress. HEENT: Pupils are reactive. Extraocular muscles are intact. No conjunctival pallor. Ears are not infected. Tongue protrudes in midline. Hydration is maintained. No posterior throat erythema. NECK: Neck movement normal. LUNGS: Clear. CVS: S1 and S2 normal. ABDOMEN: Soft and nontender. No organomegaly. Bowel sounds are present. GU: Bilateral testicular exam was performed, which is normal. Non-circumcised penis, pubic hair distribution appeared normal. Hernial sites normal. Rectal exam performed. Prostate is less than 20 g in size without any nodule. BACK: Normal. EXTREMITIES: No pedal edema. No apparent sensory or motor weakness identified.

MUSCULOSKELETAL: Normal. There are minimal arthritic charges of the right hand area. SKIN: Normal.

ASSESSMENT:
1. Complete physical exam, health maintenance exam.
2. Recent bladder infection with tachycardia. Heart evaluation normal.
3. Degenerative changes, right hand. The patient does not take any pain medication.

PLAN:
The patient was given instructions regarding health maintenance. He is fairly active at his work and at home. Seatbelt use was recommended. Dental and eye appointment was recommended. We will check PSA. Colon cancer screening was discussed at length. The patient wanted to discuss all of this with family members before making any plans. We will obtain records from his previous provider. I will be interested in seeing if they have checked his cholesterol or not. If not we may need to check it at some point. Patient understands the plan.

Codes:_____

EXAMINATION 2, REPORT 2

LOCATION: Outpatient, Hospital

CHIEF COMPLAINT: Drug overdose.

HISTORY OF PRESENT ILLNESS: This 46-year-old female presented to the emergency department brought in this morning by her mother who stated that she had taken an excess of medication of her Xanax today and now is extremely lethargic and complains of a headache. It is uncertain how many she took or even what medications she is truly prescribed. She says she had been taking Xanax. There is a paper in her chart that would indicate that she filled a prescription of Ativan within the past two weeks. It is unlikely that she is taking both. She apparently saw her psychiatrist yesterday. Today when this happened, the psychiatrist was not in the office to have this reported to or to consult with. She states she has done this because she is so sad that her husband has told her he is going to get a divorce. She has been extremely anxious and ruminating on this. She was recently at the Behavioral Center in Clarksville and was there for about 8 days, as an outpatient. She was seen by her psychiatrist in Rivertown. She was reportedly out of the office.

PAST MEDICAL HISTORY: Repeated psychiatric admissions. History of substance abuse. She had hospitalization for almost an identical thing two years ago.

PAST SURGICAL HISTORY: Laparoscopy. Tonsillectomy. She has had a cholecystectomy. In August, she had a head on crash; she was intoxicated; fractured her hip. At this point she is pretty well healed up from that. It occasionally gives her some trouble.

CURRENT MEDICATIONS: She says that she has taken Seroquel 200 mg in the morning and 1000 mg at bedtime. Trileptal 300 mg twice daily and Xanax. Lorazepam 1 mg three times daily. She also says she has taken some Hydroxyzine 50 mg two of them 3 times daily and recently started on Lamictral 25 mg. She has taken two tablets.

SOCIAL HISTORY: She is married. She smokes a pack of cigarettes a day. She has a son who is about 10. She apparently has three older daughters with children. She occasionally drinks alcohol. She says she does not get drunk.

FAMILY HISTORY: Father had laryngeal cancer. I believe is still living. Mother is still living and brought her in today. Family history of colon cancer with paternal grandfather and uterine cancer with paternal grandmother.

REVIEW OF SYSTEMS: She says she is just really feeling bad and down in the dumps and crying all the time. She says she had been losing weight.
   HEENT: She has difficulty reading up close even though she has reading glasses, otherwise unremarkable. CHEST: Negative. RESPIRATORY: Negative. HEART: Negative. GI: She had an episode of constipation here within the past few weeks, treated in the emergency department. GENITOURINARY: She has a lot of premenstrual symptoms. She says she had some voiding difficulty. NEUROLOGIC: Headache currently. MUSCULOSKELETAL: Occasionally right hip pain, but not bothering her near as much as it was in the past. PSYCHIATRIC: Longstanding history. Please see above.

PHYSICAL EXAMINATION: APPEARANCE: Patient is slightly unkempt, appears older than her stated age. VITAL SIGNS: When she came in was a little hypotensive. BP has been stable since that time. HEENT: Pupils equal, round and reactive to light. Conjunctiva is normal. Extraocular movements intact. Nose, mouth, throat, and tympanic membranes are normal. A little cracking at the left side of her lip. NECK: Supple. No jugular venous distension, thyromegaly or bruits. No lymphadenopathy. CHEST: Clear to auscultation. HEART: Regular rate and rhythm without murmurs or gallops. ABDOMEN: flat, soft, non-tender. No hepatosplenomegaly or masses noted. EXTREMITIES: Full range of motion of her hips. No real tenderness. She says she walks with a limp, but I did not have her get up and walk. She has normal peripheral pulses. Normal muscle stretch reflexes in her lower extremities. NEUROLOGICALLY: No lateralizing findings noted. LABORATORY EXAMINATION: Pretty much normal. Nothing else in her drug screen.

ASSESSMENT/PLAN: Xanax overdose has not had a lot of effects other than the extreme lethargy. She has gotten IM Haldol a couple of times to quiet her down. Will admit the patient to observation and probably wait until tomorrow to do anything else until her system has had time to clear some. Estimated observation stay, 20-24 hours.

Codes:_____

EXAMINATION 2, REPORT 3

LOCATION: Emergency Department

The emergency department paged me to take over care of a 22-month-old male after falling from second floor balcony. After getting briefed by the emergency department physician I immediately order a CT of the patient's head for injury. I accompanied the patient to x-ray and went over the films with the radiologist. Patient has a hematoma and a slight fracture of the skull with cerebral contusion. I contacted the Children's Trauma Center for air flight to their neurosurgeon. I prepped the patient for transport and escorted the patient to life flight with patient's records. Total time spent with the patient was 75 minutes.

Codes:_____

EXAMINATION 2, REPORT 4

LOCATION: Emergency Department

CHIEF COMPLAINT: Chest pain and shortness of breath.

HISTORY OF PRESENT ILLNESS
This is a 65-year-old white male whose initial history is somewhat limited due to his distress. Apparently, the patient has had some intermittent exertional, at rest chest discomfort, and shortness of breath over the past week which is worsening today at which time he had to stop several times walking around due to shortness of breath. He states an hour prior to arrival, he had heavy chest discomfort, shortness of breath, and neck and left shoulder discomfort as well. He presents immediately from triage.

PMH: Atrial fibrillation, CAD, silent MI, CHF, CVA, diabetes, hypercholesterolemia, hypertension. PSH: Pilonidal cyst and remote history of a cardiac catheterization.

SH: He quit tobacco and alcohol 20 years ago. No drugs. He is married and lives with his wife. FH: Positive for heart disease with father and brother. ROS: Negative except for pertinent positives listed above.

ALLERGIES: See nursing notes.

MEDICATION(S): See nursing notes.

PHYSICAL EXAMINATION
Vital signs per nursing notes. He is awake. He is pale, diaphoretic, and in acute distress. Head is normocephalic, atraumatic. Pupils are reactive. Extraocular muscles are full. No icterus or pallor. Nares patent. Pharynx clear. Mucous membranes are moist. Neck is supple, no JVD. Trachea is midline. No meningeal signs or stridor. Lungs are with bibasilar rales. He is tachypneic. Heart is irregular and tachycardic. He has faint peripheral pulses. There is no acute abnormality of the abdominal aorta. Abdomen is soft, mildly obese, nondistended, nontender. No rigidity, rebound, tenderness, or guarding. No peritoneal signs or organomegaly. No pulsatile masses or bruits. Musculoskeletal exam: Equal strength and tone of the extremities. Skin: Cool diaphoretic, pale. There is no cyanosis, clubbing, or edema. There is no calf asymmetry, induration, palpable cords, or signs of DVT.

Neurologically, he is alert and oriented x3 with no focal or lateralizing deficits. Vascular exam shows somewhat weakened, but equal peripheral pulses.

DIAGNOSTIC STUDIES

LABORATORY/PATHOLOGY: Routine laboratory studies obtained showed grossly normal electrolytes. His glucose was 432 for which he was given 6 units of subcu Humulin R. CBC shows WBC 12.6, hemoglobin 17.6. INR did come back as the patient was leaving for the cath laboratory at 1.5. His initial myoglobin was 60 and troponin I 0.81 and this was before any cardioversion attempts were made. Triglyceride levels were elevated at 183. Initial digoxin level 0.4.

EKG: EKG was obtained initially at arrival which showed a tachycardic rhythm. There does appear to be intermittent T waves. This is likely a flutter with 2 : 1 block. However, the patient was noted at the end of the EKG tracing to go into ventricular tachycardia. EKG was repeated with patient's rhythm at approximately 112. This did appear to be a sinus mechanism. There is poor R wave progression across the precordial leads and there is deep T-wave inversion in the lateral leads consistent with subendocardial involvement.

EMERGENCY DEPARTMENT COURSE

The patient is evaluated by myself immediately upon arrival to the ED room. IV O2 monitor were started including 2 large bore IVs. A monitor showed what appeared to be atrial fibrillation/flutter with variable response which ran anywhere from 110 to 150. However, the patient did intermittently run episodes of V-tach. He was given aspirin. He was placed on a nitroglycerin drip. He was placed with defibrillator pads and was given 60 mg of Lasix IV push. The patient continued to have runs of ventricular tachycardia. Therefore, he was given 150 mg of amiodarone IV. This was repeated. He continued to run intermittent ventricular tachycardia. He did have an episode where he became unconscious. He was shocked on a nonsynchronized mode at 200 joules, which the patient immediately woke back up and he returned to what appeared to be a sinus rhythm in the 110 range. The patient was given morphine for pain control. The patient had further episodes of ventricular tachycardia, which he became symptomatic for and was shocked an additional time at 200 joules. The patient was started on nitroglycerin and amiodarone drips. Cardiology was called on a STAT basis. Portable chest x-ray was obtained which shows cardiomegaly and pulmonary edema. I held beta blockers due to the fact that he clinically and radiologically is in pulmonary edema and I had held Integrilin and heparin as his INR was not immediately available. Cardiology did see the patient in the department and is taking the patient to the catheter laboratory. At the time of transfer, the patient's vital signs were stable. He was alert and appropriate and neurovascularly intact. I did discuss the case with the patient's family at bedside as well.

PROVISIONAL DIAGNOSIS/DIAGNOSES

1. Recurrent symptomatic ventricular tachycardia.
2. EKG evidence of subendocardial myocardial infarction.
3. Hyperlipidemia.
4. History of atrial fibrillation/flutter.
5. Diabetes uncontrolled.
6. History of previous cerebrovascular accident.
7. Remote history of tobacco and alcohol abuse.

DISPOSITION

Admit to catheter laboratory, cardiology in guarded condition. I spent 130 minutes of critical care time at patient's bedside independent of any procedures.

Codes:_____

EXAMINATION 2, REPORT 5

LOCATION: NICU, Inpatient

S: No desats or bradys, no significant residuals

O: Resp: Rate: 43-82
CV: Rate: 126-162   Map: 33-39
Exam: RRR, no M/GIR
FEN/GI: I: 222   TF: 151   Wt: 1470
            O: 138
            Exam: Soft, NT/ND, +BS
HEME:
ID: Temp Max: 37.4
Cultures: none
NEURO: vigorous
            Exam: moves all ext

A/P: 6 day old female, 32 week premie, with respiratory distress. Continue to wean flow as indicated, stop caffeine. Increase feeding by 3 cc. Stop phototherapy, check bilirubin in the morning. Continue to monitor neuro.

Codes:_____

EXAMINATION 2, REPORT 6

LOCATION: Outpatient, Clinic

A 44-year-old woman with a very complex history of pancreatitis. She has an infected pseudocyst complicated by a pulmonary embolus with a long period of time in the hospital requiring a long-term intubation and tracheostomy. She has controlled diabetes mellitus Type II and controlled mild hypertension. She was on Coumadin and had a very large splenic bleed, which required admission to the hospital. Her oral intake was compromised at this time, but she slowly got to where she was eating regular food. She comes in today, still on Coumadin. She complains of weight loss and occasional diarrhea. She is still using a walker. On exam, she looks good to me. BP: 130/96. She has some left upper quadrant tenderness. I reviewed the CT scan and dictation, which shows a decrease in the size of both the splenic hematoma and her pancreatic pseudocyst.

ASSESSMENT AND PLAN: A 44-year-old woman with resolving splenic hematoma and decreasing pseudocyst. She is still having pain, but it is slowly improving. I will telephone in a renewal of her oral Dilaudid for 30 tablets and I will see her again in two months. She will see me earlier if she has any troubles. Given her large splenic hematoma and the fact that she has a vena caval filter in place, I do not believe we should resume her Coumadin. ABC/def.

Codes:_____

EXAMINATION 2, REPORT 7

LOCATION: Shady Lane Rest Home

This is a 62-year-old male, who resides in a rest home, being evaluated today for a sore on his left upper thigh. He has had this for about a week. Triple antibiotic ointment has been applied with no change in the status of the wound. Nursing indicates that he has not been following his diet. He eats very freely despite his blood sugars going up and has a significant amount of water retention. He refuses to sign the diet waiver even considering his diabetes. He understands his diet is detrimental to his health and well being. He insists that he will eat whenever and whatever he wants.

OBJECTIVE: The sore on his leg was evaluated. It is small with some swelling and redness at the sight. Based on the looks of it, it is a spider bite. We will continue daily dressings with triple antibiotic ointment. We will keep an eye on it for infection and complication due to the patient's diabetic status.

ASSESSMENT:
1. Spider bite, left leg.
2. Dietary noncompliance.

PLAN: No change in care plans or medications at this time.

Codes:_____

EXAMINATION 2, REPORT 8

LOCATION: Francis Hill Group Home
This is a 46-year-old mentally disabled male who is currently living in a group home here in town. The resident was getting more aggressive and having outbursts that led to destruction of furniture in the group home. After consulting with the staff and charge nurse at the group home the decision was made to increase his Tegratol. It has been approximately 3 weeks now and the resident seems to be leveling off at the current dosage. The resident is otherwise healthy. All other medications will be kept at their current dosage. Total time spent this month evaluating and implementing care plan was 50 minutes.

Codes:_____

EXAMINATION 2, REPORT 9

LOCATION: Patient's home

CHART NOTE
This patient is a 63-year-old female who is seen at home today for follow-up of her chronic headaches. She is lying in bed. The chart is reviewed along with the nursing notes. Advanced directives are in place. The graphic chart is also reviewed.

S: No fevers or chills. No chest pain or shortness of breath.

O: This well-developed, well-nourished lady is sitting without distress. HEENT-normocephalic and atraumatic. Neck is supple. Lungs—clear to auscultation.

A: Chronic headaches.
Bipolar disorder.
Hypertension.
Tardive dyskinesia secondary to antipsychotics.
Urinary incontinence.

P: 1. The patient has chronic headaches for which she has been taking Fioricet as needed, but I will go ahead and start her on Topamaz for preventive measures, 25 mg one po qHS for 10 days and then one po bid for 10 days and then one in the AM and two at H.S. for 10 days. Then, we will start 50 mg po bid. Reassess in four weeks.
In the meantime, the case was discussed with the home nurse and patient's spouse; and I advised that the Topamaz may cause a little increased fatigue and

hypersomnolence; but if it is clinically significant, we might have to decrease the doses.

Further recommendations to follow as necessary

Codes:_____

EXAMINATION 2, REPORT 10

LOCATION: Inpatient, Hospital

I was asked to see this patient in consultation.

HISTORY OF PRESENT ILLNESS: Mrs. Q. is 92-year-old, right handed, female who fell with an episode of syncope. She is admitted for workup of her fainting. She injured both wrists. I have been asked to render an opinion in regards to her injured wrists by the admitting physician. She was seen in the emergency department and splinted for bilateral distal radius fractures. She feels well today. She is oriented ×3. She has no pain in the wrists. She was seen in the past with a medical history of bilateral severe carpal tunnel syndrome. She also has a cyst on her pancreas and a cataract in the right eye.

REVIEW OF SYSTEMS: Review of systems shows chronic neck aching for which she was treated by a chiropractor and she says this help her tingling in her hand from the carpal tunnel syndrome, as well. She was seen by me last year for carpal tunnel syndrome after referral by her primary doctor, from Henry Ford Hospital and the patient decided on non-operative treatment with carpal tunnel syndrome having gotten better from her chiropractic manipulations.

SOCIAL HISTORY: She is a retired hearing and speech therapist. She has hobbies of piano and photography.

PAST SURGICAL HISTORY: Uterine cancer excised. Cataract excision of the left eye.

PAST MEDICAL HISTORY: She also has arthritis.

PHYSICAL EXAMINATION: Physical examination shows that she has bilateral palmar plaster splints on, fitting well. She has circulation intact to the hands. Sensation is intact with numbness in the median distribution. Her neck shows mild limitation at the extremes of motion with no pain. She has no pain in the elbow or shoulder. No lower extremity pain. The hands show PIP joint arthrosis with Heberden's nodes on the DIP joints.

RADIOLOGY: The x-ray shows that she has bilateral distal radius fractures. On the left wrist, it is a Smith-type fracture with some palmar translation of an articular fragment on the oblique view but, on the lateral view, there is no change in the inclination of the articular surface and no gross radial shortening. On the right wrist, there is a distal radius fracture, with comminution and shortening with extension at the fracture site of 30 degrees. The skin is intact. There is no irritation of the skin by her splints.

IMPRESSION: Bilateral distal radius fractures.

RECOMMENDATIONS: We discussed the treatment options and the potential risks and benefits of each. Mrs. Q elected closed treatment of both fractures wanting to avoid surgery, understanding that she was accepting some deformity and some stiffness in the wrists by not having reduction and fixation. I think it is reasonable because she is willing to accept the deformity and she has very low functional demands at this point. In terms of weight bearing, once she has her workup finished, if she is cleared to walk but may need a walker with bilateral forearm supports to avoid putting excessive weight on the wrists with crutches or a regular walker. Therefore at this point, she elects short arm casts for both distal radius fractures and she will follow-up next week in the office for an x-ray of both wrists in the casts.

Codes:_____

EXAMINATION 2, REPORT 11

LOCATION: Hospital, Inpatient

PROGRESS NOTE

CC: Tachycardia

The patient was seen multiple times today. His blood pressure came down to the 80s to 90s. I was called by the nursing staff to see him. I decided to take his dialysis catheter out right away. We took him down to interventional radiology. I evaluated him there. He was not in any respiratory distress. He was tachycardic and blood pressure was on the low side. We took his tunneled dialysis catheter out and we placed a temporary dialysis catheter. We transferred him to the floor afterwards. His blood pressure came up. His heart rate was in the 130s. It slowed down to the 110s after 4 liters of fluid. I gave him 1 dose of 5 mg of Decadron intravenously, since the patient has been on chronic steroids.

His blood cultures later on grew gram-positive cocci in clusters.

The patient was seen multiple times throughout the day and also at night. He was feeling better. Temperature was down. I put him on acetaminophen as well, and also in the morning I started him on Zosyn 4.5 gm IV every 12 hours.

EXAMINATION: He has a newly placed left internal jugular (IJ) temporary dialysis catheter. His right tunneled dialysis catheter was taken out. His LUNGS are clear. He is tachycardic with sinus tachycardia. ABDOMEN is soft and non-tender. He has no edema. He is thirsty and has dry mucous membranes.

IMPRESSION:
1. Tachycardia.
2. Probably sepsis.
3. Probably *Staphylococcus aureus* bacteremia.
4. End stage renal disease, on hemodialysis.

PLAN:
1. Decadron 5 mg IV times one.
2. Normal saline 4 liters were given.
3. CBC and basic panel in the morning.
4. Vancomycin and Gentamicin to be followed by pharmacy.
5. Continue with Zosyn.
6. Hold dialysis for now.
7. Acetaminophen 650 mg p.o. q.4-6h. p.r.n.
8. We will get another set of blood cultures done for his newly placed central line.

I was called by the nursing staff indicating the patient had a heart rate of 190, supraventricular tachycardia. I ordered on the telephone 6 mg of adenosine STAT. The patient converted back to sinus tachycardia at around 110 per minute. He was seen afterwards. He came out of SVT and felt better. He had no chest pain or shortness of breath with that. Later throughout the day I hep-locked his IV.

Total time spent directly face-to-face with the patient today was 1 hour and 15 minutes.

Codes:_____

EXAMINATION 2, REPORT 12

LOCATION: Rehabilitation Clinic

DISABILITY ASSESSMENT

DIAGNOSIS: Work-related low back injury due to heavy lifting.

S   This 28-year-old male was referred to complete a disability assessment. He did receive physical therapy services, although has been discharged at this time. At this time, he reports there is chronic pain in his low back region.

O   The client's abilities on this date are as follows:
Activity:
Bending – unable to without discomfort. Twisting – very painful.
Kneeling—2 minutes – constantly, with troubles getting up and down.
Standing, walking and sitting—10 minutes—constantly.

A   Overall, the client does demonstrate cooperative behavior. Performance was consistent among test items. Initial and final pain level was 7 out of 10.

P   The client will continue with the prescribed recommendation from primary physician along with further therapy. The client will be seeing his doctor on this date for re-evaluation.
   Thank you for the opportunity to evaluate this patient. If I could be of further assistance, please contact me.

Codes:_____

EXAMINATION 2, REPORT 13

I was called in for standby by the primary OB/GYN for a 32-year-old patient who's admitted for delivery for possible cesarean delivery. The patient has had a complicated pregnancy due to hypertension. Labor has been progressing slowly and the patient's blood pressure continues to rise. After 70 minutes on standby, the patient delivered vaginally without my assistance.

Codes:_____

EXAMINATION 2, REPORT 14

LOCATION: Office
   Case Management
   I had a lengthy, 65 minutes, conversation with the two daughters on Friday along with an interdisciplinary team of 5. Their father is on dialysis for his end stage renal disease. We explained to them that the patient is having dementia and keeps yelling in the dialysis unit. He is always forgetful. His blood pressure dropped to the 60 systolic range and he was hypoxic. They decided to make him code level III and not take him to the hospital, which we all agreed with. We discussed stopping dialysis and it was the team's impression that he would be off dialysis. However, one of his daughters called me Friday night indicating that there was misunderstanding on her part and that she wants him to continue on dialysis.
   During the team conference, we had discussed with her and her other sister the quality of life of the patient in that dialysis is not really doing anything and it is probably inadequate anyway. They wanted to continue with dialysis; therefore, the patient had a dialysis treatment on Saturday. In general, his blood pressure was better and he was not hypoxic.

I left it to them to decide when to stop dialysis, but at this time we will continue current dialysis prescription.

Codes:_____

EXAMINATION 2, REPORT 15

LOCATION: Inpatient, Hospital

CHIEF COMPLAINT: Weakness.

HISTORY OF PRESENT ILLNESS: This is a 47-year-old gentleman who came in for increasing weakness and emesis. He vomited one time. It started six days ago and has gotten worse. He is unable to hold anything down. No fever. No abdominal pain. No shortness of breath. No chest pain. The patient is awake, disoriented, a poor historian, and does not speak English fluently. He has some dry cough. No sore throat. No earache. Questionable vague abdominal pain, denies any palpitations. No chest pain. No dyspnea. He drinks about a pint of vodka a day.

PAST MEDICAL HISTORY: History of smoking about one pack every day. Past medical history none.

ALLERGIES: NO KNOWN DRUG ALLERGIES.

MEDICATIONS: None.

SOCIAL HISTORY: As above.

FAMILY HISTORY: Noncontributory.

REVIEW OF SYSTEM: CONSTITUTIONAL: A lot of weight loss for the last few months. HEENT: No double vision, no loss of vision. CARDIOVASCULAR: No chest pain or shortness of breath. No paroxysmal nocturnal dyspnea or orthopnea. GI: As above. No melena. GU: No dysuria, no hematuria, no frequency. PULMONARY: Some dry cough, no hemoptysis, no fever. NEUROLOGICAL: No history of stroke, no seizures, no weakness. ENDOCRINE: No history of diabetes mellitus, no history of thyroid disease. No history of IV drug abuse.

PHYSICAL EXAMINATION:
VITAL SIGNS: Blood pressure on admission was 126/79, temperature 98.5, pulse of 112, respiratory rate 20, saturating at 95%. Cachectic. HEENT: Extraocular muscles are intact. Mouth dry mucosa. NECK: Supple, no JVD, no bruit, no thyromegaly. HEART: S1 and S2 with a 1/6 systolic ejection murmur at the left sternal border. LUNGS: Clear to auscultation bilaterally (no wheezing). RECTAL: Rectal exam in the emergency department nontender without any masses. Hemoccult negative. EXTREMITIES: No edema, x4. NEUROLOGICAL: Awake. Moves all extremities.

LABORATORY/X-RAY DATA: Laboratories on admission: Calcium S.3, ST 190, ALT 75, indirect bilirubin 3.7, direct bilirubin 0.4, sodium 130, potassium 3.9, BUN 23, creatinine 2.2, glucose 319, anion gap 36, carbon dioxide 11, lipase 186, WBC 16.3. hemoglobin 11.0, hematocrit 32.11, platelets 284. Ketones positive at 132. OA negative. ABG: pH 7.23, PC02 11 PO2 137, 99% on three liters. Chest x-ray: Normal, no effusion.

ASSESSMENT:
1. Diabetic ketoacidosis.
2. Probable pancreatitis.

3. Elevated liver enzymes, most likely secondary to the cirrhosis.
4. Malnutrition.
5. Metabolic acidosis.
6. Renal insufficiency, most likely secondary to dehydration.
7. Leukocytosis.
8. Anemia.
9. Tobacco Use Disorder.
10. Alcoholism.

PLAN:
1. Admit to hospital.
2. IV fluids.
3. Insulin
4. Tequin prophylactically.
5. Blood cultures.
6. Sputum cultures.
7. Urine cultures.
8. Ultrasound of the liver in the morning.
9. Folic acid. Multiple vitamin and thiamine.
10. Monitor for alcohol withdrawal.
11. Repeat potassium is 6.8. The patient is to be started Kayexalate 30 gm p.o. now. One amp potassium chloride.
12. His sugar this morning is 124. We will change his fluid to D-5 normal saline 250.

Codes:_____

EXAMINATION 2, REPORT 16

LOCATION: Office

Subject: Discussion with patient's family. Patient resides in a Nursing Facility.

I had a lengthy discussion with the patient's primary physician, her son, and her daughter (has power of attorney) about the patient's progression of her kidney disease, edema, CHF, and her left renal artery re-stenosis. I have discussed with them in detail the pathology and pathophysiology of renal artery stenosis and its effect on renal function, LV function and HTN. I have discussed also in detail the procedure of renal angiography and its possible complications including acute renal failure from contrast nephropathy that may require either temporary or permanent dialysis. The patient has significant left renal artery re-stenosis on renal arterial Doppler with possible progression of her right renal artery stenosis. We discussed also the possibility of renal artery rupture and bleeding complications. Her primary physician, son, and daughter had many questions, all of them were very appropriate questions and all of those questions were answered. We spent quite a bit of time discussing dialysis both hemodialysis and peritoneal dialysis. I have asked the primary physician and the family to keep their minds open about dialysis. She had bypass surgery already and other than having a CVA, there is no contraindication for dialysis at this time, if she ever needs it. Of course I discussed with them in details IV hydration and minimal contrast in an attempt to avoid contrast nephropathy. I have indicated that I would never recommend renal artery bypass and she is better off with interventional radiology. We discussed expectations after the procedure and the possibility of re-stenosis again in the future. They understand that there is no guarantee that her left renal artery will remain open but we will monitor it with renal arterial Doppler at 6 weeks and 3 months after the procedure.

In addition to all of the above, I have indicated the objectives of performing renal angiography, which are to preserve and hopefully improve her renal function first and improve her BP control second. Unfortunately, the patient is drinking a lot of water to help her kidney function, despite our discussions about this in the past. I have strongly advised to limit her fluid intake to 1.5 L a day, avoid salty food and increase her Bumex to 2 mg PO BID to help with her edema and dyspnea. Patient's primary physician, her son, and her daughter (the power of attorney) seemed very satisfied with the service and the discussion today. They seem to understand all the aspects of renal artery stenosis, chronic renal failure and CHF and the potential benefits and complications of renal angiography. They all agreed with the above plan.

Total time spent in care conference today was 75 minutes; all the time was spent in counseling.

Codes:_____

EXAMINATION 2, REPORT 17

LOCATION: Emergency Department

CHIEF COMPLAINT: Chest pain.

HISTORY OF PRESENT ILLNESS
This is a 42-year-old with a history of celiac disease, anemia. She is adopted. She does not know if she has a family history of cardiac disease. She has no history of diabetes, hypercholesterolemia or hypertension. The patient states she awoke this morning, noted constant aching chest pain, substernal, nonradiating, that had been constant until her evaluation tonight at 6 PM when it resolved. She has not had any cough, shortness of breath. No history of pulmonary embolism or DVT. No recent travel. She is not on birth control pills. The patient, at the present time, has not had any prolonged travel.

MED: Iron is her only medication.

SH: She is adopted.

PMH/ROS: She is still menstruating. Ophthalmolgic, otolaryngologic, lymphatic, respiratory, GI, GU, neurologic, endocrine, integumentary, and immunologic were all negative.

PHYSICAL EXAMINATION
On my exam, she is awake and alert. Conjunctivae clear. Sclerae are pale. Neck is supple, no nuchal rigidity. Trachea is midline. Breath sounds are equal and clear. Heart: Regular without murmur or extra heart sounds. Abdomen: Soft and nontender, no organomegaly or mass. She has good distal pulses. No skin rash.

EMERGENCY DEPARTMENT COURSE
Hemoglobin is 10, which is up from her last at 8. Her D-dimer and troponin are normal. Chest x-ray is without evidence of pneumothorax or pneumonia.

The patient is being discharged. She is in improved condition. She was given a chest pain instruction sheet of uncertain cause. She is going to follow up at the Community Clinic as well as with Dr C.

PROVISIONAL DIAGNOSIS/DIAGNOSES: Evaluation for chest pain.

Codes:_____

EXAMINATION 2, REPORT 18

LOCATION: Shady Lane Nursing Home

This patient is being seen for possible discharge. Advance directives are in place.

S   The patient has severe osteoarthritis and a history of cerebrovascular accident and neurogenic bladder with other multiple medical issues who has finished going through physical therapy and occupational therapy. Discharge planning has been made. No fevers or chills. No chest pain or shortness of breath.

O   This well-developed, well-nourished lady is sitting without distress. HEENT—normocephalic and atraumatic. Neck is supple. Lungs—clear to auscultation.

A   1. History of cerebrovascular accident.
2. Osteoarthritis.
3. Hypertension.
4. Gastroesophageal reflux disease.
5. Neurogenic bladder secondary to number one.

P   1. As the patient is stable, the patient will be discharged home with the current treatment plan.

Codes:_____

UNIT III

Answers

● UNIT I ANSWERS

PRACTICE 1, OFFICE OR OTHER OUTPATIENT SERVICES

Practice 1, Report A

Rationale:
A. Incorrect because the key components of this evaluation consist of an expanded problem focused (EPF) history, detailed examination and low medical decision making (MDM). **99212** would be undercoding.
B. Incorrect because even though **99213** is the correct service code, the diagnosis of cough (**786.2**) would not be coded because it is a symptom of the bronchitis.
C. Correct because the service code is for an established office service, which consists of an EPF history, detailed examination, and low MDM. Office and Other Outpatient Services codes require 2 of the 3 key components to qualify for assignment and the documentation supports assignment of this code. The diagnosis is correct with 490 (Bronchitis, not specified as acute or chronic) reported for the bronchitis since the documentation does not specify the type.
D. Incorrect because **99202** is for a new patient, and this note states that the patient is established.

Practice 1, Report B

Professional Services: **99212** (Evaluation and Management, Office and Other Outpatient); **577.0** (Pancreatitis); **577.2** (Pseudocyst, pancreas); **789.00** (Pain, abdomen, unspecified site)

Rationale: The patient is an established patient. The history of present illness (HPI) includes the location (abdomen), duration (4 months), and associated signs and symptoms (fever) for a total of 3, which is a level 2 or EPF HPI. One review of systems (ROS) (gastrointestinal) was performed for a level 1 ROS. Only the patient's past medical history was discussed for a level 3 past, family, and social history (PFSH). All 3 elements of a patient's history have to be at the same level or higher when choosing the level of history. This documentation contained a level 2 HPI, a level 1 ROS and a level 3 PFSH. The history level would therefore be a level 1 or problem focused (PF) history because the lowest level is 1.

The examination included only 1 element of constitutional element (general appearance) for 1 body area/organ system (BA/OS). The abdomen was soft for 1 BA. No organ systems were examined. This is an EPF examination.

The MDM consisted of limited diagnoses, limited data was reviewed, and the patient has a moderate risk of complication (established problem, not improving). To qualify for a given level of MDM complexity, 2 of 3 elements must be met or exceeded. The levels were 2 or EPF HPI; level 2 or EPF examination, and a level 3 or low MDM. Because this is an established patient, only 2 of the 3 key components need to be met or exceeded to assign the code. The documentation qualifies for assignment of **99213**.

The primary reason for the office service is the persisting abdominal pain (**789.00**) the fifth digit of 0, unspecified site, would be assigned because no specific location of the pain is given. A pseudocyst of the pancreas (**577.2**) was found on CT scan. The pancreatitis (**577.0**) would also be reported.

Practice 1, Report B

HISTORY ELEMENTS	Documented
HISTORY OF PRESENT ILLNESS (HPI)	
1. Location (site on body)	✗
2. Quality (characteristic: throbbing, sharp)	
3. Severity (1/10 or how intense)	
4. Duration (how long for problem or episode)	✗
5. Timing (when it occurs)	
6. Context (under what circumstances does it occur)	
7. Modifying factors (what makes it better or worse)	
8. Associated signs and symptoms (what else is happening when it occurs)	✗
TOTAL	3
LEVEL	2
REVIEW OF SYSTEMS (ROS)	Documented
1. Constitutional (e.g., weight loss, fever)	
2. Ophthalmologic (eyes)	
3. Otolaryngologic (ears, nose, mouth, throat)	
4. Cardiovascular	
5. Respiratory	
6. Gastrointestinal	✗
7. Genitourinary	
8. Musculoskeletal	
9. Integumentary (skin and/or breasts)	
10. Neurologic	
11. Psychiatric	
12. Endocrine	
13. Hematologic/Lymphatic	
14. Allergic/Immunologic	
TOTAL	1
LEVEL	1
PAST, FAMILY, AND/OR SOCIAL HISTORY (PFSH)	Documented
1. Past illness, operations, injuries, treatments, and current medications	✗
2. Family medical history for heredity and risk	
3. Social activities, both past and present	
TOTAL	1
LEVEL	3

History Level	1	2	3	
	Problem Focused	Expanded Problem Focused	Detailed	Comprehensive
HPI	Brief 1-3	Brief 1-3	Extended 4+	Extended 4+
ROS	None	Problem Pertinent	Extended 2-9	Complete 10+
PFSH	None	None	Pertinent 1	Complete 2-3
			HISTORY LEVEL	1

EXAMINATION ELEMENTS	Documented
CONSTITUTIONAL	
1. Blood pressure, sitting	
2. Blood pressure, lying	
3. Pulse	
4. Respirations	
5. Temperature	
6. Height	
7. Weight	
8. General appearance	✗
NUMBER	1
BODY AREAS (BA)	Documented
1. Head (including face)	
2. Neck	
3. Chest (including breasts and axillae)	
4. Abdomen	
5. Genitalia, groin, buttocks	
6. Back (including spine)	
7. Each extremity	
NUMBER	1
ORGAN SYSTEMS (OS)	Documented
1. Ophthalmologic (eyes)	
2. Otolaryngologic (ears, nose, mouth, throat)	
3. Cardiovascular	
4. Respiratory	
5. Gastrointestinal	
6. Genitourinary	
7. Musculoskeletal	
8. Integumentary	
9. Neurologic	
10. Psychiatric	
11. Hematologic/Lymphatic/Immunologic	
NUMBER	0
TOTAL BA/OS	2

Exam Level	1	2	3	
	Problem Focused	Expanded Problem Focused	Detailed	Comprehensive
	Limited to affected BA/OS	Limited to affected BA/OS & other related OSs	Extended of affected BA & other related OSs	General multi-system or complete single OS
# of OS or BA	1	2-7 limited	2-7 extended	8+
			EXAMINATION LEVEL	2

MDM ELEMENTS	Documented
# OF DIAGNOSIS/MANAGEMENT OPTIONS	
1. Minimal	
2. Limited	✗
3. Multiple	
4. Extensive	
LEVEL	2
AMOUNT OR COMPLEXITY OF DATA TO REVIEW	Documented
1. Minimal/None	
2. Limited	
3. Moderate	
4. Extensive	
LEVEL	2
RISK OF COMPLICATION OR DEATH IF NOT TREATED	Documented
1. Minimal	
2. Low	
3. Moderate	✗
4. High	
LEVEL	3

MDM*	1	2	3	4
	Straightforward	Low	Moderate	High
Number of DX or management options	Minimal	Limited	Multiple	Extensive
Amount or complexity of data	Minimal/None	Limited	Moderate	Extensive
Risks	Minimal	Low	Moderate	High
			MDM LEVEL	2

*To qualify for a given type of MDM complexity, 2 of 3 elements in the table must be met or exceeded.

History: Expanded Problem Focused
Examination: Problem Focused
MDM: Low

Number of Key Components: 2 of 3

99213

PRACTICE 2, HOSPITAL OBSERVATION SERVICES

Practice 2, Report A

Rationale:

A. Incorrect because the elements documented do not support a **99220** level of service. Diagnosis coding is correct.

B. Incorrect because prolonged service exclusions do not permit assignment of **99354** and **99355** with **99218**. Diagnosis coding is correct.

C. Incorrect because the cough **786.2** and abnormal findings on radiological examination (**793.1**) are missing and a CT scan was ordered for next week to assess these two conditions. CPT coding is correct.

D. Correct answer. The patient presents with end stage renal disease (585.6) and uncontrolled type 2 diabetes (250.82). Normal blood sugar is 110 mg/dl and a diagnosis of diabetes is made with a blood sugar of 126 mg/dl or higher. This patient's blood sugar was initially 895 mg/dl and went up to 1468 mg/dl, and the documentation states that the patient is going to be admitted for observation primarily to control his blood sugar levels. The patient has a cough (786.2) and bilateral lung infiltrates on chest x-ray (793.1), and a CT is to be scheduled the following week to assess both of these conditions. Also noted in the report is the elevated protein (790.99) and low albumin (790.99). The code is only reported once, 790.99. The leg edema (782.3) and depression (311) may be reported but no specific indications were given as to a treatment for either of these conditions.

Practice 2, Report B

Professional Services: **99217** (Evaluation and Management, Hospital Service, Observation Care); **403.90** (Disease, renovascular); **585.9** (CKD); **440.1** (Stenosis, renal artery); **280.0** (Anemia, due to, blood loss); **458.9** (Hypotension); **997.72** (Complication, surgical procedures, vascular, renal artery)

Rationale: There is no audit form with this case because the hospital observation discharge service is not based on the key components of history, exam, and MDM. There is only one CPT code for a hospital observation discharge—**99217**.

The primary reason the service was provided was renovascular disease and secondary to this is the chronic renal failure and renovascular disease. According to the Official Guidelines for Coding and Reporting, Section I.C.7.a.3: "Assign codes from category 403, Hypertensive chronic kidney disease, when conditions classified to categories 585-587 are present. Unlike hypertension with heart disease, ICD-9-CM presumes a cause-and-effect relationship and classifies chronic kidney disease (CKD) with hypertension as hypertensive chronic kidney disease. Fifth digits for category 403 should be assigned as follows: 0 with CKD stage I through stage IV, or unspecified. 1 with CKD stage V or end stage renal disease. The appropriate code from category 585, Chronic kidney disease, should be used as a secondary code with a code from category 403 to identify the stage of chronic kidney disease." Therefore, the renovascular disease is reported with **403.90**, with fifth digit 0 to indicate unspecified or chronic kidney disease stages I through IV. **585.9** is reported for the CRF (chronic renal failure).

The renal stenosis is reported with **440.1**, anemia with **280.0**, and hypotension with **458.9**. Also reported are the complications of the vascular renal artery surgery (**997.72**).

PRACTICE 3, HOSPITAL INPATIENT SERVICES

Practice 3, Report A

Rationale:

A. This choice is incorrect because **99205**, initial office service, would not be reported, because only one E/M service is billable per provider per day, and the service provided by the physician in the office would be "bundled" into the documentation for the initial hospital service.

B. **Is correct. 99223 is reported because the office visit and all services provided in that setting are considered when choosing the hospital admission code. To assign a code from this subcategory all three key components must meet or exceed the level in the code. The history and examination were comprehensive and the MDM was high.**

C. This choice is incorrect. CPT **99215** is for an established patient office service and would not be reported because only one E/M service is billable per provider per day and the work done by the physician in the office would be "bundled" into the documentation for the initial hospital service.

D. This choice is incorrect. **99221** is for a level 1 initial hospital service. The history and exam are comprehensive, but the MDM documented is high, rather than straightforward or low, making this incorrect.

Practice 3, Report B

Professional Services: **99238** (Evaluation and Management, Hospital, Discharge); **458.9** (Bleeding, gastrointestinal); **285.1** (Anemia, due to blood loss, acute); **414.00** (Arteriosclerosis, coronary, artery); **443.9** (Disease, peripheral vascular); **496** (Disease, lung, obstructive (chronic), COPD); **V45.82** (Status (post), angioplasty, percutaneous transluminal, coronary)

Rationale: Hospital discharges are based on time. If the documentation does not specify time spent discharging the patient, then the lowest level code must be assigned (**99238**). No audit form is needed with time based codes. The service may or may not include an examination of the patient.

The diagnoses are stated in the final diagnosis area of the discharge summary. The acute GI bleed (**458.9**) and anemia due to blood loss (**285.1**) would be reported even though they are listed as stable, which means that the condition is under control. When referencing the Index of the ICD, under "Disease, artery, coronary," the coder is directed to "see Arteriosclerosis, coronary" (**414.00**). The fifth digit of 0 would be assigned because the documentation does not state if this disease is in the patient's native vessel or in a previously grafted vessel. The PVD (peripheral vascular disease) (**443.9**), COPD (**496**) and the post-procedural status of stent placement (**V45.82**) would also be reported.

PRACTICE 4, CONSULTATIONS

Practice 4, Report A

Rationale:
A. **Is the correct answer. The service is a consultation, based on the opening statement thanking for the referral and the reason for it. The consultation codes require 3 of 3 elements. This case had a detailed history and physical exam and moderate MDM, a level 3 consultation. To assign the level 4 requires a comprehensive history and physical exam components.**
B. This choice is incorrect. CPT **99244** requires a comprehensive history and physical exam and the documentation in this scenario did not meet those criteria. The decision making is moderate and meets this level, but 3 of 3 key components must be met or exceeded to select a level and only MDM meets this level.
C. This choice is incorrect. CPT **99203** is for a new patient office service, and this scenario is for a consultation.
D. This choice is incorrect. CPT **99215** is for an established patient office service, and this scenario is for a consultation.

Practice 4, Report B

Professional Services: **99253** (Evaluation and Management, Consultation); **787.01** (Nausea, with vomiting); **789.00** (Pain, abdomen, unspecified site); **790.4** (Elevated, transaminase (level)); **250.00** (Diabetes, type II, or unspecified)

Rationale: The physician has been asked to evaluate the patient for possible cause of her nausea, vomiting, and abdominal pain. There are 4 elements of HPI, location (abdomen), duration (2 days), context (has had moderate p.o. intake), and associated signs and symptoms (constipation) for a level 4 or comprehensive HPI. Five systems were reviewed, constitutional, cardiovascular, respiratory, gastrointestinal, and genitourinary for a level 3, detailed ROS. The documentation included 3 of 3 PFSH for a level or comprehensive PFSH. All 3 elements of history must qualify for level selection. The HPI and the PFSH are comprehensive (level 4) but the ROS is only detailed (level 3) so the level of history is a level 3, or detailed.

The examination consisted of 4 constitutional elements (temperature, pulse, blood pressure, general appearance) that count as 1 BA/OS. The BAs that were examined include neck, abdomen, and all 4 extremities for a total of 6 BAs. A total of 6 OSs, ophthalmologic, otolaryngologic, cardiovascular, respiratory, gastrointestinal, and neurologic were examined. This is a total of 13 BA/OS for a level 4, or comprehensive, examination.

Extensive diagnosis/management options, moderate data were reviewed, and the patient has moderate risk of death or complication that makes the level of MDM moderate.

The first diagnosis under the physician's impression states that these symptoms could represent diabetic gastroparesis, which is also known as delayed gastric emptying due to paralysis of the stomach muscles. At the time of the report, diabetic gastroparesis represents a suspected diagnosis, which is not reported in the outpatient setting. Rather, the symptoms would be reported as nausea, with vomiting (**787.01**) and abdominal pain (**789.00**). The fifth digit on abdominal pain (**789.00**) would be "0" for unspecified abdominal pain because no further indication of location was documented. Also reported is the elevated trasaminase (**790.4**). The diabetes is reported with **250.00**, Diabetes mellitus without mention of complication, with a fifth digit to indicate "unspecified, not stated as uncontrolled."

Practice 4, Report B

HISTORY ELEMENTS			Documented
HISTORY OF PRESENT ILLNESS (HPI)			
1. Location (site on body)			X
2. Quality (characteristic: throbbing, sharp)			
3. Severity (1/10 or how intense)			
4. Duration (how long for problem or episode)			X
5. Timing (when it occurs)			
6. Context (under what circumstances does it occur)			X
7. Modifying factors (what makes it better or worse)			
8. Associated signs and symptoms (what else is happening when it occurs)			X
		TOTAL	4
		LEVEL	4

REVIEW OF SYSTEMS (ROS)			Documented
1. Constitutional (e.g., weight loss, fever)			X
2. Ophthalmologic (eyes)			
3. Otolaryngologic (ears, nose, mouth, throat)			
4. Cardiovascular			X
5. Respiratory			X
6. Gastrointestinal			X
7. Genitourinary			X
8. Musculoskeletal			
9. Integumentary (skin and/or breasts)			
10. Neurologic			
11. Psychiatric			
12. Endocrine			
13. Hematologic/Lymphatic			
14. Allergic/Immunologic			
		TOTAL	5
		LEVEL	3

PAST, FAMILY, AND/OR SOCIAL HISTORY (PFSH)			Documented
1. Past illness, operations, injuries, treatments, and current medications			X
2. Family medical history for heredity and risk			X
3. Social activities, both past and present			X
		TOTAL	3
		LEVEL	4

History Level	1	2	3	
	Problem Focused	Expanded Problem Focused	Detailed	Comprehensive
HPI	Brief 1-3	Brief 1-3	Extended 4+	Extended 4+
ROS	None	Problem Pertinent	Extended 2-9	Complete 10+
PFSH	None	None	Pertinent 1	Complete 2-3
			HISTORY LEVEL	3

EXAMINATION ELEMENTS		Documented
CONSTITUTIONAL		
1. Blood pressure, sitting		
2. Blood pressure, lying		X
3. Pulse		X
4. Respirations		
5. Temperature		X
6. Height		
7. Weight		
8. General appearance		X
	NUMBER	1

BODY AREAS (BA)		Documented
1. Head (including face)		
2. Neck		X
3. Chest (including breasts and axillae)		X
4. Abdomen		X
5. Genitalia, groin, buttocks		
6. Back (including spine)		
7. Each extremity		XXXX
	NUMBER	6

ORGAN SYSTEMS (OS)		Documented
1. Ophthalmologic (eyes)		X
2. Otolaryngologic (ears, nose, mouth, throat)		X
3. Cardiovascular		X
4. Respiratory		X
5. Gastrointestinal		X
6. Genitourinary		
7. Musculoskeletal		
8. Integumentary		
9. Neurologic		X
10. Psychiatric		
11. Hematologic/Lymphatic/Immunologic		
	NUMBER	6
	TOTAL BA/OS	13

Exam Level	1	2	3	
	Problem Focused	Expanded Problem Focused	Detailed	Comprehensive
	Limited to affected BA/OS	Limited to affected BA/OS & other related OSs	Extended of affected BA & other related OSs	General multi-system or complete single OS
# of OS or BA	1	2-7 limited	2-7 extended	8+
			EXAMINATION LEVEL	4

MDM ELEMENTS		Documented
# OF DIAGNOSIS/MANAGEMENT OPTIONS		
1. Minimal		
2. Limited		
3. Multiple		
4. Extensive		X
	LEVEL	4

AMOUNT OR COMPLEXITY OF DATA TO REVIEW		Documented
1. Minimal/None		
2. Limited		
3. Moderate		X
4. Extensive		
	LEVEL	3

RISK OF COMPLICATION OR DEATH IF NOT TREATED		Documented
1. Minimal		
2. Low		
3. Moderate		X
4. High		
	LEVEL	3

MDM*	1	2	3	4
	Straightforward	Low	Moderate	High
Number of DX or management options	Minimal	Limited	Multiple	Extensive
Amount or complexity of data	Minimal/None	Limited	Moderate	Extensive
Risks	Minimal	Low	Moderate	High
			MDM LEVEL	3

*To qualify for a given type of MDM complexity, 2 of 3 elements in the table must be met or exceeded.

History: Detailed
Examination: Comprehensive
MDM: Moderate

Number of Key Components: 3 of 3

99253

PRACTICE 5, EMERGENCY DEPARTMENT SERVICES

Practice 5, Report A

Rationale:

A. **This is the correct answer. This is an ED encounter (99284) and the highest level of service was the administration of intravenous (IV) medications, level 4, point 10. 789.09 is assigned to report the abdominal pain with fifth digit 9 to indicate other specified site, because patient's complaint and examination indicate upper abdominal, diffuse and right upper quadrant. The nausea is reported with 787.02 and the diarrhea with 787.91. Note that the viral syndrome (079.99) is not reported because provider indicated this as "probable" diagnosis and probable diagnoses are not reported in the outpatient setting. Also not reported were the asthma, hypertension, depression, migraines, esophageal reflux, or arthritis, because none of these conditions were treated or were documented to affect treatment.**

B. This choice is incorrect. 99285 requires a level of service as indicated on the acuity sheet and the highest level of service in this case was level 4, point 10, administration of IV medication. The diagnosis is also incorrect as 789.00 reports abdominal pain of an unspecified site and the report indicated upper abdominal pain (fifth digit 9). 079.9, viral syndrome, is incorrect because the diagnostic statement indicated the viral syndrome was a probable diagnosis. Also missing from this selection is the nausea reported with 787.02 and the diarrhea reported with 787.91.

C. This choice is incorrect. 99283 is too low a level of service because level 4, point 10 specifies administration of an IV medication and the documentation in this case indicated that level of service. Also documented was the level 3, point 4 service of prescription medication administration, but code selection should always be the highest code available that is supported by the provider's documentation or the service is undercoded. Diagnosis of 789.00 (abdominal pain, unspecified site) is incorrect, because the documentation indicates specific points of pain, 789.09. Also missing from this selection is the nausea reported with 787.02 and the diarrhea reported with 787.91.

D. This choice is incorrect. Although 99284 is correct with 789.09 (abdominal pain, other specified site), 079.99 (unspecified viral infection) is not reported because it is documented as "probable," and probable diagnoses are not reported in the outpatient setting. Also missing from this selection is the nausea reported with 787.02 and the diarrhea reported with 787.91.

Practice 5, Report B

Professional Services: 99283 (Evaluation and Management, Emergency Department); 845.00 (Sprain, strain, ankle); E885.2 (Fall, from, off, skateboard)

Rationale: The patient presents to the emergency room complaining of ankle pain due to a fall. The highest level of service is level 3, point 3, x-ray of one area, reported with 99283.

The ankle was not fractured, but sprained (845.00). The external cause of the injury was a fall from a skateboard (E885.2).

PRACTICE 6, PEDIATRIC CRITICAL CARE PATIENT TRANSPORT

Practice 6, Report A

Rationale:

A. Incorrect because the critical care time at the initial facility (**99291** and **99292**) is bundled into the total time for transport.

B. Incorrect because the multiple units for **99290** should have been 5, not 4.

C. Incorrect because the critical care time at the initial facility (**99291**) is bundled into the total time for transport.

D. Correct because the 99289 is correct and the multiplier for 99290 should be 5. Total time is $1^1/_2$ hours of critical care (90 minutes) and 2 hours of transport time (120 minutes), which are added together for a total of 210 minutes. From the total of 210, subtract the 74 minutes of the initial transport (99289), with 136 remaining. From 136, subtracting increments of 30 minutes (99290) equals 106, subtracting another 30 minutes (99290) equals 76, subtracting another 30 minutes (99290) equals 46, subtracting another 30 minutes (99290) equals 16 minutes remaining. The last 16 minutes would be reported with one more unit of 99290 for a total of 5 units.

Practice 6, Report B

Professional Services: **99289** (Evaluation and Management, Pediatric Interfacility Transport); **99290** × 3 (Evaluation and Management, Pediatric Interfacility Transport); **949.0** (Burn, unspecified); **785.50** (Shock); **E899** (Burning, burns)

Rationale: This documentation is very vague. The coder should discuss with the physician the need for more detailed documentation to ensure proper coding and achievement of the highest level of specificity.

The time given in this documentation is 2 hours and 40 minutes, or 160 minutes. **99289** is reported for the first 30-74 minutes. **99290** is an add-on code and is used in conjunction with **99289** to report each additional 30 minutes of time after the first 74 minutes. The additional time after the first 74 minutes is 86 minutes, or **99290** × 3. No audit form is needed when assigning codes from this subcategory because the codes are time based and not based on key components.

This is an 18-month-old who was burned and has gone into shock. The body area and severity of the burn is not specified in this documentation. Neither is the cause of the burn. The diagnosis would be reported as **949.0**, burn of unspecified area and unspecified degree. The report states the patient went into shock, which is reported with **785.50**. Additionally an E code is assigned to report an unspecified burning, **E899**.

PRACTICE 7, CRITICAL CARE SERVICES

Practice 7, Report A

Rationale:

A. This choice is incorrect. **99291** is correct for the critical care service, based on time documented. Diagnosis **806.00** (fracture, C1-C4 with unspecified spinal cord injury) is incorrect because there is no documentation of spinal cord injury. Diagnosis **E888.8** would not be reported because there is no clear documentation of what happened and the injury was likely the result of a medical condition (syncopal episode) versus an "accident." **780.09** (other alteration of consciousness) is incorrect because the documentation indicates syncope (**780.2**).

B. This choice is incorrect. **99221** reports an initial hospital service. When critical care is part of the initial visit by the same provider, the work for the admission is "bundled" into the critical care service code and not reported separately. **E888.8** would not be reported because there is no clear documentation of what happened, and the injury was likely the result of a medical condition (syncopal episode) versus an "accident." The remaining diagnoses are correct.

C. **Is the correct answer. Only 99291 can be assigned because the nonspecific statement of "Total critical care time did exceed 30 minutes" was the only documentation. 805.04 is the correct code for a closed cervical 4 fracture without any indication of spinal cord injury; 780.2 is correct for the syncope because there is no further information available. An E code is not assigned because the fracture was a result of the fall from the syncope, not an actual accident.**

D. This choice is incorrect. **99221** is for an initial hospital service. When critical care is part of the initial visit by the same provider, the work for the admission is "bundled" into the critical care service code and not separately reported. Diagnosis coding is correct.

Practice 7, Report B

Professional Services: **99291** (Evaluation and Management, Critical Care); **780.99** (Change (of), mental status/NEC); **465.9** (Infection, respiratory, upper, acute, infectious); **796.3** (Hypotension, transient); **599.0** (Urosepsis); **412** (Infarction, myocardial, healed or old, currently presenting no symptoms); **V10.51** (History (personal) of, malignant neoplasm, bladder); **V58.61** (Long-term (current) drug use, anticoagulants); **E888.9** (E code index, Fall, same level NEC); **E849.0** (E code index, Accident, occurring, home)

Rationale: This is a critical care service, which is based on the time spent with the patient, not the usual key components. At the end of the documentation it states that the physician spent 30 minutes of critical care time on the patient. When billing for critical care, the table in the E/M section of your CPT manual is helpful. The table indicates that for 30-74 minutes code **99291** is to be assigned.

The patient presents with an altered level of consciousness, **780.99**. On further testing he was found to have urosepsis, **599.0**, an upper respiratory infection, **465.9**, and transient hypotension, **796.3**. The patient also has a history of bladder cancer, **V10.51** and long term use of anticoagulants, **V58.61**. The instructions at the beginning of the E code chapter in the ICD-9-CM direct the coder to assign E codes to identify the cause of the injury. In this case, the patient was at home (**E849.0**) when he fell (**E888.9**).

PRACTICE 8, INPATIENT NEONATAL AND PEDIATRIC CRITICAL CARE SERVICES (99293-99300)

Practice 8, Report A

Rationale:

A. Incorrect because there is no indication that the neonatal intensive care physician was the surgeon. Critical care providers do not generally perform surgical procedures, other than those necessary to maintain the patient's viability, such as intubation.

B. Incorrect because the patient is in the NICU (Neonatal Intensive Care Unit) and vitals are being monitored continuously, and this is not a subsequent hospital service reported with **99231**. Also incorrect in this selection is the diagnosis code of **764.09**, Light for date, because there is no indication of the birthweight. **V45.89** reports a postprocedural state for the hernia repair, when this admission was for the surgery and none of the conditions were documented to be a result of surgery. The **550.10** to report the inguinal hernia is correct.

C. **This is the correct choice because the infant weighed 4696 grams and this was a subsequent care indicated by the title of the report "Progress Note" and the content of the note indicating previous studies and care; therefore, the service was reported with 99300. The patient was admitted for repair of a unilateral inguinal hernia (550.10) and developed acute lung congestion (486). The bradycardia is reported with 427.89.**

D. Incorrect because **V45.89** reports a postprocedural state for the hernia repair, when this admission was for the surgery and none of the conditions were documented to be a result of surgery. The remaining codes are correct.

Practice 8, Report B

Professional Services: **99299** (Evaluation and Management, Low Birthweight Infant); **765.15** (Premature, birth NEC); **765.26** (Weeks of gestation)

Rationale: Codes **99298, 99299** and **99300** are used to report physician services on days other than the day of admit, for infants of very low birth weight (VLBW) (infants weighing less than 1500 grams), low birth weight (LBW) (1500-2500 grams), or normal weight (2501-5000 grams) who do not meet the definition of critically ill but still require intensive services. These infants are recovering. Code selection depends on the weight of the infant. The infant in this documentation is 2100 grams with stable respiratory status. The correct code to assign is **99299**.

The patient is a premature underweight infant (**765.18** with a fifth digit of 8 to represent the weight of the infant) delivered at 27 weeks gestation (**765.24**). The current weight of the infant is represented by the selection of the fifth digit. Coding guidelines for code range 765.xx also indicate to "use additional code for weeks of gestation (**765.20-765.29**)."

PRACTICE 9, NURSING FACILITY SERVICES

Practice 9, Report A

Rationale:
A. This choice is incorrect because **296.90** reports an unspecified episodic mood disorder when a bipolar disorder was documented (**296.80**). The other codes are correct.

B. This choice is incorrect because **99308** is for a subsequent nursing facility service requiring EPF history and exam with a low MDM. Two of three key components are required and the EPF history, detailed exam, and moderate MDM documented support a higher level code (**99309**). Diagnosis **401.1** is incorrect, because the documentation does not specify benign hypertension. The other diagnoses are correct.

C. This choice is incorrect because **99336** is for an established patient service in a domiciliary, rest home, or custodial care setting and this patient is a resident in a nursing home. **296.90** (unspecified episodic mood disorder) is incorrect because a bipolar disorder was documented and is reported with **296.80**. **969.3** is incorrect because there is no current "poisoning" from a medication documented. The correct code should be **333.82** (tardive dyskinesia). The remaining codes are correct.

D. Is the correct answer. 99309 is correct because the patient is a resident in a nursing home and this is a subsequent service. As a subsequent service, 2 of 3 key components are required to select a level of service. The documentation supports an EPF history, a detailed exam, and moderate MDM. 784.0 reports the headaches; 296.80 reports unspecified bipolar disorder; 401.9 reports unspecified hypertension; 333.82 reports tardive dyskinesia and requires the corresponding E code, E939.3, to indicate the cause of condition as adverse effects of antidepressants. Also reported is 788.30 for the urinary incontinence.

Practice 9, Report B

Professional Services: 99307 (Evaluation and Management, Nursing Facility, Subsequent Care); **331.0** (Disease, Alzheimer's); **298.9** (Psychosis, atypical); **297.9** (Delusions, paranoid)

Rationale: The first line of the note states that this is a routine nursing facility service, which indicates this is an established patient. The only element of the HPI is the statement about frequent delusions for a level 1 HPI. The ROS consisted of constitutional, cardiovascular, and respiratory for a level 3, or detailed, ROS. No elements of PFSH for a level 2, or EPF, PFSH. The history is a level 1, PF history.

The examination consisted of only one constitutional element (general appearance), so this would qualify as a one BA/OS. Only 2 BAs were examined, the head and neck. The 3 OSs that were examined are ophthalmologic, otolaryngologic, and respiratory for a total of 6 BA/OS, which is a level 3 or detailed examination.

The MDM consisted of a limited number of diagnosis/management options, minimal data to review, and minimal risk of death for straightforward decision making.

A problem focused history, detailed examination, and straightforward MDM qualifies as a **99307**.

The documentation indicates the diagnosis of Alzheimer's (**331.0**). The patient is also experiencing atypical psychosis (**298.9**) and paranoid delusions (**297.9**).

Practice 9, Report B

HISTORY ELEMENTS	Documented
HISTORY OF PRESENT ILLNESS (HPI)	
1. Location (site on body)	
2. Quality (characteristic: throbbing, sharp)	
3. Severity (1/10 or how intense)	
4. Duration (how long for problem or episode)	✗
5. Timing (when it occurs)	
6. Context (under what circumstances does it occur)	
7. Modifying factors (what makes it better or worse)	
8. Associated signs and symptoms (what else is happening when it occurs)	
TOTAL	1
LEVEL	1

REVIEW OF SYSTEMS (ROS)	Documented
1. Constitutional (e.g., weight loss, fever)	✗
2. Ophthalmologic (eyes)	
3. Otolaryngologic (ears, nose, mouth, throat)	
4. Cardiovascular	✗
5. Respiratory	✗
6. Gastrointestinal	
7. Genitourinary	
8. Musculoskeletal	
9. Integumentary (skin and/or breasts)	
10. Neurologic	
11. Psychiatric	
12. Endocrine	
13. Hematologic/Lymphatic	
14. Allergic/Immunologic	
TOTAL	3
LEVEL	3

PAST, FAMILY, AND/OR SOCIAL HISTORY (PFSH)	Documented
1. Past illness, operations, injuries, treatments, and current medications	
2. Family medical history for heredity and risk	
3. Social activities, both past and present	
TOTAL	0
LEVEL	2

History Level		1	2	3	
		Problem Focused	Expanded Problem Focused	Detailed	Comprehensive
HPI		Brief 1-3	Brief 1-3	Extended 4+	Extended 4+
ROS		None	Problem Pertinent	Extended 2-9	Complete 10+
PFSH		None	None	Pertinent 1	Complete 2-3
				HISTORY LEVEL	1

EXAMINATION ELEMENTS	Documented
CONSTITUTIONAL	
1. Blood pressure, sitting	
2. Blood pressure, lying	
3. Pulse	
4. Respirations	
5. Temperature	
6. Height	
7. Weight	
8. General appearance	✗
NUMBER	1

BODY AREAS (BA)	Documented
1. Head (including face)	✗
2. Neck	✗
3. Chest (including breasts and axillae)	
4. Abdomen	
5. Genitalia, groin, buttocks	
6. Back (including spine)	
7. Each extremity	
NUMBER	2

ORGAN SYSTEMS (OS)	Documented
1. Ophthalmologic (eyes)	✗
2. Otolaryngologic (ears, nose, mouth, throat)	✗
3. Cardiovascular	
4. Respiratory	✗
5. Gastrointestinal	
6. Genitourinary	
7. Musculoskeletal	
8. Integumentary	
9. Neurologic	
10. Psychiatric	
11. Hematologic/Lymphatic/Immunologic	
NUMBER	3
TOTAL BA/OS	6

Exam Level	1	2	3	
	Problem Focused	Expanded Problem Focused	Detailed	Comprehensive
	Limited to affected BA/OS	Limited to affected BA/OS & other related OSs	Extended of affected BA & other related OSs	General multi-system or complete single OS
# of OS or BA	1	2-7 limited	2-7 extended	8+
			EXAMINATION LEVEL	3

MDM ELEMENTS	Documented
# OF DIAGNOSIS/MANAGEMENT OPTIONS	
1. Minimal	
2. Limited	✗
3. Multiple	
4. Extensive	
LEVEL	2
AMOUNT OR COMPLEXITY OF DATA TO REVIEW	Documented
1. Minimal/None	✗
2. Limited	
3. Moderate	
4. Extensive	
LEVEL	1
RISK OF COMPLICATION OR DEATH IF NOT TREATED	Documented
1. Minimal	✗
2. Low	
3. Moderate	
4. High	
LEVEL	1

MDM*	1	2	3	4
	Straightforward	Low	Moderate	High
Number of DX or management options	Minimal	Limited	Multiple	Extensive
Amount or complexity of data	Minimal/None	Limited	Moderate	Extensive
Risks	Minimal	Low	Moderate	High
			MDM LEVEL	1

*To qualify for a given type of MDM complexity, 2 of 3 elements in the table must be met or exceeded.

History: Problem Focused
Examination: Detailed
MDM: Straightforward

Number of Key Components: 2 of 3

99307

PRACTICE 10, DOMICILIARY, REST HOME (E.G., BOARDING HOME), OR CUSTODIAL CARE SERVICES, AND DOMICILIARY, REST HOME (E.G., ASSISTED LIVING FACILITY), OR HOME CARE PLAN OVERSIGHT SERVICES (99324-99340)

Practice 10, Report A

Rationale:

A. This is the correct choice because this is an established patient in a custodial care facility. The documentation supports an EPF history, a PF exam, and low complexity MDM. This category requires 2 out of 3 key elements to assign a code, so the correct code is 99325. The diagnosis is correctly reported as a rash (782.1).

B. Incorrect choice because 99307 is for an established patient in a nursing facility not a custodial care facility. The diagnosis is correct.

C. Incorrect choice because 99347 is for an established patient home service, not a custodial care center. The diagnosis is correct.

D. Incorrect diagnosis code of 780.52 because the sleep disturbance noted is not being treated or addressed in the care plan, so it would not be reported. The diagnosis correctly reported as a rash (782.1). 99325 is incorrect because it is for a new patient and this patient is established.

Practice 10, Report B

Professional Services: 99336 (Evaluation and Management, Domiciliary or Rest Home, Established Patient); 599.0 (Infection, urinary tract); V47.4 (Problems, urinary NEC)

Rationale: This service is an established patient service at the rest home where the patient resides. The HPI consists of the location (urinary system), quality (painful), severity (5 out of 10), and associated signs and symptoms (fever, abdominal pain) for 4 HPI or comprehensive HPI. The ROS included 4 systems, constitutional, cardiovascular, respiratory, and psychiatric, for a level 3 or detailed ROS. The history consisted of the patient's past medical history with review of his indwelling suprapubic catheter and social history (resides in a rest home) for a level 4 or comprehensive PFSH. Level selection of history must match all three areas to qualify for level selection. This documentation contained comprehensive HPI, detailed ROS, and a comprehensive PFSH for level 3 or detailed history.

The examination consisted of no constitutional items, 5 body areas, including the abdomen and all 4 extremities and 4 organ systems, cardiovascular, respiratory, integumentary, and psychiatric, for a total of 9 BA/OS and a level 4, or comprehensive, examination.

The MDM entailed multiple diagnosis/management options (new problem), no data were reviewed, and there is moderate risk (prescription drug management). This is a level 3, or moderate, MDM.

A detailed history, comprehensive examination, and moderate MDM is assigned 99336.

The diagnosis is UTI, reported with 599.0. The fever and abdominal pain would not be reported because they are symptoms of the UTI. V47.4 would be reported to indicate the status of the suprapubic catheter, because the status is related to the organ system being treated.

Practice 10, Report B

HISTORY ELEMENTS	Documented
HISTORY OF PRESENT ILLNESS (HPI)	
1. Location (site on body)	✗
2. Quality (characteristic: throbbing, sharp)	✗
3. Severity (1/10 or how intense)	✗
4. Duration (how long for problem or episode)	
5. Timing (when it occurs)	
6. Context (under what circumstances does it occur)	
7. Modifying factors (what makes it better or worse)	
8. Associated signs and symptoms (what else is happening when it occurs)	✗
TOTAL	4
LEVEL	4
REVIEW OF SYSTEMS (ROS)	Documented
1. Constitutional (e.g., weight loss, fever)	✗
2. Ophthalmologic (eyes)	
3. Otolaryngologic (ears, nose, mouth, throat)	
4. Cardiovascular	✗
5. Respiratory	✗
6. Gastrointestinal	
7. Genitourinary	
8. Musculoskeletal	
9. Integumentary (skin and/or breasts)	
10. Neurologic	
11. Psychiatric	✗
12. Endocrine	
13. Hematologic/Lymphatic	
14. Allergic/Immunologic	
TOTAL	4
LEVEL	3
PAST, FAMILY, AND/OR SOCIAL HISTORY (PFSH)	Documented
1. Past illness, operations, injuries, treatments, and current medications	✗
2. Family medical history for heredity and risk	
3. Social activities, both past and present	✗
TOTAL	2
LEVEL	4

History Level	1	2	3	4
	Problem Focused	Expanded Problem Focused	Detailed	Comprehensive
HPI	Brief 1-3	Brief 1-3	Extended 4+	Extended 4+
ROS	None	Problem Pertinent	Extended 2-9	Complete 10+
PFSH	None	None	Pertinent 1	Complete 2-3
			HISTORY LEVEL	3

EXAMINATION ELEMENTS	Documented
CONSTITUTIONAL	
1. Blood pressure, sitting	
2. Blood pressure, lying	
3. Pulse	
4. Respirations	
5. Temperature	
6. Height	
7. Weight	
8. General appearance	
NUMBER	0
BODY AREAS (BA)	Documented
1. Head (including face)	
2. Neck	
3. Chest (including breasts and axillae)	
4. Abdomen	✗
5. Genitalia, groin, buttocks	
6. Back (including spine)	
7. Each extremity	✗✗✗✗
NUMBER	5
ORGAN SYSTEMS (OS)	Documented
1. Ophthalmologic (eyes)	
2. Otolaryngologic (ears, nose, mouth, throat)	
3. Cardiovascular	✗
4. Respiratory	✗
5. Gastrointestinal	
6. Genitourinary	
7. Musculoskeletal	
8. Integumentary	✗
9. Neurologic	
10. Psychiatric	✗
11. Hematologic/Lymphatic/Immunologic	
NUMBER	4
TOTAL BA/OS	9

Exam Level	1	2	3	4
	Problem Focused	Expanded Problem Focused	Detailed	Comprehensive
	Limited to affected BA/OS	Limited to affected BA/OS & other related OSs	Extended of affected BA & other related OSs	General multi-system or complete single OS
# of OS or BA	1	2-7 limited	2-7 extended	8+
			EXAMINATION LEVEL	4

MDM ELEMENTS	Documented
# OF DIAGNOSIS/MANAGEMENT OPTIONS	
1. Minimal	
2. Limited	
3. Multiple	✗
4. Extensive	
LEVEL	3
AMOUNT OR COMPLEXITY OF DATA TO REVIEW	Documented
1. Minimal/None	✗
2. Limited	
3. Moderate	
4. Extensive	
LEVEL	1
RISK OF COMPLICATION OR DEATH IF NOT TREATED	Documented
1. Minimal	
2. Low	
3. Moderate	✗
4. High	
LEVEL	3

MDM*	1	2	3	4
	Straightforward	Low	Moderate	High
Number of DX or management options	Minimal	Limited	Multiple	Extensive
Amount or complexity of data	Minimal/None	Limited	Moderate	Extensive
Risks	Minimal	Low	Moderate	High
			MDM LEVEL	3

*To qualify for a given type of MDM complexity, 2 of 3 elements in the table must be met or exceeded.

History: Detailed
Examination: Comprehensive
MDM: Moderate

Number of Key Components: 2 of 3

99336

PRACTICE 11, HOME SERVICES

Practice 11, Report A

Rationale:

A. This is an incorrect choice because **99343** is for a new patient home visit rather than an established patient home visit. Diagnosis code **491.0** (chronic bronchitis) is incorrect because documentation did not specify acute or chronic. The osteoarthritis (**715.9**), multiple decubiti of unspecified site (**707.00**), and pitting edema (**782.3**) were correctly reported.

B. This is an incorrect choice because **99343** is for a new patient home visit rather than an established patient home visit. Diagnosis codes are correct based on the documentation in the report as bronchitis (**490**), osteoarthritis (**715.9**), multiple decubiti of unspecified site (**707.00**), and pitting edema (**782.3**).

C. **This is the correct choice because 99349 is for an established patient for a home service. Diagnosis codes are correct based on the documentation in the report as bronchitis (490), osteoarthritis (715.9), multiple decubiti of unspecified site (707.00), and pitting edema (782.3).**

D. This is an incorrect choice because the bronchitis was not documented as acute or chronic (**491.0**) and as such should have been reported with **490**. The osteoarthritis (**715.9**), multiple decubiti of unspecified site (**707.00**), and pitting edema (**782.3**) were correctly reported. **99349** is correct for an established patient home service.

Practice 11, Report B

Professional Services: 99349 (Evaluation and Management, Home Services); **490** (Bronchitis); **428.0** (Failure, heart, congestive); **332.0** (Parkinsonism)

Rationale: This is a home service, which is based on the whether the patient is new or established and the key components.

The HPI consists of 4 elements, location (lung), quality (productive), duration (since Monday), and modifying factor (Robitussin). This qualifies as a level 4 or comprehensive HPI. The patient was not able to answer questions for the ROS due to his condition so this would then qualify for a level 4 or comprehensive ROS. The patient's past medical history is reviewed, for a level 3 or detailed history. This documentation contains a comprehensive HPI, a comprehensive ROS and a detailed PFSH for a level 3 or detailed history.

The examination contains 3 constitutional elements of blood pressure, respirations, and temperature that qualify as 1 BA/OS. The BAs examined are head, abdomen, and all 4 extremities, for a total of 6 BAs. Only 2 OSs were examined, cardiovascular and respiratory. The total of BA/OS is 9 for a level 4 or comprehensive examination.

The MDM contains a multiple number of diagnosis and management options, minimal/no data to review and moderate risk. This qualifies as a level 3 or moderate MDM.

The primary diagnosis for this home service would be the bronchitis (**490**). The cough would not need to be coded according to Section II.A. of the Official Guidelines for Coding and Reporting, which indicates that codes for symptoms (such as the cough) are not reported when a more definitive diagnosis has been established (bronchitis). The patient also has CHF (**428.0**) and Parkinson's disease (**332.0**). The osteoarthritis (**715.90**) would not have to be reported as the condition was not treated.

Practice 11, Report B

HISTORY ELEMENTS	Documented
HISTORY OF PRESENT ILLNESS (HPI)	
1. Location (site on body)	X
2. Quality (characteristic: throbbing, sharp)	X
3. Severity (1/10 or how intense)	
4. Duration (how long for problem or episode)	X
5. Timing (when it occurs)	
6. Context (under what circumstances does it occur)	X
7. Modifying factors (what makes it better or worse)	X
8. Associated signs and symptoms (what else is happening when it occurs)	
TOTAL	4
LEVEL	4
REVIEW OF SYSTEMS (ROS)	Documented
1. Constitutional (e.g., weight loss, fever)	
2. Ophthalmologic (eyes)	
3. Otolaryngologic (ears, nose, mouth, throat)	
4. Cardiovascular	
5. Respiratory	
6. Gastrointestinal	
7. Genitourinary	
8. Musculoskeletal	
9. Integumentary (skin and/or breasts)	
10. Neurologic	
11. Psychiatric	
12. Endocrine	
13. Hematologic/Lymphatic	
14. Allergic/Immunologic	
TOTAL	Unobtainable
LEVEL	4
PAST, FAMILY, AND/OR SOCIAL HISTORY (PFSH)	Documented
1. Past illness, operations, injuries, treatments, and current medications	X
2. Family medical history for heredity and risk	
3. Social activities, both past and present	
TOTAL	1
LEVEL	3

History Level	1	2	3	4
	Problem Focused	Expanded Problem Focused	Detailed	Comprehensive
HPI	Brief 1-3	Brief 1-3	Extended 4+	Extended 4+
ROS	None	Problem Pertinent	Extended 2-9	Complete 10+
PFSH	None	None	Pertinent 1	Complete 2-3
HISTORY LEVEL			3	

EXAMINATION ELEMENTS	Documented
CONSTITUTIONAL	
1. Blood pressure, sitting	
2. Blood pressure, lying	X
3. Pulse	
4. Respirations	X
5. Temperature	X
6. Height	
7. Weight	
8. General appearance	
NUMBER	1
BODY AREAS (BA)	Documented
1. Head (including face)	X
2. Neck	
3. Chest (including breasts and axillae)	
4. Abdomen	X
5. Genitalia, groin, buttocks	
6. Back (including spine)	
7. Each extremity	XXXX
NUMBER	6
ORGAN SYSTEMS (OS)	Documented
1. Ophthalmologic (eyes)	
2. Otolaryngologic (ears, nose, mouth, throat)	
3. Cardiovascular	X
4. Respiratory	X
5. Gastrointestinal	
6. Genitourinary	
7. Musculoskeletal	
8. Integumentary	
9. Neurologic	
10. Psychiatric	
11. Hematologic/Lymphatic/Immunologic	
NUMBER	2
TOTAL BA/OS	9

Exam Level	1	2	3	Comprehensive
	Problem Focused	Expanded Problem Focused	Detailed	
	Limited to affected BA/OS	Limited to affected BA/OS & other related OSs	Extended of affected BA & other related OSs	General multi-system or complete single OS
# of OS or BA	1	2-7 limited	2-7 extended	8+
EXAMINATION LEVEL				4

MDM ELEMENTS	Documented
# OF DIAGNOSIS/MANAGEMENT OPTIONS	
1. Minimal	
2. Limited	
3. Multiple	X
4. Extensive	
LEVEL	3
AMOUNT OR COMPLEXITY OF DATA TO REVIEW	Documented
1. Minimal/None	X
2. Limited	
3. Moderate	
4. Extensive	
LEVEL	1
RISK OF COMPLICATION OR DEATH IF NOT TREATED	Documented
1. Minimal	
2. Low	
3. Moderate	X
4. High	
LEVEL	3

MDM*	1	2	3	4
	Straightforward	Low	Moderate	High
Number of DX or management options	Minimal	Limited	Multiple	Extensive
Amount or complexity of data	Minimal/None	Limited	Moderate	Extensive
Risks	Minimal	Low	Moderate	High
MDM LEVEL			3	

*To qualify for a given type of MDM complexity, 2 of 3 elements in the table must be met or exceeded.

History: Detailed
Examination: Comprehensive
MDM: Moderate

Number of Key Components: 2 of 3

99349

PRACTICE 12A, PROLONGED SERVICES WITH OR WITHOUT DIRECT PATIENT CONTACT

Practice 12A, Report A

Rationale:

A. This is the correct choice because the documentation supported a comprehensive history and exam with a moderate complexity of MDM. As an established patient, 2 of 3 key components are required for determining a level of service, so this service qualifies for 99215. The additional 40 minutes would be reported with the prolonged service code 99354, which is direct face-to-face care of a patient in an outpatient setting. The diagnosis is reported with 403.90, hypertensive kidney disease, even though the report did not state that there was a correlation between the hypertension and kidney disease because the guidelines (Section 1, 7.a.3.) direct the coder to assume a causal relationship between the two conditions and report a 403 code rather than 401.9 (hypertension). Also to be reported is the stage of the kidney disease, which in this case is 585.9, unspecified CKD. The history of present illness indicates that the patient was started on an Advair inhaler but by another physician, and there is no documentation that this physician treated the breathing problem, and as such the condition is not reported. V45.89, Other postprocedural status, is correct to report the previous renal artery stenting.

B. This is an incorrect choice because the level of service is too low and no prolonged service code is used. Diagnosis coding is correct.

C. This is an incorrect choice because the level of service is too low and the code **99358** is for non-direct face-to-face care. Also incorrect are the **401.9** and **585.9** to report the hypertension and chronic kidney disease because according to the guidelines (Section 1, 7.a.3.) the coder is to assign a 403 category code to report kidney disease and renal failure by assuming a causal relationship between the two. The **440.1** is incorrect because the renal artery stenosis has already been stented.

D. This is an incorrect choice because of **401.9** and **585.9** reporting the hypertension and chronic kidney disease. According to the guidelines (Section 1, 7.a.3.) the coder is to assign a 403 category code to report kidney disease and renal failure by assuming a causal relationship between the two. The **V45.89** is correct. The CPT coding is correct.

Practice 12A, Report B

See audit form on following page.

Professional Services: 99233 (Evaluation and Management, Hospital); **99356** (Evaluation and Management, Prolonged Services); **99357 × 2** (Evaluation and Management, Prolonged Services); **584.9** (Failure, renal, acute); **599.60** (Uropathy, obstructive); **585.9** (Failure, renal, chronic); **591** (Hydronephrosis); **276.1** (Hyponatremia); **276.6** (Overload, fluid)

Rationale: This is a document that represents prolonged service of care. When billing for prolonged services an E/M code from the accurate subcategory would first be selected using the key components of the documentation. The time allotted for that E/M level would be subtracted from the total time of the service and the remaining time would be reported with a prolonged service code. Prolonged service codes are add-on codes and would never be reported alone.

This patient is acutely ill and is being followed for his acute renal failure. There are 4 elements of HPI, location (kidney), quality (worsening), severity (lab findings), and associated signs and symptoms (bloody urine) for a level 4 or comprehensive HPI. Only two systems were reviewed, cardiovascular and respiratory, for a level 3 or detailed ROS. The documentation included only the post history element of PFSH for a level 3, or detailed, PFSH. A comprehensive HPI, detailed ROS, and detailed PFSH qualifies as a detailed history.

The constitutional examination consisted of 3 elements, blood pressure (lying down), pulse, and temperature, to qualify as 1 BA/OS. No BAs were examined. Two OSs were examined, cardiovascular and respiratory, for a total of 2 OSs. The exam performed on this patient entailed 3 BA/OS and qualifies as a level 3 or detailed examination.

Extensive diagnosis/management options, limited data was reviewed, and the patient has a high risk of death, which make this level of MDM high. The level of service would be **99233**. This code is allotted 35 minutes. At the end of this documentation it states that 2 hours and 25 minutes were spent with the patient. The total in minutes is 145 minutes. Subtract the 35 minutes for the initial code **99233**, which would leave 110 minutes of time to bill for prolonged services. The prolonged services are categorized by either face-to-face direct contact or without face-to-face direct contact. The direct face-to-face codes are further divided by whether the service took place in an outpatient or inpatient setting. The prolonged service codes that accompany **99233** are **99356** for the first 74 minutes of prolonged time and **99357 × 2** for the additional 36 minutes. The prolonged service table in your CPT manual is a good tool to aid in code selection for time.

The patient is being evaluated for acute renal failure (**584**). The other diagnoses are obstructive uropathy (**599.60**), chronic renal failure (**585.9**), hydronephrosis (**591**), hyponatremia (**276.1**) and fluid overload (**276.6**). All of these diagnoses would be assigned because all are being treated and each may affect the others.

Practice 12A, Report B

HISTORY ELEMENTS				Documented
HISTORY OF PRESENT ILLNESS (HPI)				
1. Location (site on body)				✗
2. Quality (characteristic: throbbing, sharp)				✗
3. Severity (1/10 or how intense)				✗
4. Duration (how long for problem or episode)				
5. Timing (when it occurs)				
6. Context (under what circumstances does it occur)				
7. Modifying factors (what makes it better or worse)				
8. Associated signs and symptoms (what else is happening when it occurs)				✗
			TOTAL	4
			LEVEL	4

REVIEW OF SYSTEMS (ROS)				Documented
1. Constitutional (e.g., weight loss, fever)				
2. Ophthalmologic (eyes)				
3. Otolaryngologic (ears, nose, mouth, throat)				
4. Cardiovascular				✗
5. Respiratory				✗
6. Gastrointestinal				
7. Genitourinary				
8. Musculoskeletal				
9. Integumentary (skin and/or breasts)				
10. Neurologic				
11. Psychiatric				
12. Endocrine				
13. Hematologic/Lymphatic				
14. Allergic/Immunologic				
			TOTAL	2
			LEVEL	3

PAST, FAMILY, AND/OR SOCIAL HISTORY (PFSH)				Documented
1. Past illness, operations, injuries, treatments, and current medications				✗
2. Family medical history for heredity and risk				
3. Social activities, both past and present				
			TOTAL	1
			LEVEL	3

History Level	1	2	3	4
	Problem Focused	Expanded Problem Focused	Detailed	Comprehensive
HPI	Brief 1-3	Brief 1-3	Extended 4+	Extended 4+
ROS	None	Problem Pertinent	Extended 2-9	Complete 10+
PFSH	None	None	Pertinent 1	Complete 2-3
			HISTORY LEVEL	3

EXAMINATION ELEMENTS	Documented
CONSTITUTIONAL	
1. Blood pressure, sitting	
2. Blood pressure, lying	✗
3. Pulse	✗
4. Respirations	
5. Temperature	✗
6. Height	
7. Weight	
8. General appearance	
NUMBER	1

BODY AREAS (BA)	Documented
1. Head (including face)	
2. Neck	
3. Chest (including breasts and axillae)	
4. Abdomen	
5. Genitalia, groin, buttocks	
6. Back (including spine)	
7. Each extremity	
NUMBER	0

ORGAN SYSTEMS (OS)	Documented
1. Ophthalmologic (eyes)	
2. Otolaryngologic (ears, nose, mouth, throat)	
3. Cardiovascular	✗
4. Respiratory	✗
5. Gastrointestinal	
6. Genitourinary	
7. Musculoskeletal	
8. Integumentary	
9. Neurologic	
10. Psychiatric	
11. Hematologic/Lymphatic/Immunologic	
NUMBER	2
TOTAL BA/OS	3

Exam Level	1	2	3	Comprehensive
	Problem Focused	Expanded Problem Focused	Detailed	
	Limited to affected BA/OS	Limited to affected BA/OS & other related OSs	Extended of affected BA & other related OSs	General multi-system or complete single OS
# of OS or BA	1	2-7 limited	2-7 extended	8+
			EXAMINATION LEVEL	3

MDM ELEMENTS				Documented
# OF DIAGNOSIS/MANAGEMENT OPTIONS				
1. Minimal				
2. Limited				
3. Multiple				
4. Extensive				✗
			LEVEL	4

AMOUNT OR COMPLEXITY OF DATA TO REVIEW				Documented
1. Minimal/None				
2. Limited				✗
3. Moderate				
4. Extensive				
			LEVEL	2

RISK OF COMPLICATION OR DEATH IF NOT TREATED				Documented
1. Minimal				
2. Low				
3. Moderate				
4. High				✗
			LEVEL	4

MDM*	1	2	3	4
	Straightforward	Low	Moderate	High
Number of DX or management options	Minimal	Limited	Multiple	Extensive
Amount or complexity of data	Minimal/None	Limited	Moderate	Extensive
Risks	Minimal	Low	Moderate	High
			MDM LEVEL	4

*To qualify for a given type of MDM complexity, 2 of 3 elements in the table must be met or exceeded.

History: Detailed
Examination: Detailed
MDM: High

Number of Key Components: 2 of 3

99233, 99356, 99357 × 2

PRACTICE 12B, STANDBY SERVICES

Practice 12B, Report A

Rationale:

A. Correct because the total time of standby was 25 minutes. The 6 minutes on the telephone regarding another patient cannot be included in the standby time. Per guidelines, standby time of less than 30 minutes cannot be separately reported.

B. Incorrect because the total time was less than 30 minutes, so no code would be assigned.

C. Incorrect because modifier -80 indicates assistant at surgery and the provider was not scrubbed or assisting in the surgery.

D. Incorrect because modifier -52 cannot be appended to an E/M service and the service cannot be reported as it was less than 30 minutes.

Practice 12B, Report B

Professional Services: 99360 × 3 (Evaluation and Management, Physician Standby Services); **656.81** (Distress, fetal, affecting management of pregnancy or childbirth, antepartum condition or complication)

Rationale: This is a document that represents physician standby services. There is only one code in this subcategory and it is reported in units depending on the length of time the physician is standing by. The requirements for this code are as follows, the standby service has to be requested by another physician, no face-to-face contact is made with the patient, and the physician standing by cannot be providing care to any other patient during that time. If the standby time is less than 30 minutes, the time is not reported. Unlike some of the other E/M codes, the unit of time for standby services must be a full 30 minutes. It is very important to read and understand the guidelines that precede this subcategory before assigning the code.

This documentation indicates 1 hour and 40 minutes of standby or 100 minutes, requested by the patient's OB/GYN physician, due to increased fetal distress. **99360** would be assigned with 3 units (×3), for 90 minutes of the 100 minutes spent in standby. The extra 10 minutes cannot be reported because it is not a full 30 minutes.

The diagnosis is the reason the attending physician requested the physician for whom services are being reported to standby. In this case, the standby was requested for fetal distress that was affecting the management of childbirth—**656.81**. The fifth digit of 1 would be assigned because the physician was present until the patient delivered.

PRACTICE 13A, CASE MANAGEMENT SERVICES (99363-99368)

Practice 13A, Report A

Rationale:

A. This choice is incorrect because **V66.7** is for an encounter for palliative care and the patient was not seen during this service. **V65.49** is appropriate for counseling the family on the options for care. The remaining diagnosis codes are correct. The CPT code is correct.

B. This choice is incorrect because **99367** is for a conference in which neither the patient nor the family are present. Diagnosis codes are correct.

C. This choice is incorrect because **99368** is for a team conference of 3 that neither the family nor patient attend and without the physician leading the team. **V66.7** is incorrect because it is for an encounter for palliative care and the patient was not seen during this service. **V65.49** is appropriate for counseling the family on the options for care. The remaining diagnosis codes are correct.

D. **This is the correct choice with both the diagnoses and service code correct. V65.49 reports consulting, which was the primary reason for the service. The patient's diagnoses are stomach cancer (primary) 151.9; secondary lung cancer (197.0); congestive heart failure (428.0); and chronic pneumonia (515).**

Practice 13A, Report B

Professional Services: **99367** (Evaluation and Management, Case Management); **583.9** (Nephritis); **585.6** (ESRD); **V49.75** (Status post below knee amputation); **V45.1** (Status, dialysis)

Rationale: Case management is when the physician is responsible for the direct care of the patient and for coordinating the care and needs of the patient with other health care services that the patient needs. **99367** is correct to assign because the time spent was 60 minutes and no family was present.

The diagnoses would be nephritis (**583.9**), end stage renal disease (**585.6**), the patient's postoperative amputation status (**V49.75**), and the renal dialysis status (**V45.1**).

PRACTICE 13B, ANTICOAGULANT MANAGEMENT

Practice 13B, Report A

A. **Is correct because it reports a 90-day period of anticoagulant management with 99363.**

B. This choice is incorrect because although it reports **99363** correctly for the initial 90 days of management, **99364** is not to have been reported.

C. This choice is incorrect because it reports a subsequent 90 days with **99364** and this patient service was an initial 90 days of management.

D. This choice is incorrect because it reports a subsequent 90 days with **99364** and initial days with **99363**.

Practice 13B, Report B

Professional Services: **99364** (Anticoagulant Management); **453.42** (Thrombosis, vein)

Rationale: This code is correct because it reports a subsequent 90 days of anticoagulant management that contained at least 3 INR measurements. **453.42** reports deep vein thrombosis of the lower leg.

PRACTICE 14, CARE PLAN OVERSIGHT SERVICES

Practice 14, Report A

Rationale:

A. Incorrect because a medical team conference was not provided. Care Plan Oversight service (**99380**) is correct. Diagnosis coding is correct.

B. **Correct because both the diagnosis and service coding are correct. The physician for whom services are being reported are not the physician in charge of chemotherapy administration because the patient's gynecologist is overseeing that treatment. This physician is providing a care plan oversight for the patient's total care. When the patient presents for chemotherapy, the gynecologist would report the chemotherapy encounter code V58.11. The patient's diagnoses are primary ovarian cancer (183.0), neoplasm-related pain (338.3), and edema (782.3).**

C. Incorrect because **99308** is for a subsequent service, and in this scenario the provider is managing the plan by telephone and is not present at the facility. The diagnosis coding is correct except for the **V58.11**. This physician is providing a care plan oversight for the patient's total care. When the patient presents for chemotherapy, the gynecologist would report the chemotherapy encounter code **V58.11**.

D. Incorrect because the diagnosis for pain management and edema are missing and they should be reported because these conditions are being managed. This physician is providing a care plan oversight for the patient's total care. When the patient presents for chemotherapy, the gynecologist would report the chemotherapy encounter code **V58.11**. The CPT code is correct.

Practice 14, Report B

Professional Services: **99378** (Evaluation and Management, Care Plan Oversight Services); **162.5** (Neoplasm, lung, lower lobe); **338.3** (Pain, neoplasm related)

Rationale: Care plan oversight services reflect a supervisory role of the physician over the patient's care. The patient is not present when the physician is performing the service. Codes entail development or revision of a care plan, review of reports of patient status, communication with other health care professionals, and review of any lab or tests that may have been performed. These codes may only be reported once for every 30-day period. Codes are divided by whether the patient is receiving care from a home health agency, hospice, or a nursing facility. The codes are further categorized based on physician time spent in care plan oversight. **99378** would be the correct code to report this service because the patient is receiving hospice care and the documented time was longer than 30 minutes.

The diagnoses would be lower lobe lung cancer (**162.5**) and **338.3** to report the pain due to the malignancy.

PRACTICE 15, PREVENTIVE MEDICINE SERVICES

Practice 15, Report A

Rationale:

A. Correct because this is a yearly physical examination of a 43-year-old established patient. 99396 is a preventive medicine code for an established patient between the ages of 40 and 64 years. The diagnoses would be V70.0 (Routine medical exam) and V72.31 (Routine GYN exam) for the health checkup. No other diagnoses are needed because the patient is not being treated at this time for her weight gain or depression.

B. Incorrect because 99213 is an E/M code for an office service of an established patient that is used for diagnosis of a new problem or followup care of an existing problem, not for yearly physicals. The diagnosis code 783.1, weight gain, would not be coded because it is not being treated during this evaluation.

C. Incorrect because 99386 is for a new patient preventive medicine service and this is an established patient. The diagnosis of weight gain (783.1) and depression (311) would not be coded because these are not being treated by this physician.

D. Incorrect because the age range for this code is 18-39 years and this patient is 43 years old.

Practice 15, Report B

Professional Services: 99396 (Evaluation and Management, Preventive Services); V70.0 (Checkup, health); V72.31 (Gynecological exam); 305.1 (Abuse, tobacco)

Rationale: Preventive medicine services are for physicals. Codes are selected based on patient age—unlike other E/M codes that are based on time or key components. Codes are further divided by whether the patient is new or established.

This documentation is of a 44-year-old established patient. The correct code for the preventive medicine service is 99396.

The assessment contains 3 diagnoses, yearly physical performed today, gynecological exam, and tobacco abuse. When coding the diagnosis on preventive examinations the first code assigned would be V70.0 for the health checkup followed by the code to report the gynecological exam. Only code the other diagnoses if there is an indication in the plan that these diagnoses are going to be treated or followed up. The physician is recommending smoking cessation, so the abuse of tobacco, 305.1, could be reported. It is important to familiarize yourself with the guidelines that precede the preventive medicine category because these guidelines explain the requirements for reporting both a preventive medicine code and an E/M service on the same day.

PRACTICE 16, NEWBORN CARE

Practice 16, Report A

Rationale:

A. Incorrect because diagnosis **V30.1** is for an infant born outside of the hospital. This infant was born in the hospital as evidenced by the exact time of birth noted and the APGAR scores reported. Diagnosis **779.3** would not be reported because "disorganized suck" alone in a newborn is not indicative of a feeding disorder. It is noted that once the infant is able to latch, 10-20 cc are being taken per feeding. CPT **99435** is correct.

B. Incorrect because **99234** is reported for observation and discharge on the same date, which fits this scenario. However this would be incorrect because there is a code for Newborn Admitted and Discharged on the same date, which is more appropriate for the patient involved. Diagnosis **V30.1** is incorrect because it is for an infant born outside of the hospital. This infant was born in the hospital as evidenced by the exact time of birth noted and the APGAR scores reported.

C. Incorrect because **99234** is reported for observation and discharge on the same date, which fits this scenario. However this would be incorrect because there is a code for Newborn Admitted and Discharged on the same date, which is more appropriate for the patient involved. Diagnosis **779.3** would not be reported because "disorganized suck" alone in a newborn is not indicative of a feeding disorder. It is noted that once the infant is able to latch, 10-20 cc are being taken per feeding. Diagnosis **V30.00** is correct.

D. **Correct because 99435 correctly reports the admission and discharge of a normal newborn on the same date. Diagnosis V30.00 is correct because it reports a single liveborn infant, born in a hospital without mention of cesarean section.**

Practice 16, Report B

Professional Services: 99433 (Evaluation and Management, Newborn Care); **767.19** (Birth, injury, scalp).

Rationale: The patient is a normal newborn, born in the hospital with a multiple day stay. CPT **99433** is reported for the subsequent hospital care of the newborn, per day. There are no elements or key components to be considered when assigning this code.

Diagnosis **767.19** is still reported because the condition is re-evaluated on examination ("exam is unchanged"). Note that diagnosis code **V30.00** is not reported for services other than the initial admission (see newborn guidelines, Section I.C.15).

PRACTICE 17, NON-FACE-TO-FACE PHYSICIAN SERVICES; SPECIAL E/M SERVICES; AND OTHER E/M SERVICES

Practice 17, Report A

Rationale:

A. Incorrect because diagnoses **846.8** and **E819.9** are for current injuries, rather than late effects. The CPT code is correct because special evaluation management services report basic life and/or disability evaluations or work-related medical disability evaluations. This evaluation is for disability resulting from an automobile accident. The treating physician is performing the evaluation. Diagnosis codes **723.1** (neck pain) and **724.2** (back pain) are correct because these represent the residual effects of the previous injury. **99455** is correct because the evaluation is being performed by the treating physician, as indicated by the statement "patient will continue with prescribed pain management regimen."

B. Incorrect because **99456** is for evaluation by other than treating physician, which was not the case in this scenario. Diagnosis coding is correct except code **338.21** is missing to report the chronic pain.

C. Incorrect because **99456** is for evaluation by other than treating physician, which was not the case in this scenario. The diagnoses **846.8** and **E819.9** are for current injuries, rather than late effects. Diagnosis codes **723.1** (neck pain) and **724.2** (back pain) are correct because they report the residual effects of previous injury. Code **338.21** is missing to report the chronic pain.

D. **Correct, because 99455 reports the evaluation done by the treating physician, as indicated by the statement "patient will continue with prescribed pain management regimen." Diagnosis codes 723.1 (neck pain) and 724.2 (back pain) are correct because they report the residual effects of previous injury. Code 338.21 is assigned to report the chronic pain (see Section I.C.6.a. of the guidelines). Diagnoses 905.7 and E929.0 are for the late effects of previously sustained injury.**

Practice 17, Report B

Professional Services: **99455** (Evaluation and Management, Insurance Examination); **354.0** (Syndrome, carpal tunnel); **338.21** (Pain, chronic)

Rationale: Special evaluation management services are for basic life and/or disability evaluations or work-related medical disability evaluations. This evaluation is for disability resulting from a work-related injury. The treating physician is performing the evaluation and correctly reporting the service with **99455**. The diagnoses are carpal tunnel syndrome (**354.0**) and chronic pain due to injury (**338.21**).

Examination 1 Answers

● EXAMINATION 1 ANSWERS, RATIONALES, AND AUDIT FORMS

Professional Services: 99304 (Evaluation and Management, Nursing Facility, Initial Care); **331.0** (Alzheimer's); **294.11** (Dementia); **332.0** (Parkinsonism); **250.00** (Diabetes, type II or unspecified type not stated as uncontrolled); **414.00** (Arteriosclerosis, coronary artery); **412** (History of, myocardial infarction); **788.30** (Urine, urinary, incontinence); **706.3** (Seborrhea); **702.0** (Keratosis, actinic); **443.9** (Disease, peripheral, vascular)

Rationale: The first line of the note states that this is a nursing facility admission. This would be reported as an initial service in the nursing facility and would be reported in the range of **99304-99306**.

The history contained 4 elements of HPI, location (brain), severity (worsened), duration (6 years), and associated signs and symptoms (assaultive) for a comprehensive HPI. A detailed ROS that consisted of cardiovascular, respiratory, gastrointestinal, genitourinary, musculoskeletal, neurologic, and allergic. All 3 elements of PFSH were stated for a level 4 or comprehensive PFSH. The history level for this documentation would be a level 3 or detailed history.

The examination consisted of only one constitutional element (general appearance), so this would qualify as 1 BA/OS. A total of 5 BAs were examined: head, neck, abdomen, and lower extremities. The 9 OSs that were examined are ophthalmologic, otolaryngologic, cardiovascular, respiratory, gastrointestinal, genitourinary, neurologic, psychiatric, and lymphatic for a total of 15 BA/OS, which is a level 4 or comprehensive examination.

The MDM consisted of an extensive number of diagnosis/management options, moderate data to review, and high risk of death for moderate decision making

A detailed history, comprehensive examination and moderate MDM qualifies as a **99304**. If the ROS had contained 3 more elements, this documentation would have qualified for a higher level.

The patient has the primary diagnosis of Alzheimer's (**331.0**). Code **294.11** would also be reported since the patient is having behavioral disturbances related to the Alzheimer's disease. The patient also has Parkinson's (**332.0**). The other listed diagnoses would be reported because they may have to be managed while the patient is in the nursing home. These include, diabetes, type II (**250.00**); arteriosclerotic heart disease (**414.00**); history of an MI (**412**), urinary incontinence (**788.30**); seborrhea (**706.3**); actinic keratosis (**702.0**); and peripheral vascular disease (PVD) (**443.9**).

Examination 1, Report 1

HISTORY ELEMENTS	Documented
HISTORY OF PRESENT ILLNESS (HPI)	
1. Location (site on body)	x
2. Quality (characteristic: throbbing, sharp)	
3. Severity (1/10 or how intense)	x
4. Duration (how long for problem or episode)	x
5. Timing (when it occurs)	
6. Context (under what circumstances does it occur)	
7. Modifying factors (what makes it better or worse)	
8. Associated signs and symptoms (what else is happening when it occurs)	x
TOTAL	4
LEVEL	4

REVIEW OF SYSTEMS (ROS)	Documented
1. Constitutional (e.g., weight loss, fever)	
2. Ophthalmologic (eyes)	
3. Otolaryngologic (ears, nose, mouth, throat)	
4. Cardiovascular	x
5. Respiratory	x
6. Gastrointestinal	x
7. Genitourinary	x
8. Musculoskeletal	x
9. Integumentary (skin and/or breasts)	
10. Neurologic	x
11. Psychiatric	
12. Endocrine	
13. Hematologic/Lymphatic	
14. Allergic/Immunologic	x
TOTAL	7
LEVEL	3

PAST, FAMILY, AND/OR SOCIAL HISTORY (PFSH)	Documented
1. Past illness, operations, injuries, treatments, and current medications	x
2. Family medical history for heredity and risk	x
3. Social activities, both past and present	x
TOTAL	3
LEVEL	4

History Level	1	2	3	4
	Problem Focused	Expanded Problem Focused	Detailed	Comprehensive
HPI	Brief 1-3	Brief 1-3	Extended 4+	Extended 4+
ROS	None	Problem Pertinent	Extended 2-9	Complete 10+
PFSH	None	None	Pertinent 1	Complete 2-3
			HISTORY LEVEL	3

EXAMINATION ELEMENTS	Documented
CONSTITUTIONAL	
1. Blood pressure, sitting	
2. Blood pressure, lying	
3. Pulse	
4. Respirations	
5. Temperature	
6. Height	
7. Weight	
8. General appearance	x
NUMBER	1

BODY AREAS (BA)	Documented
1. Head (including face)	x
2. Neck	x
3. Chest (including breasts and axillae)	
4. Abdomen	x
5. Genitalia, groin, buttocks	
6. Back (including spine)	
7. Each extremity	xx
NUMBER	5

ORGAN SYSTEMS (OS)	Documented
1. Ophthalmologic (eyes)	x
2. Otolaryngologic (ears, nose, mouth, throat)	x
3. Cardiovascular	x
4. Respiratory	x
5. Gastrointestinal	x
6. Genitourinary	x
7. Musculoskeletal	
8. Integumentary	
9. Neurologic	x
10. Psychiatric	x
11. Hematologic/Lymphatic/Immunologic	x
NUMBER	9
TOTAL BA/OS	15

Exam Level	1	2	3	4
	Problem Focused	Expanded Problem Focused	Detailed	Comprehensive
	Limited to affected BA/OS	Limited to affected BA/OS & other related OSs	Extended of affected BA & other related OSs	General multi-system or complete single OS
# of OS or BA	1	2-7 limited	2-7 extended	8+
			EXAMINATION LEVEL	4

MDM ELEMENTS	Documented
# OF DIAGNOSIS/MANAGEMENT OPTIONS	
1. Minimal	
2. Limited	
3. Multiple	
4. Extensive	x
LEVEL	4
AMOUNT OR COMPLEXITY OF DATA TO REVIEW	Documented
1. Minimal/None	
2. Limited	
3. Moderate	x
4. Extensive	
LEVEL	3
RISK OF COMPLICATION OR DEATH IF NOT TREATED	Documented
1. Minimal	
2. Low	
3. Moderate	
4. High	x
LEVEL	4

MDM*	1	2	3	4
	Straightforward	Low	Moderate	High
Number of DX or management options	Minimal	Limited	Multiple	Extensive
Amount or complexity of data	Minimal/None	Limited	Moderate	Extensive
Risks	Minimal	Low	Moderate	High
			MDM LEVEL	4

*To qualify for a given type of MDM complexity, 2 of 3 elements in the table must be met or exceeded.

History: Detailed
Examination: Comprehensive
MDM: High

Number of Key Components: 3 of 3

99304

Examination 1, Report 2

Professional Services: **99218** (Evaluation and Management, Hospital Service, Observation Care); **794.39** (Findings, abnormal, without diagnosis, stress test); **414.00** (Arteriosclerosis, coronary artery); **V45.81** (Status (post), coronary artery bypass or shunt)

Rationale: The patient has been admitted to observation to have an angiogram. There are 4 elements of HPI, location (heart), duration (August), context (exercise), associated signs and symptoms (fatigue) for a level 4, or comprehensive, HPI. The ROS consisted of only 2 systems, cardiovascular and respiratory, for a level 3, or detailed, ROS. The documentation included 1 of 3 PFSH for a level 3, or detailed, PFSH. The level of history would be detailed based on a comprehensive HPI, detailed ROS, and detailed PFSH.

The examination consisted of 5 constitutional elements, blood pressure (lying down), pulse, respirations, temperature, and general appearance. This would qualify as 1 BA/OS. A total of 2 BAs were examined, including head and abdomen. A total of 5 OS were examined, including ophthalmologic, otolaryngologic, cardiovascular, respiratory, and lymphatic. This would be a total of 8 BA/OS. This qualifies as a level 4, or comprehensive, examination.

Extensive diagnosis/management options, moderate data were reviewed, and the patient has moderate risk of death or complication makes the level of MDM moderate.

The primary diagnosis is the abnormal stress test (**794.39**). The coronary arteriosclerosis is reported with **414.00**, with the fifth digit of zero to indicate unspecified type of vessel (native or graft). The status post bypass would also be reported (**V45.81**).

Examination 1, Report 2

HISTORY ELEMENTS			Documented
HISTORY OF PRESENT ILLNESS (HPI)			
1. Location (site on body)			✗
2. Quality (characteristic: throbbing, sharp)			
3. Severity (1/10 or how intense)			
4. Duration (how long for problem or episode)			✗
5. Timing (when it occurs)			
6. Context (under what circumstances does it occur)			✗
7. Modifying factors (what makes it better or worse)			
8. Associated signs and symptoms (what else is happening when it occurs)			✗
		TOTAL	4
		LEVEL	4

REVIEW OF SYSTEMS (ROS)			Documented
1. Constitutional (e.g., weight loss, fever)			
2. Ophthalmologic (eyes)			
3. Otolaryngologic (ears, nose, mouth, throat)			
4. Cardiovascular			✗
5. Respiratory			✗
6. Gastrointestinal			
7. Genitourinary			
8. Musculoskeletal			
9. Integumentary (skin and/or breasts)			
10. Neurologic			
11. Psychiatric			
12. Endocrine			
13. Hematologic/Lymphatic			
14. Allergic/Immunologic			
		TOTAL	2
		LEVEL	3

PAST, FAMILY, AND/OR SOCIAL HISTORY (PFSH)			Documented
1. Past illness, operations, injuries, treatments, and current medications			✗
2. Family medical history for heredity and risk			
3. Social activities, both past and present			
		TOTAL	1
		LEVEL	3

History Level	1	2	3	4
	Problem Focused	Expanded Problem Focused	Detailed	Comprehensive
HPI	Brief 1-3	Brief 1-3	Extended 4+	Extended 4+
ROS	None	Problem Pertinent	Extended 2-9	Complete 10+
PFSH	None	None	Pertinent 1	Complete 2-3
			HISTORY LEVEL	3

EXAMINATION ELEMENTS			Documented
CONSTITUTIONAL			
1. Blood pressure, sitting			
2. Blood pressure, lying			✗
3. Pulse			✗
4. Respirations			✗
5. Temperature			✗
6. Height			
7. Weight			
8. General appearance			✗
		NUMBER	1

BODY AREAS (BA)			Documented
1. Head (including face)			✗
2. Neck			
3. Chest (including breasts and axillae)			
4. Abdomen			✗
5. Genitalia, groin, buttocks			
6. Back (including spine)			
7. Each extremity			
		NUMBER	2

ORGAN SYSTEMS (OS)			Documented
1. Ophthalmologic (eyes)			✗
2. Otolaryngologic (ears, nose, mouth, throat)			✗
3. Cardiovascular			✗
4. Respiratory			✗
5. Gastrointestinal			
6. Genitourinary			
7. Musculoskeletal			
8. Integumentary			
9. Neurologic			
10. Psychiatric			
11. Hematologic/Lymphatic/Immunologic			✗
		NUMBER	5
		TOTAL BA/OS	8

Exam Level	1	2	3	4
	Problem Focused	Expanded Problem Focused	Detailed	Comprehensive
	Limited to affected BA/OS	Limited to affected BA/OS & other related OSs	Extended of affected BA & other related OSs	General multi-system or complete single OS
# of OS or BA	1	2-7 limited	2-7 extended	8+
			EXAMINATION LEVEL	4

MDM ELEMENTS		Documented
# OF DIAGNOSIS/MANAGEMENT OPTIONS		
1. Minimal		
2. Limited		
3. Multiple		
4. Extensive		✗
	LEVEL	4
AMOUNT OR COMPLEXITY OF DATA TO REVIEW		Documented
1. Minimal/None		
2. Limited		
3. Moderate		✗
4. Extensive		
	LEVEL	3
RISK OF COMPLICATION OR DEATH IF NOT TREATED		Documented
1. Minimal		
2. Low		
3. Moderate		✗
4. High		
	LEVEL	3

MDM*	1	2	3	4
	Straightforward	Low	Moderate	High
Number of DX or management options	Minimal	Limited	Multiple	Extensive
Amount or complexity of data	Minimal/None	Limited	Moderate	Extensive
Risks	Minimal	Low	Moderate	High
			MDM LEVEL	3

*To qualify for a given type of MDM complexity, 2 of 3 elements in the table must be met or exceeded.

History: Detailed
Examination: Comprehensive
MDM: Moderate

Number of Key Components: 3 of 3

99218

Examination 1, Report 3

Professional Services: 99243 (Evaluation and Management, Consultation); 836.1 (Tear, meniscus, lateral); 836.0 (Tear, meniscus, medial); 715.36 (Osteoarthrosis, lower leg); 401.9 (Hypertension); 736.42 (Genu varus deformity); 414.00 (Arteriosclerosis, coronary artery); 272.0 (Hypercholesterolemia)

Rationale: The physician has been asked to evaluate the patient and render his or her opinion regarding the knee pain. There are 4 elements of HPI, location (knee), duration (a few months), context (when he came out of the truck), and associated signs and symptoms (buckling) for a level 4 or comprehensive HPI. Four systems were reviewed, cardiovascular, GI, GU, and neurologic and the physician documented the remainder of the ROS negative for a level 4, complete ROS. The documentation included 1 of 3 PFSH for a level 3 or detailed PFSH. All 3 elements of history must qualify for level selection. The HPI and ROS are comprehensive and the PFSH qualifies as detailed so this is a detailed history.

The examination consisted of 7 constitutional elements for 1 BA/OS. The only BAs examined were the 2 lower extremities. Only 2 of the 4 extremities would count because there is no mention of the upper extremities. A total of 2 OSs, musculoskeletal and neurologic, were examined. This is a total of 5 BA/OS. This qualifies as a level 3 or detailed examination.

Extensive diagnosis/management options, limited data were reviewed, and the patient has moderate risk of death or complication makes this a level 3 or moderate MDM.

Modifier -57 would not be added to the code 99243 because the documentation indicates the patient first needs medical clearance and to discontinue taking his Coumadin 1 to 2 days prior to the procedure. Modifier -57 is only assigned when the E/M was performed the day of or the day before the procedure.

During the course of the consultation the patient was diagnosed with lateral (836.1) and medial (836.0) meniscus tear. The documentation indicates the patient has degenerative joint disease and when referencing the index of the ICD-9-CM under the main term "Degeneration, joint disease," the coder is directed to "see Osteoarthrosis." Osteoarthrosis of the knee, which is considered part of the lower leg, is reported with 715.36 (per Coding Clinic, Vol 20, No 4, 4th Quarter, 2003). 401.9 reports the essential hypertension. Also noted on review of the x-rays was genu varus deformity (bow legged) of the right knee, 736.42. The coronary artery disease (414.00) and hypercholesterolemia (272.0) would also be reported.

Examination 1, Report 3

HISTORY ELEMENTS			Documented
HISTORY OF PRESENT ILLNESS (HPI)			
1. Location (site on body)			X
2. Quality (characteristic: throbbing, sharp)			
3. Severity (1/10 or how intense)			
4. Duration (how long for problem or episode)			X
5. Timing (when it occurs)			
6. Context (under what circumstances does it occur)			X
7. Modifying factors (what makes it better or worse)			
8. Associated signs and symptoms (what else is happening when it occurs)			X
		TOTAL	4
		LEVEL	4

REVIEW OF SYSTEMS (ROS)			Documented
1. Constitutional (e.g., weight loss, fever)			X
2. Ophthalmologic (eyes)			X
3. Otolaryngologic (ears, nose, mouth, throat)			X
4. Cardiovascular			X
5. Respiratory			X
6. Gastrointestinal			X
7. Genitourinary			X
8. Musculoskeletal			X
9. Integumentary (skin and/or breasts)			X
10. Neurologic			X
11. Psychiatric			X
12. Endocrine			X
13. Hematologic/Lymphatic			X
14. Allergic/Immunologic			X
		TOTAL	14
		LEVEL	4

PAST, FAMILY, AND/OR SOCIAL HISTORY (PFSH)			Documented
1. Past illness, operations, injuries, treatments, and current medications			X
2. Family medical history for heredity and risk			
3. Social activities, both past and present			
		TOTAL	1
		LEVEL	3

History Level	1	2	3	
	Problem Focused	Expanded Problem Focused	Detailed	Comprehensive
HPI	Brief 1-3	Brief 1-3	Extended 4+	Extended 4+
ROS	None	Problem Pertinent	Extended 2-9	Complete 10+
PFSH	None	None	Pertinent 1	Complete 2-3
			HISTORY LEVEL	3

EXAMINATION ELEMENTS	Documented
CONSTITUTIONAL	
1. Blood pressure, sitting	
2. Blood pressure, lying	X
3. Pulse	X
4. Respirations	X
5. Temperature	X
6. Height	X
7. Weight	X
8. General appearance	X
NUMBER	1

BODY AREAS (BA)	Documented
1. Head (including face)	
2. Neck	
3. Chest (including breasts and axillae)	
4. Abdomen	
5. Genitalia, groin, buttocks	
6. Back (including spine)	
7. Each extremity	XX
NUMBER	2

ORGAN SYSTEMS (OS)	Documented
1. Ophthalmologic (eyes)	
2. Otolaryngologic (ears, nose, mouth, throat)	
3. Cardiovascular	
4. Respiratory	
5. Gastrointestinal	
6. Genitourinary	
7. Musculoskeletal	X
8. Integumentary	
9. Neurologic	X
10. Psychiatric	
11. Hematologic/Lymphatic/Immunologic	
NUMBER	2
TOTAL BA/OS	5

Exam Level	1	2	3	
	Problem Focused	Expanded Problem Focused	Detailed	Comprehensive
	Limited to affected BA/OS	Limited to affected BA/OS & other related OSs	Extended of affected BA & other related OSs	General multi-system or complete single OS
# of OS or BA	1	2-7 limited	2-7 extended	8+
			EXAMINATION LEVEL	3

MDM ELEMENTS				Documented
# OF DIAGNOSIS/MANAGEMENT OPTIONS				
1. Minimal				
2. Limited				
3. Multiple				
4. Extensive				X
			LEVEL	4
AMOUNT OR COMPLEXITY OF DATA TO REVIEW				Documented
1. Minimal/None				
2. Limited				X
3. Moderate				
4. Extensive				
			LEVEL	2
RISK OF COMPLICATION OR DEATH IF NOT TREATED				Documented
1. Minimal				
2. Low				
3. Moderate				X
4. High				
			LEVEL	3

MDM*	1	2	3	4
	Straightforward	Low	Moderate	High
Number of DX or management options	Minimal	Limited	Multiple	Extensive
Amount or complexity of data	Minimal/None	Limited	Moderate	Extensive
Risks	Minimal	Low	Moderate	High
			MDM LEVEL	3

*To qualify for a given type of MDM complexity, 2 of 3 elements in the table must be met or exceeded.

History: Detailed
Examination: Detailed
MDM: Moderate

Number of Key Components: 3 of 3

99243

Examination 1, Report 4

Professional Services: **99282** (Evaluation and Management, Emergency Department); **462** (Pharyngitis)

Rationale: The patient presents to the emergency room complaining of a sore throat. The highest level of service was level 2, point 1, administration of over-the-counter medication (Motrin), assigned **99282**.

The patient was diagnosed with pharyngitis (**462**). The patient also has bipolar disorder, but that would not have to be reported here because it is not being treated and does not affect the outcome of the patient's diagnosis.

Examination 1, Report 5

Professional Services: **99291** (Evaluation and Management, Critical Care); **99292** (Evaluation and Management, Critical Care); **780.97** (Change (of), mental status/NEC); **584.9** (Failure, renal, acute); **486** (Pneumonia); **410.91** (Infarction, myocardial, initial episode); **799.0** (Hypoxemia); **790.99** (Findings, abnormal, without diagnosis, serum, blood)

Rationale: This is a critical care service, which is based on the time spent with the patient, not the usual key components. At the end of the documentation it states that the physician spent 90 minutes of critical care time on the patient. When billing for critical care, the table in the E/M section of your CPT is helpful. The table states that for 75-104 minutes you would use codes **99291** and **99292**.

The patient presents with acute mental status changes, **780.97**. On further testing he was found to be in acute renal failure, **584.9**; acute MI, **410.91**; pneumonia, **486**; and hypoxemia, **799.0**. The patient was also found to have elevated BNP, **790.99**. BNP stands for Brain Natriuretic Peptide. This is a lab that is performed on the plasma of the blood that aids in diagnosing symptoms of CHF.

Examination 1, Report 6

Professional Services: **99349** (Evaluation and Management, Home Services); **496** (Disease, pulmonary, obstructive diffuse (chronic)); **332.0** (Parkinsonism); **715.36** (Osteoarthrosis, lower leg)

Rationale: This is a home service, which is based on whether the patient is new or established and the key components.

The HPI consisted of 3 elements, location (lung), modifying factors (nebulizer), and associated signs and symptoms (coughing spells). This qualifies as a level 2, or EPF, HPI. The ROS consisted of constitutional (good appetite), cardiovascular (edema), and psychiatric (anxiety) for a level 3, or detailed, ROS. The PFSH contained the past and social history of the patient for a level 4, or comprehensive, history. This documentation contains an EPF HPI, a detailed ROS, and a comprehensive PFSH for a level 2, or EPF, history.

The examination contains 4 constitutional elements (blood pressure (lying), pulse, respirations, and general appearance) that qualify as 1 BA/OS. The BAs examined are abdomen and all 4 extremities, for a total of 5 BAs. Only 2 OSs were examined, cardiovascular and respiratory. The total of BA/OS is 8 for a level 4 or comprehensive examination.

The MDM contains multiple diagnosis and management options, minimal/no data to review, and moderate risk. This qualifies as a level 3, or moderate, MDM.

The primary diagnosis for this home service is maintenance of the patient's COPD (**496**). The patient also has Parkinson's disease (**332.0**) and has severe osteoarthritis of his knees (**715.36**).

Examination 1, Report 6

HISTORY ELEMENTS				Documented
HISTORY OF PRESENT ILLNESS (HPI)				
1. Location (site on body)				X
2. Quality (characteristic: throbbing, sharp)				
3. Severity (1/10 or how intense)				
4. Duration (how long for problem or episode)				
5. Timing (when it occurs)				
6. Context (under what circumstances does it occur)				
7. Modifying factors (what makes it better or worse)				X
8. Associated signs and symptoms (what else is happening when it occurs)				X
			TOTAL	3
			LEVEL	2

REVIEW OF SYSTEMS (ROS)				Documented
1. Constitutional (e.g., weight loss, fever)				X
2. Ophthalmologic (eyes)				
3. Otolaryngologic (ears, nose, mouth, throat)				
4. Cardiovascular				X
5. Respiratory				
6. Gastrointestinal				
7. Genitourinary				
8. Musculoskeletal				
9. Integumentary (skin and/or breasts)				
10. Neurologic				
11. Psychiatric				X
12. Endocrine				
13. Hematologic/Lymphatic				
14. Allergic/Immunologic				
			TOTAL	3
			LEVEL	3

PAST, FAMILY, AND/OR SOCIAL HISTORY (PFSH)				Documented
1. Past illness, operations, injuries, treatments, and current medications				X
2. Family medical history for heredity and risk				
3. Social activities, both past and present				X
			TOTAL	2
			LEVEL	4

History Level	1	2	3	4
	Problem Focused	Expanded Problem Focused	Detailed	Comprehensive
HPI	Brief 1-3	Brief 1-3	Extended 4+	Extended 4+
ROS	None	Problem Pertinent	Extended 2-9	Complete 10+
PFSH	None	None	Pertinent 1	Complete 2-3
			HISTORY LEVEL	2

EXAMINATION ELEMENTS			Documented
CONSTITUTIONAL			
1. Blood pressure, sitting			
2. Blood pressure, lying			X
3. Pulse			X
4. Respirations			X
5. Temperature			
6. Height			
7. Weight			
8. General appearance			X
		NUMBER	1

BODY AREAS (BA)			Documented
1. Head (including face)			
2. Neck			
3. Chest (including breasts and axillae)			
4. Abdomen			X
5. Genitalia, groin, buttocks			
6. Back (including spine)			
7. Each extremity			XXX
		NUMBER	5

ORGAN SYSTEMS (OS)			Documented
1. Ophthalmologic (eyes)			
2. Otolaryngologic (ears, nose, mouth, throat)			
3. Cardiovascular			X
4. Respiratory			X
5. Gastrointestinal			
6. Genitourinary			
7. Musculoskeletal			
8. Integumentary			
9. Neurologic			
10. Psychiatric			
11. Hematologic/Lymphatic/Immunologic			
		NUMBER	2
		TOTAL BA/OS	8

Exam Level	1	2	3	4
	Problem Focused	Expanded Problem Focused	Detailed	Comprehensive
	Limited to affected BA/OS	Limited to affected BA/OS & other related OSs	Extended of affected BA & other related OSs	General multi-system or complete single OS
# of OS or BA	1	2-7 limited	2-7 extended	8+
			EXAMINATION LEVEL	4

MDM ELEMENTS				Documented
# OF DIAGNOSIS/MANAGEMENT OPTIONS				
1. Minimal				
2. Limited				
3. Multiple				X
4. Extensive				
			LEVEL	3
AMOUNT OR COMPLEXITY OF DATA TO REVIEW				Documented
1. Minimal/None				X
2. Limited				
3. Moderate				
4. Extensive				
			LEVEL	1
RISK OF COMPLICATION OR DEATH IF NOT TREATED				Documented
1. Minimal				
2. Low				
3. Moderate				X
4. High				
			LEVEL	3

MDM*	1	2	3	4
	Straightforward	Low	Moderate	High
Number of DX or management options	Minimal	Limited	Multiple	Extensive
Amount or complexity of data	Minimal/None	Limited	Moderate	Extensive
Risks	Minimal	Low	Moderate	High
			MDM LEVEL	3

*To qualify for a given type of MDM complexity, 2 of 3 elements in the table must be met or exceeded.

History: Expanded Problem Focused
Examination: Comprehensive
MDM: Moderate

Number of Key Components: 2 of 3

99349

Examination 1, Report 7

Professional Services: **99233** (Evaluation and Management, Hospital); **99356** (Evaluation and Management, Prolonged Services); **99357** (Evaluation and Management, Prolonged Services); **423.9** (Effusion, pericardial); **584.9** (Failure, failed, renal, acute); **276.1** (Hyponatremia); **275.41** (Hypocalcemia); **288.60** (Leukocytosis); **599.0** (Infection, urinary tract); **288.0** (Anemia, due to blood loss); **790.6** (Findings, liver function test)

Rationale: This is a document that represents prolonged service of care. The time allotted for that E/M level would be subtracted from the total time of the service and the remaining time would be reported with a prolonged service code. Prolonged service codes are add-on codes and are only reported in addition to another code.

This patient is acutely ill with renal failure and now has developed a pericardial effusion, which is an accumulation of blood in the sac that surrounds the heart. There is only 1 element of HPI, location (heart), for a level 2, or EPF, HPI. Two systems were reviewed, constitutional and cardiovascular, for a level 3, or detailed, ROS. No elements of PFSH were performed for a level 2, or EPF, PFSH. Two elements of the history are EPF and one element is detailed, so this will be an EPF history.

The examination consisted of the constitutional elements of general appearance and blood pressure (lying down), for 1 BA/OS. The abdomen is the only BA examined and 2 OSs were examined, cardiovascular and respiratory, for a total of 4 BA/OS. The exam qualifies as a level 3, or detailed, examination.

There are extensive diagnosis/management options, moderate data were reviewed, and the patient has a high risk of death makes this level of MDM high. The level of service would be **99233**. This code is allotted 35 minutes. At the end of this documentation it states that 1 hour and 55 minutes was spent with the patient. The total in minutes is 115 minutes. Subtract the 35 minutes included in the initial code **99233**, leaving 80 minutes of time to report as prolonged services. The prolonged services are categorized by either face-to-face direct contact or without face-to-face direct contact. The direct face-to face codes are further categorized by whether the service took place in an outpatient or inpatient setting. The prolonged service codes that would accompany **99233** are **99356** for the first 74 minutes of prolonged time and **99357** for the additional 6 minutes. The prolonged service table in your CPT is a good tool to aid in code selection for time.

The patient has the new acute problem of pericardial effusion (**423.9**). The other diagnoses to use would be the acute renal failure (**584.9**), hyponatremia (**276.1**), hypocalcemia (**275.41**), leukocytosis (**288.60**), UTI (**599.0**), anemia due to blood loss (**280.0**) and the abnormal liver function test (**790.6**). All of these diagnoses are being treated and each may affect the others.

ment options | Minimal | Limited | Multiple | Extensive |
Amount or complexity of data	Minimal/None	Limited	Moderate	Extensive
Risks	Minimal	Low	Moderate	High
			MDM LEVEL	4

*To qualify for a given type of MDM complexity, 2 of 3 elements in the table must be met or exceeded.

History: Expanded Problem Focused
Examination: Detailed
MDM: High

Number of Key Components: 2 of 3

99232, 99356, 99357

Examination 1, Report 8

Professional Services: 99360 (Evaluation and Management, Physician Standby Services); 724.02 (Stenosis, spinal, lumbar, lumbosacral)

Rationale: This is a document that represents physician standby services for which there is only one code—99360. The code is reported in units depending on the time the physician provided standby service. The standby must have been requested by another physician, no face-to-face contact was made with the patient, and the physician standing by was not providing care to any other patient during the standby time. If the standby time is less than 30 minutes, the service is not reported. Unlike some of the other E/M codes, the unit of time for standby services must be a full 30 minutes. It is very important to read and understand the guidelines in the CPT that apply to standby service.

The time in the documentation was from 8:45 AM to 9:25 AM, or 40 minutes of standby time requested by the neurosurgeon. Code 99360 would be used for 30 minutes of the 40 minutes. The extra 10 minutes cannot be reported because it is not a full 30 minutes.

The diagnosis would be the reason the physician was asked to stand by. In this case it was the reason the patient is having surgery, lumbar stenosis, 724.02.

Examination 1, Report 9

Professional Services: 99367 (Evaluation and Management, Case Management); 786.2 (Cough); 793.1 (Findings, abnormal, without diagnosis, radiologic (x-ray); lung)

Rationale: Case management is when the physician is responsible for the direct care of the patient and for coordinating the care and needs of the patient with other health care services to meet the needs of the patient. These services may be provided by means of a medical team conference. The code description for 99367 states without the patient present in a conference that lasted 30 minutes or more.

The diagnoses are cough, 786.2, and abnormal chest x-ray, 793.1.

Examination 1, Report 10

Professional Services: **99395** (Evaluation and Management, Preventive Services); **V70.0** (Checkup, health); **V72.31** (Gynecologic, exam), **623.8** (Bleeding, vaginal)

Rationale: Preventive medicine services are for timely evaluations, yearly physicals. Codes are selected by patient age, unlike other E/M codes that are selected by time or key components. Codes are further categorized by whether the patient is new or established.

This documentation is of an established patient who is 39 years old. The correct code for the preventive medicine service would be **99395**.

The assessment contains 3 diagnoses: gynecologic examination with pap, vaginal tenderness and slight vaginal bleeding, and health maintenance issues. When reporting the diagnosis on preventive examinations the first code would be **V70.0** for the health checkup followed by **V72.31** for the gynecological exam. Only code the other diagnoses if there is an indication in the plan that they will be treated or followed up on. The Premarin cream was prescribed to decrease vaginal bleeding, so the bleeding is reported with **623.8**. It is important to familiarize yourself with the guidelines that precede the preventive medicine codes in the CPT because they explain the requirements for reporting a preventive medicine code and an E/M service on the same day.

Examination 1, Report 11

Professional Services: **99450** (Evaluation and Management, Work-Related and/or Medical Disability Evaluation); **V70.3** (Examination, insurance certification), **V77.99** (Basic Metabolic Panel), **V81.6** (Urinalysis)

Rationale: Special evaluation management services are for basic life and/or disability evaluations or work-related medical disability evaluations. This evaluation is a life insurance examination. The correct code would be **99450**. The diagnosis would be a V code to indicate that this was an insurance evaluation, **V70.3**. The notes following the heading for V70 indicate to "Use additional code(s) to identify any special screening examinations performed (**V73.0-V82.9**)."

Examination 1, Report 12

Professional Services: **99300** (Evaluation and Management, Infant); **550.90** (Hernia, inguinal, unilateral or unspecified); **V45.89** (Status (post), postoperative NEC)

Rationale: Codes **99298**, **99299**, and **99300** are used to report physician services on days other than the day of admit for infants of VLBW (infants weighing less than 1500 grams), LBW (1500-2500 grams), or normal weight (2501-5000 grams) who are not critically ill but do still require intensive services. These infants are recovering. Code selection depends on the weight of the infant. The infant in this documentation is 4725 grams now working on increasing weight, reported with **99300**.

Patient has scrotal hernia, **550.90**, and is status post supraglottoplasty, **V45.89**.

Examination 1, Report 13

Professional Services: **99377** (Evaluation and Management, Care Plan Oversight Services); **585.4** (Disease, kidney, chronic, stage IV); **496** (Disease, lung, obstructive (chronic)); **331.0** (Disease, Alzheimer's); **V45.1** (Dialysis, status)

Rationale: Care plan oversight services reflect a supervisory role of the physician to the patient. The patient is not present when the physician is performing the service. Codes include development or revision of a care plan, review of reports of patient status, communication with other health care professionals, and review of any lab or tests that may have been performed. These codes may only be reported once for every 30-day period. Codes are divided by where the patient is residing—home health agency, hospice, or a nursing facility—and further divided based on time. Code **99377** would be the correct CPT code to use for this documentation because the patient is receiving hospice care and the time of service was less than 30 minutes.

The diagnoses would be stage IV chronic kidney disease (**585.4**), COPD (**496**), Alzheimer's (**331.0**), and **V45.1** to report the dialysis status.

Examination 1, Report 14

Professional Services: **99340** (Evaluation and Management, Care Plan Oversight Services); **716.96** (Arthritis, lower leg); **492.8** (Emphysema); **285.9** (Anemia)

Rationale: This is a care plan oversight service where the patient resides in a rest home. The time involved was 45 minutes to formulate the plan and an additional 38 minutes discussing this with family members. The total time was 83 minutes so the correct code would be **99340**. The telephone conversation is part of the care plan oversight and that is why that time is added to the other time.

The diagnoses would be arthritis of the knees, which is reported as lower leg, **716.96**. The emphysema, **492.8**, would also be reported, and the anemia, **285.9**, with a Hgb of 9.2 and a prescription of Aranesp.

Examination 1, Report 15

See audit form on following page.

Professional Services: **99202** (Evaluation and Management, Office and Other Outpatient); **719.45** (Pain, joint, hip); **786.2** (Cough); **787.1** (Heartburn); **305.1** (Addiction, nicotine); **296.90** (Psychosis, affective); **278.00** (Obesity); **V85.3** (BMI)

Rationale: The patient is a new patient establishing with a physician. The HPI included 6 elements of location (hip), duration (3 months), timing (constant), context (standing), modifying factor (obesity, pulse, weight), and associated signs and symptoms (tingling) for a level 4, comprehensive HPI. The ROS included constitutional, otolaryngologic, cardiovascular, respiratory, gastrointestinal, genitourinary, and musculoskeletal for a total of 3 or a level 3/ detailed ROS. All three elements of the PFSH were reviewed for a level 4 PFSH. A comprehensive HPI, detailed ROS, and comprehensive PFSH is a level 3, or detailed, history.

The examination included blood pressure, pulse, weight, and general appearance for 1 BA/OS. The BAs examined were head, neck, and all 4 extremities for 6 BAs. The OSs examined were ophthalmologic, cardiovascular, respiratory, gastrointestinal, musculoskeletal, and lymphatic for 6 OSs. This is a total of 13 BA/OS for a level 4, or comprehensive, exam.

The MDM included multiple management options, minimal data were reviewed, and the patient has minimal risk of complication for a level 1, or straightforward, MDM.

Because this is a new patient, 3 of the 3 key components need to be met for level selection. This documentation qualifies for a **99202**.

The reason for the office service is to establish a new physician. The first condition listed in the assessment section of the report is the joint pain. When coding joint pain do not reference the index under "Pain, hip" but "Pain, joint, hip." The other diagnosis of cough (**786.2**), heartburn (**787.1**), and nicotine addiction (**305.1**) would also be reported. The patient also has major depressive disorder (**296.2**), but when referencing this code in the Tabular of the ICD-9-CM the manual states "single episode." This is not a single episode for this patient. When referenced under "Disorder, major depressive" the coder is directed to "see also Psychosis, affective (**296.90**)." The obesity (**278.00**) and Body Mass Index (BMI, Body Mass Index was 34) (**V85.34**) are also reported.

Examination 1, Report 15

HISTORY ELEMENTS	Documented
HISTORY OF PRESENT ILLNESS (HPI)	
1. Location (site on body)	X
2. Quality (characteristic: throbbing, sharp)	
3. Severity (1/10 or how intense)	
4. Duration (how long for problem or episode)	X
5. Timing (when it occurs)	X
6. Context (under what circumstances does it occur)	X
7. Modifying factors (what makes it better or worse)	X
8. Associated signs and symptoms (what else is happening when it occurs)	X
TOTAL	6
LEVEL	4
REVIEW OF SYSTEMS (ROS)	Documented
1. Constitutional (e.g., weight loss, fever)	X
2. Ophthalmologic (eyes)	
3. Otolaryngologic (ears, nose, mouth, throat)	X
4. Cardiovascular	X
5. Respiratory	X
6. Gastrointestinal	X
7. Genitourinary	X
8. Musculoskeletal	X
9. Integumentary (skin and/or breasts)	
10. Neurologic	
11. Psychiatric	
12. Endocrine	
13. Hematologic/Lymphatic	
14. Allergic/Immunologic	
TOTAL	7
LEVEL	3
PAST, FAMILY, AND/OR SOCIAL HISTORY (PFSH)	Documented
1. Past illness, operations, injuries, treatments, and current medications	X
2. Family medical history for heredity and risk	X
3. Social activities, both past and present	X
TOTAL	3
LEVEL	4

History Level	1	2	3	4
	Problem Focused	Expanded Problem Focused	Detailed	Comprehensive
HPI	Brief 1-3	Brief 1-3	Extended 4+	Extended 4+
ROS	None	Problem Pertinent	Extended 2-9	Complete 10+
PFSH	None	None	Pertinent 1	Complete 2-3
HISTORY LEVEL			3	

EXAMINATION ELEMENTS	Documented
CONSTITUTIONAL	
1. Blood pressure, sitting	X
2. Blood pressure, lying	
3. Pulse	X
4. Respirations	
5. Temperature	
6. Height	
7. Weight	X
8. General appearance	X
NUMBER	1
BODY AREAS (BA)	Documented
1. Head (including face)	X
2. Neck	X
3. Chest (including breasts and axillae)	
4. Abdomen	
5. Genitalia, groin, buttocks	
6. Back (including spine)	
7. Each extremity	XXXX
NUMBER	6
ORGAN SYSTEMS (OS)	Documented
1. Ophthalmologic (eyes)	X
2. Otolaryngologic (ears, nose, mouth, throat)	
3. Cardiovascular	X
4. Respiratory	X
5. Gastrointestinal	X
6. Genitourinary	
7. Musculoskeletal	X
8. Integumentary	
9. Neurologic	
10. Psychiatric	
11. Hematologic/Lymphatic/Immunologic	X
NUMBER	6
TOTAL BA/OS	13

Exam Level	1	2	3	4
	Problem Focused	Expanded Problem Focused	Detailed	Comprehensive
	Limited to affected BA/OS	Limited to affected BA/OS & other related OSs	Extended of affected BA & other related OSs	General multi-system or complete single OS
# of OS or BA	1	2-7 limited	2-7 extended	8+
EXAMINATION LEVEL				4

MDM ELEMENTS	Documented
# OF DIAGNOSIS/MANAGEMENT OPTIONS	
1. Minimal	
2. Limited	
3. Multiple	X
4. Extensive	
LEVEL	3
AMOUNT OR COMPLEXITY OF DATA TO REVIEW	Documented
1. Minimal/None	X
2. Limited	
3. Moderate	
4. Extensive	
LEVEL	1
RISK OF COMPLICATION OR DEATH IF NOT TREATED	Documented
1. Minimal	X
2. Low	
3. Moderate	
4. High	
LEVEL	1

MDM*	1	2	3	4
	Straightforward	Low	Moderate	High
Number of DX or management options	Minimal	Limited	Multiple	Extensive
Amount or complexity of data	Minimal/None	Limited	Moderate	Extensive
Risks	Minimal	Low	Moderate	High
MDM LEVEL	1			

*To qualify for a given type of MDM complexity, 2 of 3 elements in the table must be met or exceeded.

History: Detailed
Examination: Comprehensive
MDM: Straightforward

Number of Key Components: 3 of 3

99202

Examination 1, Report 16

See audit form on following page.

Professional Services: 99232 (Evaluation and Management, Hospital); **428.0** (Failure, congestive heart); **424.1** (Stenosis, aortic (valve)); **585.9** (Failure, renal, chronic); **276.6** (Overload fluid); **V45.1** (Dialysis, status)

Rationale: This is a subsequent hospital service progress note. The HPI consists of location (lung) and severity (improved) for a total of 2 HPI, or EPF. The ROS is stated as complete and negative. All systems were reviewed in the ROS for a level 4, or comprehensive, ROS. No elements of PFSH were performed for an EPF PFSH. The history levels for this progress note would be EPF.

The examination consisted of 3 elements of constitutional: temperature, weight, and general appearance for one BA/OS. The BAs examined were head, neck, abdomen, and all 4 extremities for 7 BAs. The OSs examined were ophthalmologic, otolaryngologic, cardiovascular, and neurologic for 4 OSs. This is a total of 12 BA/OS for a level 4, or comprehensive, examination.

The MDM consists of multiple diagnosis/management options, minimal data were reviewed (labs only), and a moderate risk of complication or death for a level 3 or moderate MDM.

The assessment consists of 4 diagnoses, congestive heart failure (**428.0**) and aortic stenosis (**424.1**). The stage of the CRF was not specified, so **585.9** is reported. The patient also had fluid overload reported with **276.6**. **V45.1** reports the dialysis status.

Examination 1, Report 16

HISTORY ELEMENTS	Documented
HISTORY OF PRESENT ILLNESS (HPI)	
1. Location (site on body)	✗
2. Quality (characteristic: throbbing, sharp)	
3. Severity (1/10 or how intense)	✗
4. Duration (how long for problem or episode)	
5. Timing (when it occurs)	
6. Context (under what circumstances does it occur)	
7. Modifying factors (what makes it better or worse)	
8. Associated signs and symptoms (what else is happening when it occurs)	
TOTAL	2
LEVEL	2
REVIEW OF SYSTEMS (ROS)	Documented
1. Constitutional (e.g., weight loss, fever)	✗
2. Ophthalmologic (eyes)	✗
3. Otolaryngologic (ears, nose, mouth, throat)	✗
4. Cardiovascular	✗
5. Respiratory	✗
6. Gastrointestinal	✗
7. Genitourinary	✗
8. Musculoskeletal	✗
9. Integumentary (skin and/or breasts)	✗
10. Neurologic	✗
11. Psychiatric	✗
12. Endocrine	✗
13. Hematologic/Lymphatic	✗
14. Allergic/Immunologic	✗
TOTAL	14
LEVEL	4
PAST, FAMILY, AND/OR SOCIAL HISTORY (PFSH)	Documented
1. Past illness, operations, injuries, treatments, and current medications	
2. Family medical history for heredity and risk	
3. Social activities, both past and present	
TOTAL	0
LEVEL	2

History Level	1	2	3	4
	Problem Focused	Expanded Problem Focused	Detailed	Comprehensive
HPI	Brief 1-3	Brief 1-3	Extended 4+	Extended 4+
ROS	None	Problem Pertinent	Extended 2-9	Complete 10+
PFSH	None	None	Pertinent 1	Complete 2-3
			HISTORY LEVEL	2

EXAMINATION ELEMENTS	Documented
CONSTITUTIONAL	
1. Blood pressure, sitting	
2. Blood pressure, lying	
3. Pulse	
4. Respirations	
5. Temperature	✗
6. Height	
7. Weight	✗
8. General appearance	✗
NUMBER	1
BODY AREAS (BA)	Documented
1. Head (including face)	✗
2. Neck	✗
3. Chest (including breasts and axillae)	
4. Abdomen	✗
5. Genitalia, groin, buttocks	
6. Back (including spine)	
7. Each extremity	✗✗✗✗
NUMBER	7
ORGAN SYSTEMS (OS)	Documented
1. Ophthalmologic (eyes)	✗
2. Otolaryngologic (ears, nose, mouth, throat)	✗
3. Cardiovascular	✗
4. Respiratory	
5. Gastrointestinal	
6. Genitourinary	
7. Musculoskeletal	
8. Integumentary	
9. Neurologic	✗
10. Psychiatric	
11. Hematologic/Lymphatic/Immunologic	
NUMBER	4
TOTAL BA/OS	12

Exam Level	1	2	3	4
	Problem Focused	Expanded Problem Focused	Detailed	Comprehensive
	Limited to affected BA/OS	Limited to affected BA/OS & other related OSs	Extended of affected BA & other related OSs	General multi-system or complete single OS
# of OS or BA	1	2-7 limited	2-7 extended	8+
			EXAMINATION LEVEL	4

MDM ELEMENTS	Documented
# OF DIAGNOSIS/MANAGEMENT OPTIONS	
1. Minimal	
2. Limited	
3. Multiple	✗
4. Extensive	
LEVEL	3
AMOUNT OR COMPLEXITY OF DATA TO REVIEW	Documented
1. Minimal/None	✗
2. Limited	
3. Moderate	
4. Extensive	
LEVEL	1
RISK OF COMPLICATION OR DEATH IF NOT TREATED	Documented
1. Minimal	
2. Low	
3. Moderate	✗
4. High	
LEVEL	3

MDM*	1	2	3	4
	Straightforward	Low	Moderate	High
Number of DX or management options	Minimal	Limited	Multiple	Extensive
Amount or complexity of data	Minimal/None	Limited	Moderate	Extensive
Risks	Minimal	Low	Moderate	High
			MDM LEVEL	3

*To qualify for a given type of MDM complexity, 2 of 3 elements in the table must be met or exceeded.

History: Expanded Problem Focused
Examination: Comprehensive
MDM: Moderate

Number of Key Components: 2 of 3

99232

Examination 1, Report 17

Professional Services: **99289** (Evaluation and Management, Pediatric Interfacility Transport); **99288** (Evaluation and Management, Emergency Department); **427.5** (Arrest, cardiac); **994.8** (Shock, electric); **941.20** (Burn, head, second degree); **941.23** (Burn, lips, second degree); **947.0** (Burn, mouth); **948.00** (Burn, less than 10%); **E925.9** (Electric shock, electrocution)

Rationale: Codes **99289** and **99290** are used to report the physical attendance and face-to-face care of a physician during the transport of a critically ill or injured pediatric patient. The first code, **99289**, is for the first 30-74 minutes. This documentation states that the physician spent 70 minutes in direct face-to-face care trying to stabilize the patient. Code **99290** would not be used in this case because the time is less than 74 minutes. No audit form is needed when assigning codes from this subcategory. Codes are based on time only. The physician also performed direction of advanced life support by instructing the air flight personnel on pulmonary/cardiac resuscitation during flight. Code **99288** would be the correct code to use for this.

This is a 10-month-old male who went into cardiac arrest due to electrocution after chewing through an electrical cord. The primary and most serious diagnosis would be the cardiac arrest (**427.5**). The nonfatal effects of electrocution are reported with **994.8**. There are multiple sites of burns that were second degree, lower face (**941.20**), lips (**941.23**) and mouth (**947.0**). **948.00** reports the body surface of less than 10%. The external cause of this injury is the electrical shock, reported with **E925.9**, electrocution.

Examination 1, Report 18

Professional Services: 99326 (Evaluation and Management, Domiciliary or Rest Home, New Patient); **786.2** (Cough); **786.07** (Wheezing); **462** (Pharyngitis)

Rationale: This service is a new patient service at the domiciliary home where the patient resides. The HPI consisted of the location (lung), quality (wheezing), duration (yesterday), and associated signs and symptoms (denies SOB) for 4 HPI or comprehensive HPI.

The ROS included 4 systems, constitutional, otolaryngologic, psychiatric, and lymphatic for a level 3 or detailed ROS.

Past history of pneumonia and social history (resides in domiciliary care facility) were documented for a level 4, or complete, PFSH. This documentation contained comprehensive HPI, detailed ROS, and comprehensive PFSH for level 3 or detailed history.

The examination consisted of 4 constitutional items, blood pressure (lying), pulse, respirations, and temperature for 1 BA/OS. A total of 5 BAs were examined, including the abdomen and all 4 extremities, and 1 OS, respiratory was performed for a total of 7 BA/OS and a level 3, or detailed, examination.

The MDM entailed extensive diagnosis/management options, limited data were reviewed, and there is moderate risk for a level 3, or moderate, MDM.

Because this is a new patient service all three key components must be used in level selection. This documentation contains an EPF history, detailed examination, and low MDM for a level **99326**.

This physician does not give us a definitive diagnosis and more testing is being ordered to try to determine the cause of the patient's symptoms. In this case the symptoms would be reported including the cough, **786.2**; wheezing, **786.07**; and sore throat, **462**.

Examination 1, Report 18

HISTORY ELEMENTS	Documented
HISTORY OF PRESENT ILLNESS (HPI)	
1. Location (site on body)	X
2. Quality (characteristic: throbbing, sharp)	X
3. Severity (1/10 or how intense)	
4. Duration (how long for problem or episode)	X
5. Timing (when it occurs)	
6. Context (under what circumstances does it occur)	
7. Modifying factors (what makes it better or worse)	
8. Associated signs and symptoms (what else is happening when it occurs)	X
TOTAL	4
LEVEL	4

REVIEW OF SYSTEMS (ROS)	Documented
1. Constitutional (e.g., weight loss, fever)	X
2. Ophthalmologic (eyes)	
3. Otolaryngologic (ears, nose, mouth, throat)	X
4. Cardiovascular	
5. Respiratory	
6. Gastrointestinal	
7. Genitourinary	
8. Musculoskeletal	
9. Integumentary (skin and/or breasts)	
10. Neurologic	
11. Psychiatric	X
12. Endocrine	
13. Hematologic/Lymphatic	X
14. Allergic/Immunologic	
TOTAL	4
LEVEL	3

PAST, FAMILY, AND/OR SOCIAL HISTORY (PFSH)	Documented
1. Past illness, operations, injuries, treatments, and current medications	X
2. Family medical history for heredity and risk	
3. Social activities, both past and present	X
TOTAL	2
LEVEL	4

History Level	1	2	3	
	Problem Focused	Expanded Problem Focused	Detailed	Comprehensive
HPI	Brief 1-3	Brief 1-3	Extended 4+	Extended 4+
ROS	None	Problem Pertinent	Extended 2-9	Complete 10+
PFSH	None	None	Pertinent 1	Complete 2-3
			HISTORY LEVEL	3

EXAMINATION ELEMENTS	Documented
CONSTITUTIONAL	
1. Blood pressure, sitting	
2. Blood pressure, lying	X
3. Pulse	X
4. Respirations	X
5. Temperature	X
6. Height	
7. Weight	
8. General appearance	
NUMBER	1

BODY AREAS (BA)	Documented
1. Head (including face)	
2. Neck	
3. Chest (including breasts and axillae)	
4. Abdomen	X
5. Genitalia, groin, buttocks	
6. Back (including spine)	
7. Each extremity	XXXX
NUMBER	5

ORGAN SYSTEMS (OS)	Documented
1. Ophthalmologic (eyes)	
2. Otolaryngologic (ears, nose, mouth, throat)	
3. Cardiovascular	
4. Respiratory	X
5. Gastrointestinal	
6. Genitourinary	
7. Musculoskeletal	
8. Integumentary	
9. Neurologic	
10. Psychiatric	
11. Hematologic/Lymphatic/Immunologic	
NUMBER	1
TOTAL BA/OS	7

Exam Level	1	2	3	
	Problem Focused	Expanded Problem Focused	Detailed	Comprehensive
	Limited to affected BA/OS	Limited to affected BA/OS & other related OSs	Extended of affected BA & other related OSs	General multi-system or complete single OS
# of OS or BA	1	2-7 limited	2-7 extended	8+
			EXAMINATION LEVEL	3

MDM ELEMENTS	Documented
# OF DIAGNOSIS/MANAGEMENT OPTIONS	
1. Minimal	
2. Limited	
3. Multiple	
4. Extensive	X
LEVEL	4
AMOUNT OR COMPLEXITY OF DATA TO REVIEW	Documented
1. Minimal/None	
2. Limited	X
3. Moderate	
4. Extensive	
LEVEL	2
RISK OF COMPLICATION OR DEATH IF NOT TREATED	Documented
1. Minimal	
2. Low	
3. Moderate	X
4. High	
LEVEL	3

MDM*	1	2	3	4
	Straightforward	Low	Moderate	High
Number of DX or management options	Minimal	Limited	Multiple	Extensive
Amount or complexity of data	Minimal/None	Limited	Moderate	Extensive
Risks	Minimal	Low	Moderate	High
			MDM LEVEL	3

*To qualify for a given type of MDM complexity, 2 of 3 elements in the table must be met or exceeded.

History: Detailed
Examination: Detailed
MDM: Moderate

Number of Key Components: 3 of 3

99326

Examination 2 Answers

● EXAMINATION 2 ANSWERS, RATIONALES, AND AUDIT FORMS

Examination 2, Report 1

Professional Services: **99386** (Evaluation and Management, Preventive Services); **V70.0** (Checkup, health), **V76.44** (Screening, PSA)

Rationale: Preventive Medicine services are for timely evaluations, yearly physicals. Codes are selected by patient age, unlike other E/M codes that go by time or key components. Codes are further categorized by whether the patient is new or established.

This documentation is of a new patient who is 55 years old. The correct code for the preventive med service would be **99386**.

The assessment contains diagnoses of health maintenance examination, recent bladder infection with tachycardia, and degenerative changes of hand. When reporting the diagnoses for a preventive examination the first code to report would be **V70.0** for the health checkup and **V76.44** to indicate a PSA screening. Only code the other diagnoses if there is an indication in the plan that they are going to be treated or followed up on. It is important to familiarize yourself with the guidelines that precede the preventive medicine category in the CPT. They explain the requirements for reporting both a preventive medicine code and an E/M service on the same day.

Examination 2, Report 2

Professional Services: **99219** (Evaluation and Management, Hospital Service, Observation Care); **969.0** (Table of Drugs and Chemicals, poisoning, antidepressant); **780.79** (Lethargy); **784.0** (Headache); **E980.3** (Table of Drugs and Chemicals, poisoning, antidepressants, undetermined)

Rationale: The patient has been admitted to observation following a drug overdose. Her mother brought the patient in through the ED. There are 4 elements of HPI, location (headache), quality (extreme), duration (today), and associated signs and symptoms (lethargy) for a level 4, or comprehensive, HPI. The ROS consisted of 10 systems, constitutional, ophthalmologic, otolaryngologic, cardiovascular, respiratory, gastrointestinal, genitourinary, musculoskeletal, neurologic, and psychiatric for a level 4, or comprehensive, ROS. The documentation included 3 of 3 PFSH for a level 4, or comprehensive, PFSH. All 3 elements of history were comprehensive so this would be a comprehensive HPI.

The examination consisted of 2 constitutional elements, blood pressure and general appearance, for 1 BA/OS. A total of 4 BAs were examined including, neck, abdomen, and 2 extremities (legs). A total of 8 OSs were examined, ophthalmologic, otolaryngologic, cardiovascular, respiratory, gastrointestinal, musculoskeletal, neurologic, and lymphatic, for a total of 13 BA/OS. This qualifies as a level 4, or comprehensive, examination.

There are extensive diagnosis/management options, minimal data were reviewed, and the patient has moderate risk of death or complication makes the level of MDM moderate.

When coding overdoses refer to the Guidelines, Section I.C.17.e.1, which states you should use the Table Of Drugs and Chemicals and code the poisoning first, the manifestations second, and the E code last. This patient had an overdose of Xanax, which is taken for depression. When referencing the Table of Drugs and Chemicals, there is no listing for Xanax so you would reference the term "antidepressant" and report **969.0** for the poisoning. It would be correct to also report **780.79** for the lethargy and **784.0** for the headache. The E code reports "undetermined" intent because it is not known if this was an intentional or accidental overdose (**E980.3**).

Examination 2, Report 2

HISTORY ELEMENTS	Documented
HISTORY OF PRESENT ILLNESS (HPI)	
1. Location (site on body)	✗
2. Quality (characteristic: throbbing, sharp)	✗
3. Severity (1/10 or how intense)	
4. Duration (how long for problem or episode)	✗
5. Timing (when it occurs)	
6. Context (under what circumstances does it occur)	
7. Modifying factors (what makes it better or worse)	
8. Associated signs and symptoms (what else is happening when it occurs)	✗
TOTAL	4
LEVEL	4
REVIEW OF SYSTEMS (ROS)	Documented
1. Constitutional (e.g., weight loss, fever)	✗
2. Ophthalmologic (eyes)	✗
3. Otolaryngologic (ears, nose, mouth, throat)	✗
4. Cardiovascular	✗
5. Respiratory	✗
6. Gastrointestinal	✗
7. Genitourinary	✗
8. Musculoskeletal	✗
9. Integumentary (skin and/or breasts)	
10. Neurologic	✗
11. Psychiatric	✗
12. Endocrine	
13. Hematologic/Lymphatic	
14. Allergic/Immunologic	
TOTAL	10
LEVEL	4
PAST, FAMILY, AND/OR SOCIAL HISTORY (PFSH)	Documented
1. Past illness, operations, injuries, treatments, and current medications	✗
2. Family medical history for heredity and risk	✗
3. Social activities, both past and present	✗
TOTAL	3
LEVEL	4

History Level	1	2	3	
	Problem Focused	Expanded Problem Focused	Detailed	Comprehensive
HPI	Brief 1-3	Brief 1-3	Extended 4+	Extended 4+
ROS	None	Problem Pertinent	Extended 2-9	Complete 10+
PFSH	None	None	Pertinent 1	Complete 2-3
			HISTORY LEVEL	4

EXAMINATION ELEMENTS	Documented
CONSTITUTIONAL	
1. Blood pressure, sitting	
2. Blood pressure, lying	✗
3. Pulse	
4. Respirations	
5. Temperature	
6. Height	
7. Weight	
8. General appearance	✗
NUMBER	1
BODY AREAS (BA)	Documented
1. Head (including face)	
2. Neck	✗
3. Chest (including breasts and axillae)	
4. Abdomen	✗
5. Genitalia, groin, buttocks	
6. Back (including spine)	
7. Each extremity	✗✗
NUMBER	4
ORGAN SYSTEMS (OS)	Documented
1. Ophthalmologic (eyes)	✗
2. Otolaryngologic (ears, nose, mouth, throat)	✗
3. Cardiovascular	✗
4. Respiratory	✗
5. Gastrointestinal	✗
6. Genitourinary	
7. Musculoskeletal	✗
8. Integumentary	
9. Neurologic	✗
10. Psychiatric	
11. Hematologic/Lymphatic/Immunologic	✗
NUMBER	8
TOTAL BA/OS	13

Exam Level	1	2	3	4
	Problem Focused	Expanded Problem Focused	Detailed	Comprehensive
	Limited to affected BA/OS	Limited to affected BA/OS & other related OSs	Extended of affected BA & other related OSs	General multi-system or complete single OS
# of OS or BA	1	2-7 limited	2-7 extended	8+
			EXAMINATION LEVEL	4

MDM ELEMENTS	Documented
# OF DIAGNOSIS/MANAGEMENT OPTIONS	
1. Minimal	
2. Limited	
3. Multiple	
4. Extensive	✗
LEVEL	4
AMOUNT OR COMPLEXITY OF DATA TO REVIEW	Documented
1. Minimal/None	✗
2. Limited	
3. Moderate	
4. Extensive	
LEVEL	1
RISK OF COMPLICATION OR DEATH IF NOT TREATED	Documented
1. Minimal	
2. Low	
3. Moderate	✗
4. High	
LEVEL	3

MDM*	1	2	3	4
	Straightforward	Low	Moderate	High
Number of DX or management options	Minimal	Limited	Multiple	Extensive
Amount or complexity of data	Minimal/None	Limited	Moderate	Extensive
Risks	Minimal	Low	Moderate	High
			MDM LEVEL	3

*To qualify for a given type of MDM complexity, 2 of 3 elements in the table must be met or exceeded.

History: Comprehensive
Examination: Comprehensive
MDM: Moderate

Number of Key Components: 3 of 3

99219

Examination 2, Report 3

Professional Services: **99289** (Evaluation and Management, Pediatric Interfacility Transport); **99290** (Evaluation and Management, Pediatric Interfacility Transport); **803.10** (Fracture, skull, with, contusion, cerebral); **E882** (Fall, from, off, balcony)

Rationale: Codes **99289** and **99290** are used to report the physical attendance and face-to-face care of a physician during the transport of a critically ill or injured pediatric patient. The first code **99289** is for the first 30-74 minutes. Code **99290** is an add-on code and is used in conjunction with **99289** to show each additional 30 minutes of time after the first 74 minutes. No audit form is needed when assigning codes from this subcategory. Codes are based on time only.

This is a 22-month-old male who fell from a second-floor balcony. The note states the total time spent with the patient was 75 minutes. The first 74 minutes would be reported with **99289**. The additional minute would be reported with **99290**. The Critical Care timetable is a good reference for code selection in this category.

The first stated diagnosis is hematoma of the brain. When referencing the ICD-9-CM index the entry states: "with skull fracture—*see* fracture, skull, by site." The fracture of the skull is reported with **803.10**. The fifth digit of zero would be selected because the patient's state of consciousness is not documented. This code includes the contusion, so **853.0** would to be reported in addition to the fracture code. The external cause code would be **E882**, fall from a balcony.

Examination 2, Report 4

Professional Services: **99291** (Evaluation and Management, Critical Care); **99292 × 2** (Evaluation and Management, Critical Care); **92960** (Cardioversion); **427.1** (Tachycardia, ventricular); **410.71** (Infarct, myocardial, subendocardial); **429.3** (Cardiomegaly); **514** (Edema, lung); **272.4** (Hyperlipidemia); **250.02** (Diabetes, type II or unspecified type, uncontrolled); **V12.59** (Accident, cerebrovascular, healed or old)

Rationale: This is a critical care service, which is based on the time spent with the patient, not the usual key components. The critical care time is constituted as time spent devoted to only this patient. The physician cannot be treating or evaluating any other patient during this time. The time does not have to be spent at bedside with the patient, as long as the time is spent regarding the patient. Also, the time does not have to be continuous. For example, the physician could spend 1 hour of critical care in the morning and then reevaluate the patient in the afternoon for another hour. This day of critical care would be for 2 hours, **99291** and **99292**.

In this case, at the end of the documentation it states that the physician spent 130 minutes of critical care time on the patient. When reporting for critical care the table in the E/M section of your CPT is helpful. The table indicates that for 105-134 minutes codes **99291** and **99292 × 2** are to be assigned.

The patient came in with chest pain and SOB, but on further examination and testing he is found to be in ventricular tachycardia, **427.1**, and his EKG shows a subendocardial MI. The EKG indicates cardiomegaly, **429.3** and pulmonary edema, **514**. The patient has diabetes, unspecified type, but his diabetes is stated to be uncontrolled, **250.02**. There is a history of CVA, **V12.59**. During this evaluation the patient required shocking to return his heart to normal sinus rhythm. In the guidelines that precede the critical care codes, a list of procedures bundled into the codes is listed and **92960**, external cardioversion, is not a bundled code so this would be reported separately from the critical care codes.

Examination 2, Report 5

Professional Services: **99298** (Evaluation and Management, Low Birthweight Infant); **765.15** (Premature, birth NEC); **765.26** (Weeks of gestation); **770.89** (Respiration, insufficiency, newborn NEC)

Rationale: Codes **99298**, **99299**, and **99300** are used to report physician services on days other than the day of admit for infants of VLBW (infants weighing less than 1500 grams), LBW (1500-2500 grams), or normal weight (2501-5000 grams) who are not by definition critically ill but do still require intensive services. These infants are recovering. Code selection depends on the weight of the infant. The infant in this documentation is 1470 grams and is being weaned off a respirator. The infant's respiratory status is improving, so this would be the correct area for code selection. The correct code to use would be **99298**.

The patient is a premature, underweight infant (**765.15**—fifth digit represents weight of infant), who was delivered at 32 weeks gestation (**765.26**), and in respiratory distress (**770.89**). When coding for the premature infant, the current weight of the infant is represented by the selection of the fifth digit. Coding guidelines for code range 765.xx also indicate to use an additional code for weeks of gestation (**765.20-765.29**).

Examination 2, Report 6

Professional Services: **99213** (Evaluation and Management, Office and Other Outpatient); **783.21** (Loss, weight (cause unknown)); **787.91** (Diarrhea); **865.01** (Hematoma, spleen); **577.2** (Pseudocyst, pancreas); **415.19** (Embolism, pulmonary); **401.9** (Hypertension, unspecified); **250.00** (Diabetes, Type II or unspecified type, not stated as uncontrolled)

Rationale: The patient is an established patient (noted in the heading). The HPI includes the location (pancreas, abdomen) and associated signs and symptoms (weight loss), for 2 from HPI, or EPF HPI. One system, gastrointestinal (diarrhea), was performed for 1 ROS, and only the patient's past medical history was discussed. The history for this documentation would be a level 2, or EPF, history.

The examination was minimal including 2 elements of constitutional, general appearance (looks good to me) and one vital sign (blood pressure) so this would count for 1 BA or OS. The abdomen was tender for 1 BA and no organ systems were examined. This is a total of 2 BA/OS for an EPF examination.

The MDM consisted of multiple diagnoses, moderate data were reviewed (viewed CT scan and read report), and the patient has a moderate risk of complication for a moderate level of MDM.

Because this is an established patient, only 2 of the 3 key components need to be met for level selection. This documentation qualifies for a **99213**.

The chief complaints are weight loss (**783.21**) and diarrhea (**787.91**). She is being treated for the splenic hematoma (**865.01**), pseudocyst of the pancreas (**577.2**), and pulmonary embolism (**415.19**). There are chronic conditions of hypertension (**401.9**) and type II diabetes (**250.00**).

Examination 2, Report 6

HISTORY ELEMENTS				Documented
HISTORY OF PRESENT ILLNESS (HPI)				
1. Location (site on body)				x
2. Quality (characteristic: throbbing, sharp)				
3. Severity (1/10 or how intense)				
4. Duration (how long for problem or episode)				
5. Timing (when it occurs)				
6. Context (under what circumstances does it occur)				
7. Modifying factors (what makes it better or worse)				
8. Associated signs and symptoms (what else is happening when it occurs)				x
			TOTAL	2
			LEVEL	2
REVIEW OF SYSTEMS (ROS)				Documented
1. Constitutional (e.g., weight loss, fever)				
2. Ophthalmologic (eyes)				
3. Otolaryngologic (ears, nose, mouth, throat)				
4. Cardiovascular				
5. Respiratory				
6. Gastrointestinal				x
7. Genitourinary				
8. Musculoskeletal				
9. Integumentary (skin and/or breasts)				
10. Neurologic				
11. Psychiatric				
12. Endocrine				
13. Hematologic/Lymphatic				
14. Allergic/Immunologic				
			TOTAL	1
			LEVEL	2
PAST, FAMILY, AND/OR SOCIAL HISTORY (PFSH)				Documented
1. Past illness, operations, injuries, treatments, and current medications				x
2. Family medical history for heredity and risk				
3. Social activities, both past and present				
			TOTAL	1
			LEVEL	3

History Level	1	2	3	4
	Problem Focused	Expanded Problem Focused	Detailed	Comprehensive
HPI	Brief 1-3	Brief 1-3	Extended 4+	Extended 4+
ROS	None	Problem Pertinent	Extended 2-9	Complete 10+
PFSH	None	None	Pertinent 1	Complete 2-3
			HISTORY LEVEL	2

EXAMINATION ELEMENTS				Documented
CONSTITUTIONAL				
1. Blood pressure, sitting				x
2. Blood pressure, lying				
3. Pulse				
4. Respirations				
5. Temperature				
6. Height				
7. Weight				
8. General appearance				x
			NUMBER	1
BODY AREAS (BA)				Documented
1. Head (including face)				
2. Neck				
3. Chest (including breasts and axillae)				
4. Abdomen				x
5. Genitalia, groin, buttocks				
6. Back (including spine)				
7. Each extremity				
			NUMBER	1
ORGAN SYSTEMS (OS)				Documented
1. Ophthalmologic (eyes)				
2. Otolaryngologic (ears, nose, mouth, throat)				
3. Cardiovascular				
4. Respiratory				
5. Gastrointestinal				
6. Genitourinary				
7. Musculoskeletal				
8. Integumentary				
9. Neurologic				
10. Psychiatric				
11. Hematologic/Lymphatic/Immunologic				
			NUMBER	0
			TOTAL BA/OS	2

Exam Level	1	2	3	4
	Problem Focused	Expanded Problem Focused	Detailed	Comprehensive
	Limited to affected BA/OS	Limited to affected BA/OS & other related OSs	Extended of affected BA & other related OSs	General multi-system or complete single OS
# of OS or BA	1	2-7 limited	2-7 extended	8+
			EXAMINATION LEVEL	2

MDM ELEMENTS				Documented
# OF DIAGNOSIS/MANAGEMENT OPTIONS				
1. Minimal				
2. Limited				
3. Multiple				x
4. Extensive				
			LEVEL	3
AMOUNT OR COMPLEXITY OF DATA TO REVIEW				Documented
1. Minimal/None				
2. Limited				
3. Moderate				x
4. Extensive				
			LEVEL	3
RISK OF COMPLICATION OR DEATH IF NOT TREATED				Documented
1. Minimal				
2. Low				
3. Moderate				x
4. High				
			LEVEL	3

MDM*	1	2	3	4
	Straightforward	Low	Moderate	High
Number of DX or management options	Minimal	Limited	Multiple	Extensive
Amount or complexity of data	Minimal/None	Limited	Moderate	Extensive
Risks	Minimal	Low	Moderate	High
			MDM LEVEL	3

*To qualify for a given type of MDM complexity, 2 of 3 elements in the table must be met or exceeded.

History: Expanded Problem Focused
Examination: Expanded Problem Focused
MDM: Moderate

Number of Key Components: 2 of 3

99213

Examination 2, Report 7

Professional Services: **99335** (Evaluation and Management, Domiciliary or Rest Home, Established Patient); **916.4** (Injury, superficial, leg); **250.00** (Diabetes, type II or unspecified type, not stated as uncontrolled); **V15.81** (Noncompliance with medical treatment); **E906.4** (Bite, spider, nonvenomous)

Rationale: This service is an established patient service at the rest home where the patient resides. The HPI consists of the location (upper thigh), duration (about a week), modifying factor (ointment not making it better), and associated signs and symptoms (diabetes) for a total of 4 elements for a comprehensive HPI. Two ROS are constitutional (dietary issues) and endocrine (blood sugars going up) for a level 3, or detailed, ROS. There are past medical history (diabetes) and social history (resides in rest home) for a level 4, or comprehensive, PFSH. Comprehensive HPI, detailed ROS, and comprehensive PFSH is a level 3, or detailed, history.

The examination consisted of no constitutional items, 1 body area, the left leg, and no organ systems for a total of 1 BA/OS and level 1, or PF, examination.

The MDM included multiple diagnosis/management options, because this is a new problem, no data were reviewed, and there is low risk for a level 2, or low, MDM.

A detailed history, PF examination, and low MDM would be **99335**.

The diagnosis would be the superficial injury to the leg, **916.4**. The diabetes would be reported with the fifth digit of 0 for unspecified or not stated as uncontrolled type because the documentation does not indicate the type. Even though the patient's blood sugars have been elevated, the coder cannot make the determination that the diabetes is uncontrolled. Unless documented by the provider that the diabetes is uncontrolled, it should not be reported as such. Code **V15.81** is reported to indicate the patient is being noncompliant with his diet, which relates to the control of his diabetes. The cause of the wound is reported with **E906.4**, nonvenomous spider bite.

Examination 2, Report 7

HISTORY ELEMENTS	Documented
HISTORY OF PRESENT ILLNESS (HPI)	
1. Location (site on body)	X
2. Quality (characteristic: throbbing, sharp)	
3. Severity (1/10 or how intense)	
4. Duration (how long for problem or episode)	X
5. Timing (when it occurs)	
6. Context (under what circumstances does it occur)	
7. Modifying factors (what makes it better or worse)	X
8. Associated signs and symptoms (what else is happening when it occurs)	X
TOTAL	4
LEVEL	4

REVIEW OF SYSTEMS (ROS)	Documented
1. Constitutional (e.g., weight loss, fever)	X
2. Ophthalmologic (eyes)	
3. Otolaryngologic (ears, nose, mouth, throat)	
4. Cardiovascular	
5. Respiratory	
6. Gastrointestinal	
7. Genitourinary	
8. Musculoskeletal	
9. Integumentary (skin and/or breasts)	
10. Neurologic	
11. Psychiatric	
12. Endocrine	X
13. Hematologic/Lymphatic	
14. Allergic/Immunologic	
TOTAL	2
LEVEL	3

PAST, FAMILY, AND/OR SOCIAL HISTORY (PFSH)	Documented
1. Past illness, operations, injuries, treatments, and current medications	X
2. Family medical history for heredity and risk	
3. Social activities, both past and present	X
TOTAL	2
LEVEL	4

History Level	1	2	3	4
	Problem Focused	Expanded Problem Focused	Detailed	Comprehensive
HPI	Brief 1-3	Brief 1-3	Extended 4+	Extended 4+
ROS	None	Problem Pertinent	Extended 2-9	Complete 10+
PFSH	None	None	Pertinent 1	Complete 2-3
HISTORY LEVEL			3	

EXAMINATION ELEMENTS	Documented
CONSTITUTIONAL	
1. Blood pressure, sitting	
2. Blood pressure, lying	
3. Pulse	
4. Respirations	
5. Temperature	
6. Height	
7. Weight	
8. General appearance	
NUMBER	0
BODY AREAS (BA)	Documented
1. Head (including face)	
2. Neck	
3. Chest (including breasts and axillae)	
4. Abdomen	
5. Genitalia, groin, buttocks	
6. Back (including spine)	
7. Each extremity	X
NUMBER	1
ORGAN SYSTEMS (OS)	Documented
1. Ophthalmologic (eyes)	
2. Otolaryngologic (ears, nose, mouth, throat)	
3. Cardiovascular	
4. Respiratory	
5. Gastrointestinal	
6. Genitourinary	
7. Musculoskeletal	
8. Integumentary	
9. Neurologic	
10. Psychiatric	
11. Hematologic/Lymphatic/Immunologic	
NUMBER	0
TOTAL BA/OS	1

Exam Level	1	2	3	4
	Problem Focused	Expanded Problem Focused	Detailed	Comprehensive
	Limited to affected BA/OS	Limited to affected BA/OS & other related OSs	Extended of affected BA & other related OSs	General multi-system or complete single OS
# of OS or BA	1	2-7 limited	2-7 extended	8+
EXAMINATION LEVEL				1

MDM ELEMENTS	Documented
# OF DIAGNOSIS/MANAGEMENT OPTIONS	
1. Minimal	
2. Limited	
3. Multiple	X
4. Extensive	
LEVEL	3
AMOUNT OR COMPLEXITY OF DATA TO REVIEW	Documented
1. Minimal/None	X
2. Limited	
3. Moderate	
4. Extensive	
LEVEL	1
RISK OF COMPLICATION OR DEATH IF NOT TREATED	Documented
1. Minimal	
2. Low	X
3. Moderate	
4. High	
LEVEL	2

MDM*	1	2	3	4
	Straightforward	Low	Moderate	High
Number of DX or management options	Minimal	Limited	Multiple	Extensive
Amount or complexity of data	Minimal/None	Limited	Moderate	Extensive
Risks	Minimal	Low	Moderate	High
MDM LEVEL			2	

*To qualify for a given type of MDM complexity, 2 of 3 elements in the table must be met or exceeded.

History: Detailed
Examination: Problem Focused
MDM: Low

Number of Key Components: 2 of 3

99335

Examination 2, Report 8

Professional Services: **99340** (Evaluation and Management, Care Plan Oversight Services); **319** (Retardation, mental); **312.00** (Outburst, aggressive, unspecified)

Rationale: Codes **99339** and **99340** represent the work done by the physician in overseeing a patient in a domiciliary, rest home (assisted living facility), or home care facility. They are reported once a calendar month based on the time spent by the physician providing the service. This note states that the patient resides in a group home and the plan took 50 minutes, **99340**.

The diagnoses are mental retardation, **319**, and aggressive outbursts, **312.00**. The fifth digit of 0, unspecified, would be reported because the level of outburst was not documented.

Examination 2, Report 9

Professional Services: **99348** (Evaluation and Management, Home Services); **784.0** (Headache); **296.80** (Disorder, bipolar)

Rationale: This is a home service, which is based on the whether the patient is new or established and the key components. The patient is being evaluated for chronic headaches.

The HPI consists of only location (head) for a level 1, or PF, HPI. There are 3 systems reviewed, constitutional, cardiovascular, and respiratory, for a level 3, or detailed, ROS. The patient's past medical history is reviewed, for a level 3, or detailed, history. This documentation contains a level 2, or EPF, history.

The examination contains a total of 6 BA/OS. These include the head, neck, ophthalmologic, otolaryngologic, respiratory, and psychiatric, for a level 3, or detailed, examination.

The MDM contains limited number of diagnosis and management options, limited data to review, and moderate risk. This qualifies as a level 2, or low, MDM.

There are 5 listed diagnoses but only those being treated or related to the ones being treated would need to be reported. For this service the main diagnosis would be **784.0** (headaches). Even though the headaches are listed as chronic, there is not a separate diagnosis for chronic headaches. The patient's bipolar disorder would also be reported because this may be the reason the patient is in need of home visits and may affect treatment.

Examination 2, Report 9

HISTORY ELEMENTS			Documented
HISTORY OF PRESENT ILLNESS (HPI)			
1. Location (site on body)			✗
2. Quality (characteristic: throbbing, sharp)			
3. Severity (1/10 or how intense)			
4. Duration (how long for problem or episode)			
5. Timing (when it occurs)			
6. Context (under what circumstances does it occur)			
7. Modifying factors (what makes it better or worse)			
8. Associated signs and symptoms (what else is happening when it occurs)			
		TOTAL	1
		LEVEL	2
REVIEW OF SYSTEMS (ROS)			Documented
1. Constitutional (e.g., weight loss, fever)			✗
2. Ophthalmologic (eyes)			
3. Otolaryngologic (ears, nose, mouth, throat)			
4. Cardiovascular			✗
5. Respiratory			✗
6. Gastrointestinal			
7. Genitourinary			
8. Musculoskeletal			
9. Integumentary (skin and/or breasts)			
10. Neurologic			
11. Psychiatric			
12. Endocrine			
13. Hematologic/Lymphatic			
14. Allergic/Immunologic			
		TOTAL	3
		LEVEL	3
PAST, FAMILY, AND/OR SOCIAL HISTORY (PFSH)			Documented
1. Past illness, operations, injuries, treatments, and current medications			✗
2. Family medical history for heredity and risk			
3. Social activities, both past and present			
		TOTAL	1
		LEVEL	3

History Level	1	2	3	4
	Problem Focused	Expanded Problem Focused	Detailed	Comprehensive
HPI	Brief 1-3	Brief 1-3	Extended 4+	Extended 4+
ROS	None	Problem Pertinent	Extended 2-9	Complete 10+
PFSH	None	None	Pertinent 1	Complete 2-3
			HISTORY LEVEL	2

EXAMINATION ELEMENTS			Documented
CONSTITUTIONAL			
1. Blood pressure, sitting			
2. Blood pressure, lying			
3. Pulse			
4. Respirations			
5. Temperature			
6. Height			
7. Weight			
8. General appearance			
		NUMBER	0
BODY AREAS (BA)			Documented
1. Head (including face)			✗
2. Neck			✗
3. Chest (including breasts and axillae)			
4. Abdomen			
5. Genitalia, groin, buttocks			
6. Back (including spine)			
7. Each extremity			
		NUMBER	2
ORGAN SYSTEMS (OS)			Documented
1. Ophthalmologic (eyes)			✗
2. Otolaryngologic (ears, nose, mouth, throat)			✗
3. Cardiovascular			
4. Respiratory			✗
5. Gastrointestinal			
6. Genitourinary			
7. Musculoskeletal			
8. Integumentary			
9. Neurologic			
10. Psychiatric			✗
11. Hematologic/Lymphatic/Immunologic			
		NUMBER	4
		TOTAL BA/OS	6

Exam Level	1	2	3	4
	Problem Focused	Expanded Problem Focused	Detailed	Comprehensive
	Limited to affected BA/OS	Limited to affected BA/OS & other related OSs	Extended of affected BA & other related OSs	General multi-system or complete single OS
# of OS or BA	1	2-7 limited	2-7 extended	8+
			EXAMINATION LEVEL	3

MDM ELEMENTS			Documented
# OF DIAGNOSIS/MANAGEMENT OPTIONS			
1. Minimal			
2. Limited			✗
3. Multiple			
4. Extensive			
		LEVEL	2
AMOUNT OR COMPLEXITY OF DATA TO REVIEW			Documented
1. Minimal/None			
2. Limited			✗
3. Moderate			
4. Extensive			
		LEVEL	2
RISK OF COMPLICATION OR DEATH IF NOT TREATED			Documented
1. Minimal			
2. Low			
3. Moderate			✗
4. High			
		LEVEL	3

MDM*	1	2	3	4
	Straightforward	Low	Moderate	High
Number of DX or management options	Minimal	Limited	Multiple	Extensive
Amount or complexity of data	Minimal/None	Limited	Moderate	Extensive
Risks	Minimal	Low	Moderate	High
			MDM LEVEL	2

*To qualify for a given type of MDM complexity, 2 of 3 elements in the table must be met or exceeded.

History: Expanded Problem Focused
Examination: Detailed
MDM: Low

Number of Key Components: 2 of 3

99348

Examination 2, Report 10

Professional Services: **99253** (Evaluation and Management, Consultation); **813.42** (Fracture, radius, lower end, closed); **E888.9** (Fall, same level, NEC)

Rationale: The patient has been admitted to the hospital to determine the reason for her syncope. This physician was asked to see the patient and render an opinion regarding the upper extremity fractures. There are 4 elements of HPI, location (upper extremities), severity (no pain), context (fell during episode of syncope), and modifying factors (feels better with splints) for a level 4 or comprehensive HPI. Two systems were reviewed, musculoskeletal and neurologic, for a level 3 ROS. The documentation included 2 of 3 PFSH for a level 4 or comprehensive PFSH. All 3 elements of history must qualify for level selection. The HPI and PFSH are comprehensive but the ROS only qualifies as detailed, therefore this is a detailed history.

The examination consisted of no constitutional elements. The BAs that were examined include neck and all 4 extremities for a total of 5 BAs. A total of 4 OSs, musculoskeletal, integumentary (skin intact), psychiatric (oriented ×3), and neurologic were also examined for a total of 9 BA/OS. This qualifies as a level 4, or comprehensive, examination.

There are limited diagnosis/management options, limited data were reviewed, and the patient has low risk of death or complication, which makes the level of MDM low.

This was a closed fracture of the lower radius of the right wrist, **813.42**. The external cause code is a fall, but it was not specified as to how the patient fell, **E888.9**.

Examination 2, Report 10

HISTORY ELEMENTS	Documented
HISTORY OF PRESENT ILLNESS (HPI)	
1. Location (site on body)	✗
2. Quality (characteristic: throbbing, sharp)	
3. Severity (1/10 or how intense)	✗
4. Duration (how long for problem or episode)	
5. Timing (when it occurs)	
6. Context (under what circumstances does it occur)	✗
7. Modifying factors (what makes it better or worse)	✗
8. Associated signs and symptoms (what else is happening when it occurs)	
TOTAL	4
LEVEL	4

REVIEW OF SYSTEMS (ROS)	Documented
1. Constitutional (e.g., weight loss, fever)	
2. Ophthalmologic (eyes)	
3. Otolaryngologic (ears, nose, mouth, throat)	
4. Cardiovascular	
5. Respiratory	
6. Gastrointestinal	
7. Genitourinary	
8. Musculoskeletal	✗
9. Integumentary (skin and/or breasts)	
10. Neurologic	✗
11. Psychiatric	
12. Endocrine	
13. Hematologic/Lymphatic	
14. Allergic/Immunologic	
TOTAL	2
LEVEL	3

PAST, FAMILY, AND/OR SOCIAL HISTORY (PFSH)	Documented
1. Past illness, operations, injuries, treatments, and current medications	✗
2. Family medical history for heredity and risk	
3. Social activities, both past and present	✗
TOTAL	2
LEVEL	4

History Level	1	2	3	4
	Problem Focused	Expanded Problem Focused	Detailed	Comprehensive
HPI	Brief 1-3	Brief 1-3	Extended 4+	Extended 4+
ROS	None	Problem Pertinent	Extended 2-9	Complete 10+
PFSH	None	None	Pertinent 1	Complete 2-3
			HISTORY LEVEL	3

EXAMINATION ELEMENTS	Documented
CONSTITUTIONAL	
1. Blood pressure, sitting	
2. Blood pressure, lying	
3. Pulse	
4. Respirations	
5. Temperature	
6. Height	
7. Weight	
8. General appearance	
NUMBER	0

BODY AREAS (BA)	Documented
1. Head (including face)	
2. Neck	✗
3. Chest (including breasts and axillae)	
4. Abdomen	
5. Genitalia, groin, buttocks	
6. Back (including spine)	
7. Each extremity	✗✗✗
NUMBER	5

ORGAN SYSTEMS (OS)	Documented
1. Ophthalmologic (eyes)	
2. Otolaryngologic (ears, nose, mouth, throat)	
3. Cardiovascular	
4. Respiratory	
5. Gastrointestinal	
6. Genitourinary	
7. Musculoskeletal	✗
8. Integumentary	✗
9. Neurologic	✗
10. Psychiatric	✗
11. Hematologic/Lymphatic/Immunologic	
NUMBER	4
TOTAL BA/OS	9

Exam Level	1	2	3	4
	Problem Focused	Expanded Problem Focused	Detailed	Comprehensive
	Limited to affected BA/OS	Limited to affected BA/OS & other related OSs	Extended of affected BA & other related OSs	General multi-system or complete single OS
# of OS or BA	1	2-7 limited	2-7 extended	8+
			EXAMINATION LEVEL	4

MDM ELEMENTS	Documented
# OF DIAGNOSIS/MANAGEMENT OPTIONS	
1. Minimal	
2. Limited	✗
3. Multiple	
4. Extensive	
LEVEL	2
AMOUNT OR COMPLEXITY OF DATA TO REVIEW	Documented
1. Minimal/None	
2. Limited	✗
3. Moderate	
4. Extensive	
LEVEL	2
RISK OF COMPLICATION OR DEATH IF NOT TREATED	Documented
1. Minimal	
2. Low	✗
3. Moderate	
4. High	
LEVEL	2

MDM*	1	2	3	4
	Straightforward	Low	Moderate	High
Number of DX or management options	Minimal	Limited	Multiple	Extensive
Amount or complexity of data	Minimal/None	Limited	Moderate	Extensive
Risks	Minimal	Low	Moderate	High
			MDM LEVEL	2

*To qualify for a given type of MDM complexity, 2 of 3 elements in the table must be met or exceeded.

History: Detailed
Examination: Comprehensive
MDM: Low

Number of Key Components: 3 of 3

99253

Examination 2, Report 11

Professional Services: **99233** (Evaluation and Management, Hospital); **99356** (Evaluation and Management, Prolonged Services); **785.0** (Tachycardia); **458.9** (Low, blood pressure); **585.6** (Disease, renal, end-stage); **790.7** (Findings, abnormal, without diagnosis, culture, blood); **041.89** (Infection, infected, infective, bacterial, specified NEC)

Rationale: This is a document that represents prolonged service of care. The time allotted for the E/M code assigned would be subtracted from the total time of the service and the remaining time would be reported with a prolonged service code. Prolonged service codes are add-on codes, are never reported alone and do not require a modifier.

This patient is acutely ill, is tachycardic and has developed problems due to his renal dialysis catheter.

There are 3 elements of HPI, location (heart), severity (130s), modifying factors (take dialysis catheter out) for a level 2, or EPF, HPI. Only 1 system examination was performed, respiratory, for a level 2, or EPF, ROS. The documentation included only 1 element of PFSH for a level 3, or detailed, PFSH. An EPF HPI, EPF ROS, and detailed PFSH qualifies as a EPF history.

The constitutional examination consisted of 3 elements (BP, pulse, temperature) to qualify as 1 BA/OS. One BA was examined, the abdomen. The OSs consisted of otolaryngologic, cardiovascular, and respiratory for a total of 3 OSs. The exam performed on this patient included 5 BA/OS and qualifies as a level 3, or detailed, examination.

Extensive diagnosis/management options, limited data reviewed and the patient's high risk of death make this level of MDM high. The level of service would be **99233**. This code is allotted 35 minutes. At the end of this documentation it states that 1 hour and 15 minutes were spent with the patient. The total in minutes is 75 minutes. Subtract the 35 minutes for the initial code **99233**, leaving 40 minutes of time to report for prolonged services. The prolonged services are categorized by either face-to-face direct contact or without face-to-face direct contact. The direct face-to face codes are further categorized by whether the service took place in an outpatient or inpatient setting. The prolonged service code that would accompany **99233** would be **99356**.

The patient is being evaluated for tachycardia (**785.0**), low blood pressure (**458.9**), and end-stage renal disease (**585.6**). The sepsis and staph aureus bacteremia are not reported because they are probable diagnoses. The gram-positive cocci found in the blood culture is reported with **790.7** for bacteremia and **041.89** for the cocci.

Examination 2, Report 11

HISTORY ELEMENTS	Documented
HISTORY OF PRESENT ILLNESS (HPI)	
1. Location (site on body)	✗
2. Quality (characteristic: throbbing, sharp)	
3. Severity (1/10 or how intense)	✗
4. Duration (how long for problem or episode)	
5. Timing (when it occurs)	
6. Context (under what circumstances does it occur)	
7. Modifying factors (what makes it better or worse)	✗
8. Associated signs and symptoms (what else is happening when it occurs)	
TOTAL	3
LEVEL	2

REVIEW OF SYSTEMS (ROS)	Documented
1. Constitutional (e.g., weight loss, fever)	
2. Ophthalmologic (eyes)	
3. Otolaryngologic (ears, nose, mouth, throat)	
4. Cardiovascular	
5. Respiratory	✗
6. Gastrointestinal	
7. Genitourinary	
8. Musculoskeletal	
9. Integumentary (skin and/or breasts)	
10. Neurologic	
11. Psychiatric	
12. Endocrine	
13. Hematologic/Lymphatic	
14. Allergic/Immunologic	
TOTAL	1
LEVEL	2

PAST, FAMILY, AND/OR SOCIAL HISTORY (PFSH)	Documented
1. Past illness, operations, injuries, treatments, and current medications	✗
2. Family medical history for heredity and risk	
3. Social activities, both past and present	
TOTAL	1
LEVEL	3

History Level	1	2	3	4
	Problem Focused	Expanded Problem Focused	Detailed	Comprehensive
HPI	Brief 1-3	Brief 1-3	Extended 4+	Extended 4+
ROS	None	Problem Pertinent	Extended 2-9	Complete 10+
PFSH	None	None	Pertinent 1	Complete 2-3
HISTORY LEVEL				2

EXAMINATION ELEMENTS	Documented
CONSTITUTIONAL	
1. Blood pressure, sitting	
2. Blood pressure, lying	✗
3. Pulse	✗
4. Respirations	
5. Temperature	✗
6. Height	
7. Weight	
8. General appearance	
NUMBER	1

BODY AREAS (BA)	Documented
1. Head (including face)	
2. Neck	
3. Chest (including breasts and axillae)	
4. Abdomen	✗
5. Genitalia, groin, buttocks	
6. Back (including spine)	
7. Each extremity	
NUMBER	1

ORGAN SYSTEMS (OS)	Documented
1. Ophthalmologic (eyes)	
2. Otolaryngologic (ears, nose, mouth, throat)	✗
3. Cardiovascular	✗
4. Respiratory	✗
5. Gastrointestinal	
6. Genitourinary	
7. Musculoskeletal	
8. Integumentary	
9. Neurologic	
10. Psychiatric	
11. Hematologic/Lymphatic/Immunologic	
NUMBER	3
TOTAL BA/OS	5

Exam Level	1	2	3	4
	Problem Focused	Expanded Problem Focused	Detailed	Comprehensive
	Limited to affected BA/OS	Limited to affected BA/OS & other related OSs	Extended of affected BA & other related OSs	General multi-system or complete single OS
# of OS or BA	1	2-7 limited	2-7 extended	8+
EXAMINATION LEVEL				3

MDM ELEMENTS	Documented
# OF DIAGNOSIS/MANAGEMENT OPTIONS	
1. Minimal	
2. Limited	
3. Multiple	
4. Extensive	✗
LEVEL	4

AMOUNT OR COMPLEXITY OF DATA TO REVIEW	Documented
1. Minimal/None	
2. Limited	✗
3. Moderate	
4. Extensive	
LEVEL	2

RISK OF COMPLICATION OR DEATH IF NOT TREATED	Documented
1. Minimal	
2. Low	
3. Moderate	
4. High	✗
LEVEL	4

MDM*	1	2	3	4
	Straightforward	Low	Moderate	High
Number of DX or management options	Minimal	Limited	Multiple	Extensive
Amount or complexity of data	Minimal/None	Limited	Moderate	Extensive
Risks	Minimal	Low	Moderate	High
MDM LEVEL				4

*To qualify for a given type of MDM complexity, 2 of 3 elements in the table must be met or exceeded.

History: Expanded Problem Focused
Examination: Detailed
MDM: High

Number of Key Components: 2 of 3

99233, 99356

Examination 2, Report 12

Professional Services: **99456** (Evaluation and Management, Insurance Examination); **959.19** (Injury, back); **338.21** (Pain, chronic)

Rationale: Special evaluation management services are for basic life and/or disability evaluations or work-related medical disability evaluations. This evaluation is for disability caused by a work-related injury. Someone other than the treating physician is performing the evaluation, so the correct code to use would be **99456**.

The diagnoses would be the injury to the back (**959.19**). The external cause code **E927** for the injury during lifting is not reported because this is not the initial treatment.

338.21 reports the chronic pain due to trauma.

Examination 2, Report 13

Professional Services: **99360** × 2 (Evaluation and Management, Physician Standby Services); **642.91** (Hypertension, complicating pregnancy, antepartum condition or complication)

Rationale: This is a document that represents physician standby services, which is reported in units depending on the time the physician is standing by. The requirements for this code are as follows: it has to be requested by another physician, no face-to-face contact is made with the patient, and the physician standing by cannot be providing care to any other patient during that time. If the standby time is less than 30 minutes, the service is not reported. Unlike some of the other E/M codes, the unit of time for standby services must be a full 30 minutes. It is very important to read and understand the guidelines that precede this code. This documentation is for 70 minutes of standby, requested by the patient's OB/GYN, because of the patient's severe hypertension. Code **99360** would be reported with 2 units, for 60 minutes of the 70 minutes. The extra 10 minutes cannot be reported because it is not a full 30 minutes.

The diagnosis would be reported as **642.91**. You would use the hypertension table in the ICD-9-CM and reference complication of pregnancy, unspecified, with the fifth digit of 1 because the physician was present until after the patient delivered.

Examination 2, Report 14

Professional Services: **99367** (Evaluation and Management, Case Management); **V65.49** (Counseling, specified reason NEC); **585.6** (Disease, renal, end-stage); **V45.1** (Dialysis, status)

Rationale: Case management is when the physician is responsible for the direct care of the patient and for coordinating the care and needs of the patient with other health care services that the patient needs. The team conference was without the patient but with the family. The physician was present for the conference, making **99367** the correct choice.

The diagnosis would be **V65.49** for the counseling, **585.6** for the end stage renal disease, and **V45.1** to indicate the current dialysis status.

Examination 2, Report 15

Professional Services: **99223** (Evaluation and Management, Hospital); **250.10** (Diabetes, ketoacidosis, unspecified); **790.5** (Findings, enzymes, serum NEC); **263.9** (Malnutrition); **276.2** (Acidosis, metabolic); **593.9** (Insufficiency, renal, acute); **288.60** (Leukocytosis); **285.9** (Anemia); **305.1** (Abuse, tobacco); **303.90** (Alcoholism)

Rationale: This patient is acutely ill and is being admitted to the hospital; the admitting physician's services would be reported using an initial hospital care code. There are 5 elements of HPI: location (body, abdomen), quality (increasing), severity (vomited one time), duration (6 days ago), and associated signs and symptoms (no fever) for a level 4, or comprehensive, HPI. A ROS was performed of 11 organ systems including constitutional, ophthalmologic, otolaryngologic, cardiovascular, respiratory, GI, GU, neurologic, psychiatric (disoriented), endocrine, and allergic (no known allergies) for a level 4, or comprehensive, ROS. The documentation included all 3 elements of PFSH for a level 4, or comprehensive, PFSH. Because all 3 elements of history are comprehensive this would be a comprehensive history.

The constitutional examination consisted of 4 elements (blood pressure, temp, pulse, respiration) to qualify as 1 BA/OS. The BAs that were examined include head, neck and all 4 extremities for a total of 6 BAs. The OSs consisted of ophthalmologic, otolaryngologic, cardiovascular, respiratory, gastrointestinal, and neurologic for a total of 6 OSs. The exam performed on this patient included 13 BA/OS and qualifies as a level 4, or comprehensive, examination.

Extensive diagnosis/management options, limited data reviewed and the patient's high risk of death make this level of MDM high. The level of service would be **99223**.

The CC at the beginning of the documentation is stated as weakness, but upon continuing on through the note more definitive diagnoses are made. The patient has many diagnoses and all should be reported except for the "probable pancreatitis." The diabetic ketoacidosis (**250.10**) is reported with the fifth digit of 0 because of the unspecified type of diabetes. The elevated liver enzymes (**790.5**), malnutrition (**263.9**), metabolic acidosis (**276.2**), renal insufficiency (**593.9**), leukocytosis (**288.60**), anemia (**285.9**), abuse of tobacco (**305.1**), and alcoholism (**303.90**) should all be reported.

Examination 2, Report 15

HISTORY ELEMENTS	Documented
HISTORY OF PRESENT ILLNESS (HPI)	
1. Location (site on body)	X
2. Quality (characteristic: throbbing, sharp)	X
3. Severity (1/10 or how intense)	X
4. Duration (how long for problem or episode)	X
5. Timing (when it occurs)	
6. Context (under what circumstances does it occur)	
7. Modifying factors (what makes it better or worse)	
8. Associated signs and symptoms (what else is happening when it occurs)	X
TOTAL	5
LEVEL	4

REVIEW OF SYSTEMS (ROS)	Documented
1. Constitutional (e.g., weight loss, fever)	X
2. Ophthalmologic (eyes)	X
3. Otolaryngologic (ears, nose, mouth, throat)	X
4. Cardiovascular	X
5. Respiratory	X
6. Gastrointestinal	X
7. Genitourinary	X
8. Musculoskeletal	
9. Integumentary (skin and/or breasts)	
10. Neurologic	X
11. Psychiatric	X
12. Endocrine	X
13. Hematologic/Lymphatic	
14. Allergic/Immunologic	X
TOTAL	11
LEVEL	4

PAST, FAMILY, AND/OR SOCIAL HISTORY (PFSH)	Documented
1. Past illness, operations, injuries, treatments, and current medications	X
2. Family medical history for heredity and risk	X
3. Social activities, both past and present	X
TOTAL	3
LEVEL	4

History Level	1	2	3	4
	Problem Focused	Expanded Problem Focused	Detailed	Comprehensive
HPI	Brief 1-3	Brief 1-3	Extended 4+	Extended 4+
ROS	None	Problem Pertinent	Extended 2-9	Complete 10+
PFSH	None	None	Pertinent 1	Complete 2-3
HISTORY LEVEL				4

EXAMINATION ELEMENTS	Documented
CONSTITUTIONAL	
1. Blood pressure, sitting	
2. Blood pressure, lying	X
3. Pulse	X
4. Respirations	X
5. Temperature	X
6. Height	
7. Weight	
8. General appearance	
NUMBER	1

BODY AREAS (BA)	Documented
1. Head (including face)	X
2. Neck	X
3. Chest (including breasts and axillae)	
4. Abdomen	
5. Genitalia, groin, buttocks	
6. Back (including spine)	
7. Each extremity	XXX
NUMBER	6

ORGAN SYSTEMS (OS)	Documented
1. Ophthalmologic (eyes)	X
2. Otolaryngologic (ears, nose, mouth, throat)	X
3. Cardiovascular	X
4. Respiratory	X
5. Gastrointestinal	X
6. Genitourinary	
7. Musculoskeletal	
8. Integumentary	
9. Neurologic	X
10. Psychiatric	
11. Hematologic/Lymphatic/Immunologic	
NUMBER	6
TOTAL BA/OS	13

Exam Level	1	2	3	4
	Problem Focused	Expanded Problem Focused	Detailed	Comprehensive
	Limited to affected BA/OS	Limited to affected BA/OS & other related OSs	Extended of affected BA & other related OSs	General multi-system or complete single OS
# of OS or BA	1	2-7 limited	2-7 extended	8+
EXAMINATION LEVEL				4

MDM ELEMENTS	Documented
# OF DIAGNOSIS/MANAGEMENT OPTIONS	
1. Minimal	
2. Limited	
3. Multiple	
4. Extensive	X
LEVEL	4
AMOUNT OR COMPLEXITY OF DATA TO REVIEW	Documented
1. Minimal/None	
2. Limited	X
3. Moderate	
4. Extensive	
LEVEL	2
RISK OF COMPLICATION OR DEATH IF NOT TREATED	Documented
1. Minimal	
2. Low	
3. Moderate	
4. High	X
LEVEL	4

MDM*	1	2	3	4
	Straightforward	Low	Moderate	High
Number of DX or management options	Minimal	Limited	Multiple	Extensive
Amount or complexity of data	Minimal/None	Limited	Moderate	Extensive
Risks	Minimal	Low	Moderate	High
MDM LEVEL				4

*To qualify for a given type of MDM complexity, 2 of 3 elements in the table must be met or exceeded.

History: Comprehensive
Examination: Comprehensive
MDM: High

Number of Key Components: 3 of 3

99223

Examination 2, Report 16

Professional Services: **99380** (Evaluation and Management, Care Plan Oversight Services); **428.0** (Failure, heart, congestive); **440.1** (Stenosis, renal, artery); **585.9** (Failure, renal, chronic)

Rationale: Care plan oversight services reflect a supervisory role of the physician to the patient. The patient is not present when the physician provides this service. Codes include development or revision of a care plan, reviewing reports regarding patient status, communication with other health care professionals, and review of lab or tests that may have been performed. These codes may only be reported once for every 30-day period. Codes are divided by the location in which the patient is residing, such as home health agency, hospice, or nursing facility. The codes are further divided based on the time spent providing the service. **99380** would be the correct code to report the service provided based on this documentation because the patient is residing in a nursing facility and the time spent providing the service was more than 30 minutes.

The diagnoses are CHF (**428.0**), renal artery stenosis (**440.1**), edema (**782.3**) and **585.9** for the chronic renal failure. The edema and dyspnea referenced in the second paragraph are symptoms of the CHF and as such are not reported separately.

Examination 2, Report 17

Professional Services: **99283** (Evaluation and Management, Emergency Department); **786.51** (Pain, chest, substernal)

Rationale: The patient presents to the emergency room complaining of chest pain. The highest level of service is Level 3, **99283**, point 3, x-ray of chest.

The patient's chest pain is stated as substernal (**786.51**). No cause is found for her chest pain.

Examination 2, Report 18

Professional Services: **99315** (Evaluation and Management, Nursing Facility, Discharge); **V12.59** (Accident, cerebrovascular, healed or old); **715.90** (Osteoarthrosis, site unspecified); **401.9** (Hypertension, unspecified); **530.81** (Reflux, gastroesophageal); **596.54** (Neurogenic, bladder)

Rationale: The nursing facility discharge services are based on time the physician spends in the final discharge of a patient, not the key components that other E/M services require. The service may or may not include an examination of the patient. Since the physician did not indicate the time spent in discharge of this patient the lowest level of nursing facility discharge, **99315**, is reported for the service.

The documentation does not state late effects of the cerebrovascular accident so this would be reported as a history of, **V12.59**. The site of the osteoarthritis is not specified so the fifth digit on code **715.9** would be 0, **715.90**. The hypertension is not specified as benign or malignant so **401.9** would be the correct code to use. The GERD would be reported with **530.81** and the neurogenic bladder would be **596.54**.

ICD-9-CM Official Guidelines for Coding and Reporting

Reprinted as released by the Centers for Medicare and Medicaid Services and the National Center for Health Statistics. See http://www.cdc.gov/nchs/datawh/ftpserv/ ftpicd9/ftpicd9.htm#guidelines.

**Effective October 1, 2007
Narrative changes appear in bold text
Items underlined have been moved within the guidelines since
November 15, 2006
The guidelines include the updated V Code Table**

The Centers for Medicare and Medicaid Services (CMS) and the National Center for Health Statistics (NCHS), two departments within the U. S. Federal Government's Department of Health and Human Services (DHHS) provide the following guidelines for coding and reporting using the International Classification of Diseases, 9th Revision, Clinical Modification (ICD-9-CM). These guidelines should be used as a companion document to the official version of the ICD-9-CM as published on CD-ROM by the U.S. Government Printing Office (GPO).

These guidelines have been approved by the four organizations that make up the Cooperating Parties for the ICD-9-CM: the American Hospital Association (AHA), the American Health Information Management Association (AHIMA), CMS, and NCHS. These guidelines are included on the official government version of the ICD-9-CM, and also appear in *"Coding Clinic for ICD-9-CM"* published by the AHA.

These guidelines are a set of rules that have been developed to accompany and complement the official conventions and instructions provided within the ICD-9-CM itself. These guidelines are based on the coding and sequencing instructions in Volumes I, II and III of ICD-9-CM, but provide additional instruction. Adherence to these guidelines when assigning ICD-9-CM diagnosis and procedure codes is required under the Health Insurance Portability and Accountability Act (HIPAA). The diagnosis codes (Volumes 1-2) have been adopted under HIPAA for all healthcare settings. Volume 3 procedure codes have been adopted for inpatient procedures reported by hospitals. A joint effort between the healthcare provider and the coder is essential to achieve complete and accurate documentation, code assignment, and reporting of diagnoses and procedures. These guidelines have been developed to assist both the healthcare provider and the coder in identifying those diagnoses and procedures that are to be reported. The importance of consistent, complete documentation in the medical record cannot be overemphasized. Without such documentation accurate coding cannot be achieved. The entire record should be reviewed to determine the specific reason for the encounter and the conditions treated.

The term encounter is used for all settings, including hospital admissions. In the context of these guidelines, the term provider is used throughout the guidelines to mean physician or any qualified health care practitioner who is legally accountable for establishing the patient's diagnosis. Only this set of guidelines, approved by the Cooperating Parties, is official.

The guidelines are organized into sections. Section I includes the structure and conventions of the classification and general guidelines that apply to the entire classification, and chapter-specific guidelines that correspond to the chapters as they are arranged in the classification. Section II includes guidelines for selection of principal diagnosis for non-outpatient settings. Section III includes guidelines for reporting additional diagnoses in non-outpatient settings. Section IV is for outpatient coding and reporting.

ICD-9-CM Official Guidelines for Coding and Reporting

Section I.   Conventions, general coding guidelines and chapter specific guidelines

    A. Conventions for the ICD-9-CM

        1. Format:

        2. Abbreviations

            a. Index abbreviations

            b. Tabular abbreviations

        3. Punctuation

        4. Includes and Excludes Notes and Inclusion terms

        5. Other and Unspecified codes

            a. "Other" codes

            b. "Unspecified" codes

        6. Etiology/manifestation convention ("code first", "use additional code" and "in diseases classified elsewhere" notes)

        7. "And"

        8. "With"

        9. "See" and "See Also"

    B. General Coding Guidelines

        1. Use of Both Alphabetic Index and Tabular List

        2. Locate each term in the Alphabetic Index

        3. Level of Detail in Coding

        4. Code or codes from 001.0 through V84.8

        5. Selection of codes 001.0 through 999.9

        6. Signs and symptoms

        7. Conditions that are an integral part of a disease process

        8. Conditions that are not an integral part of a disease process

        9. Multiple coding for a single condition

       10. Acute and Chronic Conditions

       11. Combination Code

12. Late Effects

13. Impending or Threatened Condition

C. Chapter-Specific Coding Guidelines

  1. Chapter 1: Infectious and Parasitic Diseases (001-139)

    a. Human Immunodeficiency Virus (HIV) Infections

    b. Septicemia, Systemic Inflammatory Response Syndrome (SIRS), Sepsis, Severe Sepsis, and Septic Shock

  2. Chapter 2: Neoplasms (140-239)

    a. Treatment directed at the malignancy

    b. Treatment of secondary site

    c. Coding and sequencing of complications

    d. Primary malignancy previously excised

    e. Admissions/Encounters involving chemotherapy, immunotherapy and radiation therapy

    f. Admission/encounter to determine extent of malignancy

    g. Symptoms, signs, and ill-defined conditions listed in Chapter 16 **associated with neoplasms**

    h. Admission/encounter for pain control/management

  3. Chapter 3: Endocrine, Nutritional, and Metabolic Diseases and Immunity Disorders (240-279)

    a. Diabetes mellitus

  4. Chapter 4: Diseases of Blood and Blood Forming Organs (280-289)

    a. Anemia of chronic disease

  5. Chapter 5: Mental Disorders (290-319)

Reserved for future guideline expansion

  6. Chapter 6: Diseases of Nervous System and Sense Organs (320-389)

    a. Pain – Category 338

  7. Chapter 7: Diseases of Circulatory System (390-459)

    a. Hypertension

    b. Cerebral infarction/stroke/cerebrovascular accident (CVA)

    c. Postoperative cerebrovascular accident

    d. Late Effects of Cerebrovascular Disease

    e. Acute myocardial infarction (AMI)

  8. Chapter 8: Diseases of Respiratory System (460-519)

    a. Chronic Obstructive Pulmonary Disease [COPD] and Asthma

    b. Chronic Obstructive Pulmonary Disease [COPD] and Bronchitis

    c. Acute Respiratory Failure

    d. Influenza due to identified avian influenza virus (avian influenza)

9. Chapter 9: Diseases of Digestive System (520-579)

Reserved for future guideline expansion

10. Chapter 10: Diseases of Genitourinary System (580-629)

   a. Chronic kidney disease

11. Chapter 11: Complications of Pregnancy, Childbirth, and the Puerperium (630-677)

   a. General Rules for Obstetric Cases

   b. Selection of OB Principal or First-listed Diagnosis

   c. Fetal Conditions Affecting the Management of the Mother

   d. HIV Infection in Pregnancy, Childbirth and the Puerperium

   e. Current Conditions Complicating Pregnancy

   f. Diabetes mellitus in pregnancy

   g. Gestational diabetes

   h. Normal Delivery, Code 650

   i. The Postpartum and Peripartum Periods

   j. Code 677, Late effect of complication of pregnancy

   k. Abortions

12. Chapter 12: Diseases Skin and Subcutaneous Tissue (680-709)

Reserved for future guideline expansion

13. Chapter 13: Diseases of Musculoskeletal and Connective Tissue (710-739)

   a. Coding of Pathologic Fractures

14. Chapter 14: Congenital Anomalies (740-759)

   a. Codes in categories 740-759, Congenital Anomalies

15. Chapter 15: Newborn (Perinatal) Guidelines (760-779)

   a. General Perinatal Rules

   b. Use of codes V30-V39

   c. Newborn transfers

   d. Use of category V29

   e. Use of other V codes on perinatal records

   f. Maternal Causes of Perinatal Morbidity

   g. Congenital Anomalies in Newborns

   h. Coding Additional Perinatal Diagnoses

   i. Prematurity and Fetal Growth Retardation

   j. Newborn sepsis

16. Chapter 16: Signs, Symptoms and Ill-Defined Conditions (780-799)

Reserved for future guideline expansion

17. Chapter 17: Injury and Poisoning (800-999)

   a. Coding of Injuries

   b. Coding of Traumatic Fractures

   c. Coding of Burns

   d. Coding of Debridement of Wound, Infection, or Burn

   e. Adverse Effects, Poisoning and Toxic Effects

   f. Complications of care

   g. SIRS due to Non-infectious Process

18. Classification of Factors Influencing Health Status and Contact with Health Service

(Supplemental V01-V84)

   a. Introduction

   b. V codes use in any healthcare setting

   c. V Codes indicate a reason for an encounter

   d. Categories of V Codes

   e. V Code Table

19. Supplemental Classification of External Causes of Injury and Poisoning

(E-codes, E800-E999)

   a. General E Code Coding Guidelines

   b. Place of Occurrence Guideline

   c. Adverse Effects of Drugs, Medicinal and Biological Substances Guidelines

   d. Multiple Cause E Code Coding Guidelines

   e. Child and Adult Abuse Guideline

   f. Unknown or Suspected Intent Guideline

   g. Undetermined Cause

   h. Late Effects of External Cause Guidelines

   i. Misadventures and Complications of Care Guidelines

   j. Terrorism Guidelines

Section II.   Selection of Principal Diagnosis

A. Codes for symptoms, signs, and ill-defined conditions

B. Two or more interrelated conditions, each potentially meeting the definition for principal diagnosis.

C. Two or more diagnoses that equally meet the definition for principal diagnosis

D. Two or more comparative or contrasting conditions.

E. A symptom(s) followed by contrasting/comparative diagnoses

F. Original treatment plan not carried out

G. Complications of surgery and other medical care

H. Uncertain Diagnosis

I. Admission from Observation Unit

1. Admission Following Medical Observation

2. Admission Following Post-Operative Observation

J. Admission from Outpatient Surgery

Section III. Reporting Additional Diagnoses

A. Previous conditions

B. Abnormal findings

C. Uncertain Diagnosis

Section IV. Diagnostic Coding and Reporting Guidelines for Outpatient Services

A. Selection of first-listed condition

1. Outpatient Surgery

2. Observation Stay

B. Codes from 001.0 through V84.8

C. Accurate reporting of ICD-9-CM diagnosis codes

D. Selection of codes 001.0 through 999.9

E. Codes that describe symptoms and signs

F. Encounters for circumstances other than a disease or injury

G. Level of Detail in Coding

1. ICD-9-CM codes with 3, 4, or 5 digits

2. Use of full number of digits required for a code

H. ICD-9-CM code for the diagnosis, condition, problem, or other reason for encounter/visit

I. Uncertain diagnosis

J. Chronic diseases

K. Code all documented conditions that coexist

L. Patients receiving diagnostic services only

M. Patients receiving therapeutic services only

N. Patients receiving preoperative evaluations only

O. Ambulatory surgery

P. Routine outpatient prenatal visits

Appendix I: Present on Admission Reporting Guidelines

SECTION I. CONVENTIONS, GENERAL CODING GUIDELINES AND CHAPTER SPECIFIC GUIDELINES

The conventions, general guidelines and chapter-specific guidelines are applicable to all health care settings unless otherwise indicated.

A. Conventions for the ICD-9-CM

The conventions for the ICD-9-CM are the general rules for use of the classification independent of the guidelines. These conventions are incorporated within the index and tabular of the ICD-9-CM as instructional notes. The conventions are as follows:

1. **Format:**

   The ICD-9-CM uses an indented format for ease in reference

2. **Abbreviations**

   a. **Index abbreviations**

   NEC   "Not elsewhere classifiable" This abbreviation in the index represents "other specified" when a specific code is not available for a condition the index directs the coder to the "other specified" code in the tabular.

   b. **Tabular abbreviations**

   NEC   "Not elsewhere classifiable" This abbreviation in the tabular represents "other specified". When a specific code is not available for a condition the tabular includes an NEC entry under a code to identify the code as the "other specified" code. *(See Section I.A.5.a. "Other" codes")*.

   NOS   "Not otherwise specified" This abbreviation is the equivalent of unspecified. *(See Section I.A.5.b., "Unspecified" codes)*

3. **Punctuation**

   [ ]   Brackets are used in the tabular list to enclose synonyms, alternative wording or explanatory phrases. Brackets are used in the index to identify manifestation codes. *(See Section I.A.6. "Etiology/manifestations")*

   ( )   Parentheses are used in both the index and tabular to enclose supplementary words that may be present or absent in the statement of a disease or procedure without affecting the code number to which it is assigned. The terms within the parentheses are referred to as nonessential modifiers.

   :   Colons are used in the Tabular list after an incomplete term which needs one or more of the modifiers following the colon to make it assignable to a given category.

4. **Includes and Excludes Notes and Inclusion terms**

   Includes: This note appears immediately under a three-digit code title to further define, or give examples of, the content of the category.

   Excludes: An excludes note under a code indicates that the terms excluded from the code are to be coded elsewhere. In some cases the codes for the excluded terms should not be used in conjunction with the code from which it is excluded. An example of this is a congenital condition excluded from an acquired form of the same condition. The congenital and acquired codes should not be used together. In other cases, the excluded terms may be used together with an excluded code. An example of this is when fractures of different bones are coded to different codes. Both codes may be used together if both types of fractures are present.

Inclusion terms: List of terms is included under certain four and five digit codes. These terms are the conditions for which that code number is to be used. The terms may be synonyms of the code title, or, in the case of "other specified" codes, the terms are a list of the various conditions assigned to that code. The inclusion terms are not necessarily exhaustive. Additional terms found only in the index may also be assigned to a code.

5. **Other and Unspecified codes**

a. **"Other" codes**

Codes titled "other" or "other specified" (usually a code with a 4th digit 8 or fifth-digit 9 for diagnosis codes) are for use when the information in the medical record provides detail for which a specific code does not exist. Index entries with NEC in the line designate "other" codes in the tabular. These index entries represent specific disease entities for which no specific code exists so the term is included within an "other" code.

b. **"Unspecified" codes**

Codes (usually a code with a 4th digit 9 or 5th digit 0 for diagnosis codes) titled "unspecified" are for use when the information in the medical record is insufficient to assign a more specific code.

6. **Etiology/manifestation convention ("code first", "use additional code" and "in diseases classified elsewhere" notes)**

Certain conditions have both an underlying etiology and multiple body system manifestations due to the underlying etiology. For such conditions, the ICD-9-CM has a coding convention that requires the underlying condition be sequenced first followed by the manifestation. Wherever such a combination exists, there is a "use additional code" note at the etiology code, and a "code first" note at the manifestation code. These instructional notes indicate the proper sequencing order of the codes, etiology followed by manifestation.

In most cases the manifestation codes will have in the code title, "in diseases classified elsewhere." Codes with this title are a component of the etiology/ manifestation convention. The code title indicates that it is a manifestation code. "In diseases classified elsewhere" codes are never permitted to be used as first listed or principal diagnosis codes. They must be used in conjunction with an underlying condition code and they must be listed following the underlying condition.

There are manifestation codes that do not have "in diseases classified elsewhere" in the title. For such codes a "use additional code" note will still be present and the rules for sequencing apply.

In addition to the notes in the tabular, these conditions also have a specific index entry structure. In the index both conditions are listed together with the etiology code first followed by the manifestation codes in brackets. The code in brackets is always to be sequenced second.

The most commonly used etiology/manifestation combinations are the codes for Diabetes mellitus, category 250. For each code under category 250 there is a use additional code note for the manifestation that is specific for that particular diabetic manifestation. Should a patient have more than one manifestation of diabetes, more than one code from category 250 may be used with as many manifestation codes as are needed to fully describe the patient's complete diabetic condition. The category 250 diabetes codes should be sequenced first, followed by the manifestation codes.

"Code first" and "Use additional code" notes are also used as sequencing rules in the classification for certain codes that are not part of an etiology/ manifestation combination.

See—Section I.B.9. "Multiple coding for a single condition".

7. "And"

The word "and" should be interpreted to mean either "and" or "or" when it appears in a title.

8. "With"

The word "with" in the alphabetic index is sequenced immediately following the main term, not in alphabetical order.

9. "See" and "See Also"

The "see" instruction following a main term in the index indicates that another term should be referenced. It is necessary to go to the main term referenced with the "see" note to locate the correct code.

A "see also" instruction following a main term in the index instructs that there is another main term that may also be referenced that may provide additional index entries that may be useful. It is not necessary to follow the "see also" note when the original main term provides the necessary code.

B. General Coding Guidelines

1. Use of Both Alphabetic Index and Tabular List

Use both the Alphabetic Index and the Tabular List when locating and assigning a code. Reliance on only the Alphabetic Index or the Tabular List leads to errors in code assignments and less specificity in code selection.

2. Locate each term in the Alphabetic Index

Locate each term in the Alphabetic Index and verify the code selected in the Tabular List. Read and be guided by instructional notations that appear in both the Alphabetic Index and the Tabular List.

3. Level of Detail in Coding

Diagnosis and procedure codes are to be used at their highest number of digits available.

ICD-9-CM diagnosis codes are composed of codes with 3, 4, or 5 digits. Codes with three digits are included in ICD-9-CM as the heading of a category of codes that may be further subdivided by the use of fourth and/or fifth digits, which provide greater detail.

A three-digit code is to be used only if it is not further subdivided. Where fourth-digit subcategories and/or fifth-digit subclassifications are provided, they must be assigned. A code is invalid if it has not been coded to the full number of digits required for that code. For example, Acute myocardial infarction, code 410, has fourth digits that describe the location of the infarction (e.g., 410.2, Of inferolateral wall), and fifth digits that identify the episode of care. It would be incorrect to report a code in category 410 without a fourth and fifth digit.

ICD-9-CM Volume 3 procedure codes are composed of codes with either 3 or 4 digits. Codes with two digits are included in ICD-9-CM as the heading of a category of codes that may be further subdivided by the use of third and/or fourth digits, which provide greater detail.

4. **Code or codes from 001.0 through V84.8**

The appropriate code or codes from 001.0 through V84.8 must be used to identify diagnoses, symptoms, conditions, problems, complaints or other reason(s) for the encounter/visit.

5. **Selection of codes 001.0 through 999.9**

The selection of codes 001.0 through 999.9 will frequently be used to describe the reason for the admission/encounter. These codes are from the section of ICD-9-CM for the classification of diseases and injuries (e.g., infectious and parasitic diseases; neoplasms; symptoms, signs, and ill-defined conditions, etc.).

6. **Signs and symptoms**

Codes that describe symptoms and signs, as opposed to diagnoses, are acceptable for reporting purposes when a related definitive diagnosis has not been established (confirmed) by the provider. Chapter 16 of ICD-9-CM, Symptoms, Signs, and Ill-defined conditions (codes 780.0—799.9) contain many, but not all codes for symptoms.

7. **Conditions that are an integral part of a disease process**

Signs and symptoms that are associated routinely with a disease process should not be assigned as additional codes, unless otherwise instructed by the classification.

8. **Conditions that are not an integral part of a disease process**

Additional signs and symptoms that may not be associated routinely with a disease process should be coded when present.

9. **Multiple coding for a single condition**

In addition to the etiology/manifestation convention that requires two codes to fully describe a single condition that affects multiple body systems, there are other single conditions that also require more than one code. "Use additional code" notes are found in the tabular at codes that are not part of an etiology/manifestation pair where a secondary code is useful to fully describe a condition. The sequencing rule is the same as the etiology/manifestation pair—, "use additional code" indicates that a secondary code should be added.

For example, for infections that are not included in chapter 1, a secondary code from category 041, Bacterial infection in conditions classified elsewhere and of unspecified site, may be required to identify the bacterial organism causing the infection. A "use additional code" note will normally be found at the infectious disease code, indicating a need for the organism code to be added as a secondary code.

"Code first" notes are also under certain codes that are not specifically manifestation codes but may be due to an underlying cause. When a "code first" note is present and an underlying condition is present the underlying condition should be sequenced first.

"Code, if applicable, any causal condition first", notes indicate that this code may be assigned as a principal diagnosis when the causal condition is unknown or not applicable. If a causal condition is known, then the code for that condition should be sequenced as the principal or first-listed diagnosis.

Multiple codes may be needed for late effects, complication codes and obstetric codes to more fully describe a condition. See the specific guidelines for these conditions for further instruction.

10. Acute and Chronic Conditions

If the same condition is described as both acute (subacute) and chronic, and separate subentries exist in the Alphabetic Index at the same indentation level, code both and sequence the acute (subacute) code first.

11. Combination Code

A combination code is a single code used to classify:

Two diagnoses, or

A diagnosis with an associated secondary process (manifestation)

A diagnosis with an associated complication

Combination codes are identified by referring to subterm entries in the Alphabetic Index and by reading the inclusion and exclusion notes in the Tabular List.

Assign only the combination code when that code fully identifies the diagnostic conditions involved or when the Alphabetic Index so directs. Multiple coding should not be used when the classification provides a combination code that clearly identifies all of the elements documented in the diagnosis. When the combination code lacks necessary specificity in describing the manifestation or complication, an additional code should be used as a secondary code.

12. Late Effects

A late effect is the residual effect (condition produced) after the acute phase of an illness or injury has terminated. There is no time limit on when a late effect code can be used. The residual may be apparent early, such as in cerebrovascular accident cases, or it may occur months or years later, such as that due to a previous injury. Coding of late effects generally requires two codes sequenced in the following order: The condition or nature of the late effect is sequenced first. The late effect code is sequenced second.

An exception to the above guidelines are those instances where the code for late effect is followed by a manifestation code identified in the Tabular List and title, or the late effect code has been expanded (at the fourth and fifth-digit levels) to include the manifestation(s). The code for the acute phase of an illness or injury that led to the late effect is never used with a code for the late effect.

13. Impending or Threatened Condition

Code any condition described at the time of discharge as "impending" or "threatened" as follows:

If it did occur, code as confirmed diagnosis.

If it did not occur, reference the Alphabetic Index to determine if the condition has a subentry term for "impending" or "threatened" and also reference main term entries for "Impending" and for "Threatened."

If the subterms are listed, assign the given code.

If the subterms are not listed, code the existing underlying condition(s) and not the condition described as impending or threatened.

C. Chapter-Specific Coding Guidelines

In addition to general coding guidelines, there are guidelines for specific diagnoses and/or conditions in the classification. Unless otherwise indicated, these guidelines apply to all health care settings. Please refer to Section II for guidelines on the selection of principal diagnosis.

1. Chapter 1: Infectious and Parasitic Diseases (001-139)

a. Human Immunodeficiency Virus (HIV) Infections

1) Code only confirmed cases

Code only confirmed cases of HIV infection/illness. This is an exception to the hospital inpatient guideline Section II, H.
     In this context, "confirmation" does not require documentation of positive serology or culture for HIV; the provider's diagnostic statement that the patient is HIV positive, or has an HIV-related illness is sufficient.

2) Selection and sequencing of HIV codes

(a) Patient admitted for HIV-related condition

If a patient is admitted for an HIV-related condition, the principal diagnosis should be 042, followed by additional diagnosis codes for all reported HIV-related conditions.

(b) Patient with HIV disease admitted for unrelated condition

If a patient with HIV disease is admitted for an unrelated condition (such as a traumatic injury), the code for the unrelated condition (e.g., the nature of injury code) should be the principal diagnosis. Other diagnoses would be 042 followed by additional diagnosis codes for all reported HIV-related conditions.

(c) Whether the patient is newly diagnosed

Whether the patient is newly diagnosed or has had previous admissions/encounters for HIV conditions is irrelevant to the sequencing decision.

(d) Asymptomatic human immunodeficiency virus

V08 Asymptomatic human immunodeficiency virus [HIV] infection, is to be applied when the patient without any documentation of symptoms is listed as being "HIV positive," "known HIV," "HIV test positive," or similar terminology. Do not use this code if the term "AIDS" is used or if the patient is treated for any HIV-related illness or is described as having any condition(s) resulting from his/her HIV positive status; use 042 in these cases.

(e) Patients with inconclusive HIV serology

Patients with inconclusive HIV serology, but no definitive diagnosis or manifestations of the illness, may be assigned code 795.71, Inconclusive serologic test for Human Immunodeficiency Virus [HIV].

(f) Previously diagnosed HIV-related illness

Patients with any known prior diagnosis of an HIV-related illness should be coded to 042. Once a patient has developed an HIV-related illness, the patient should always be assigned code 042 on every subsequent admission/encounter. Patients previously diagnosed with any HIV illness (042) should never be assigned to 795.71 or V08.

(g) HIV Infection in Pregnancy, Childbirth and the Puerperium

During pregnancy, childbirth or the puerperium, a patient admitted (or presenting for a health care encounter) because of an HIV-related illness should receive a principal diagnosis code of 647.6X, Other specified infectious and parasitic diseases in the mother classifiable elsewhere, but complicating the pregnancy, childbirth or the puerperium, followed by 042 and the code(s) for the HIV-related illness(es). Codes from Chapter 15 always take sequencing priority.

Patients with asymptomatic HIV infection status admitted (or presenting for a health care encounter) during pregnancy, childbirth, or the puerperium should receive codes of 647.6X and V08.

(h) Encounters for testing for HIV

If a patient is being seen to determine his/her HIV status, use code V73.89, Screening for other specified viral disease. Use code V69.8, Other problems related to lifestyle, as a secondary code if an asymptomatic patient is in a known high risk group for HIV. Should a patient with signs or symptoms or illness, or a confirmed HIV related diagnosis be tested for HIV, code the signs and symptoms or the diagnosis. An additional counseling code V65.44 may be used if counseling is provided during the encounter for the test.

When a patient returns to be informed of his/her HIV test results use code V65.44, HIV counseling, if the results of the test are negative.

If the results are positive but the patient is asymptomatic use code V08, Asymptomatic HIV infection. If the results are positive and the patient is symptomatic use code 042, HIV infection, with codes for the HIV related symptoms or diagnosis. The HIV counseling code may also be used if counseling is provided for patients with positive test results.

b. Septicemia, Systemic Inflammatory Response Syndrome (SIRS), Sepsis, Severe Sepsis, and Septic Shock

   1) SIRS, Septicemia, and Sepsis

   (a) The terms *septicemia* and *sepsis* are often used interchangeably by providers, however they are not considered synonymous terms. The following descriptions are provided for reference but do not preclude querying the provider for clarification about terms used in the documentation:

   (i)   Septicemia generally refers to a systemic disease associated with the presence of pathological microorganisms or toxins in the blood, which can include bacteria, viruses, fungi or other organisms.

   (ii)   Systemic inflammatory response syndrome (SIRS) generally refers to the systemic response to infection, trauma/burns, or other insult (such as cancer) with symptoms including fever, tachycardia, tachypnea, and leukocytosis.

   (iii) Sepsis generally refers to SIRS due to infection.

   (iv)   Severe sepsis generally refers to sepsis with associated acute organ dysfunction.

   (b) The Coding of SIRS, sepsis and severe sepsis

   The coding of SIRS, sepsis and severe sepsis requires a minimum of 2 codes: a code for the underlying cause (such as infection or trauma) and a code from subcategory 995.9 Systemic inflammatory response syndrome (SIRS).

   (i)   The code for the underlying cause (such as infection or trauma) must be sequenced before the code from subcategory 995.9 Systemic inflammatory response syndrome (SIRS).

   (ii)   Sepsis and severe sepsis require a code for the systemic infection (038.xx, 112.5, etc.) and either code 995.91, Sepsis, or 995.92, Severe sepsis. If the causal organism is not documented, assign code 038.9, Unspecified septicemia.

   (iii) Severe sepsis requires additional code(s) for the associated acute organ dysfunction(s).

   (iv)   If a patient has sepsis with multiple organ dysfunctions, follow the instructions for coding severe sepsis.

   (v)   Either the term sepsis or SIRS must be documented to assign a code from subcategory 995.9.

   (vi)   *See Section I.C.17.g), Injury and poisoning, for information regarding systemic inflammatory response syndrome (SIRS) due to trauma/burns and other non-infectious processes.*

   (c) Due to the complex nature of sepsis and severe sepsis, some cases may require querying the provider prior to assignment of the codes.

2) Sequencing sepsis and severe sepsis

(a) Sepsis and severe sepsis as principal diagnosis

If sepsis or severe sepsis is present on admission, and meets the definition of principal diagnosis, the systemic infection code (e.g., 038.xx, 112.5, etc) should be assigned as the principal diagnosis, followed by code 995.91, Sepsis, or 995.92, Severe sepsis, as required by the sequencing rules in the Tabular List. Codes from subcategory 995.9 can never be assigned as a principal diagnosis. A code should also be assigned for any localized infection, if present.

If the sepsis or severe sepsis is due to a postprocedural infection, see Section I.C.10 for guidelines related to sepsis due to postprocedural infection.

(b) Sepsis and severe sepsis as secondary diagnoses

When sepsis or severe sepsis develops during the encounter (it was not present on admission), the systemic infection code and code 995.91 or 995.92 should be assigned as secondary diagnoses.

(c) Documentation unclear as to whether sepsis or severe sepsis is present on admission

Sepsis or severe sepsis may be present on admission but the diagnosis may not be confirmed until sometime after admission. If the documentation is not clear whether the sepsis **or severe sepsis** was present on admission, the provider should be queried.

3) Sepsis/SIRS with Localized Infection

If the reason for admission is both sepsis, severe sepsis, or SIRS and a localized infection, such as pneumonia or cellulitis, a code for the systemic infection (038.xx, 112.5, etc) should be assigned first, then code 995.91 or 995.92, followed by the code for the localized infection. If the patient is admitted with a localized infection, such as pneumonia, and sepsis/SIRS doesn't develop until after admission, see guideline I.C.1.b2.b).

In the localized infection is postprocedural, *see Section I.C.10 for guidelines related to sepsis due to postprocedural infection.*

Note: The term urosepsis is a nonspecific term. If that is the only term documented then only code 599.0 should be assigned based on the default for the term in the ICD-9-CM index, in addition to the code for the causal organism if known.

4) Bacterial Sepsis and Septicemia

In most cases, it will be a code from category 038, Septicemia, that will be used in conjunction with a code from subcategory 995.9 such as the following:

(a) Streptococcal sepsis

If the documentation in the record states streptococcal sepsis, codes 038.0, Streptococcal septicemia, and code 995.91 should be used, in that sequence.

(b) Streptococcal septicemia

If the documentation states streptococcal septicemia, only code 038.0 should be assigned, however, the provider should be queried whether the patient has sepsis, an infection with SIRS.

5) Acute organ dysfunction that is not clearly associated with the sepsis

If a patient has sepsis and an acute organ dysfunction, but the medical record documentation indicates that the acute organ dysfunction is related to a medical condition other than the sepsis, do not assign code 995.92, Severe sepsis. An acute organ dysfunction must be associated with the sepsis in order to assign the severe sepsis code. If the documentation is not clear as to whether an acute organ dysfunction is related to the sepsis or another medical condition, query the provider.

6) Septic shock

(a) Sequencing of septic shock

Septic shock generally refers to circulatory failure associated with severe sepsis, and, therefore, it represents a type of acute organ dysfunction.

For all cases of septic shock, the code for the systemic infection should be sequenced first, followed by codes 995.92 and 785.52. Any additional codes for other acute organ dysfunctions should also be assigned. As noted in the sequencing instructions in the Tabular List, the code for septic shock cannot be assigned as a principal diagnosis.

(b) Septic Shock without documentation of severe sepsis

Septic shock indicates the presence of severe sepsis.

Code 995.92, Severe sepsis, must be assigned with code 785.52, Septic shock, even if the term severe sepsis is not documented in the record. The "use additional code" note and the "code first" note in the tabular support this guideline.

7) Sepsis and septic shock complicating abortion and pregnancy

Sepsis and septic shock **complicating** abortion, ectopic pregnancy, and molar pregnancy are classified to category codes in Chapter 11 (630-639).

See section I.C.11.

8) Negative or inconclusive blood cultures

Negative or inconclusive blood cultures do not preclude a diagnosis of septicemia or sepsis in patients with clinical evidence of the condition, however, the provider should be queried.

9) Newborn sepsis

See Section I.C.15.j for information on the coding of newborn sepsis.

10) Sepsis due to a Postprocedural Infection

(a) **Documentation of causal relationship**

As with all postprocedural complications, code assignment is based on the provider's documentation of the relationship between the infection and the procedure.

(b) **Sepsis due to postprocedural infection**

In cases of postprocedural sepsis, the complication code, such as code 998.59, Other postoperative infection, or 674.3x, Other complications of obstetrical surgical wounds should be coded first followed by the appropriate sepsis codes (systemic infection code and either code 995.91or 995.92). An additional code(s) for any acute organ dysfunction should also be assigned for cases of severe sepsis.

11) External cause of injury codes with SIRS

Refer to Section I.C.19.a.7 for instruction on the use of external cause of injury codes with codes for SIRS resulting from trauma.

12) Sepsis and Severe Sepsis Associated with Non-infectious Process

(a) **Sequencing <u>of sepsis/severe sepsis associated with non-infectious process</u>**

In some cases, a non-infectious process, such as trauma, may lead to an infection which can result in sepsis or severe sepsis. If sepsis or severe sepsis is documented as associated with a non-infectious condition, such as a burn or serious injury, and this condition meets the definition for principal diagnosis, the code for the non-infectious condition should be sequenced first, followed by the code for the systemic infection and either code 995.91, Sepsis, or 995.92, Severe sepsis. Additional codes for any associated acute organ dysfunction(s) should also be assigned for cases of severe sepsis. If the sepsis or severe sepsis meets the definition of principal diagnosis, the systemic infection and sepsis codes should be sequenced before the non-infectious condition. When both the associated non-infectious condition and the sepsis or severe sepsis meet the definition of principal diagnosis, either may be assigned as principal diagnosis.

See Section I.C.1.b.2)(a) for guidelines pertaining to sepsis or severe sepsis as the principal diagnosis.

(b) **Only one SIRS (subcategory 995.9) code should be assigned**

Only one code **from subcategory 995.9 should be assigned for SIRS associated with trauma or other non-infectious condition. Assign the SIRS code (subcategory 995.9) that corresponds to the principal diagnosis. That is, if trauma or a non-infectious condition is the underlying cause, assign code 995.93 or 995.94. If an infection is the underlying cause, assign code 995.91 or 995.92.**

See Section I.C.17.g for information on the coding of SIRS due to trauma/burns or other non-infectious disease processes.

2. Chapter 2: Neoplasms (140-239)

General guidelines

Chapter 2 of the ICD-9-CM contains the codes for most benign and all malignant neoplasms. Certain benign neoplasms, such as prostatic adenomas, may be found in the specific body system chapters. To properly code a neoplasm it is necessary to determine from the record if the neoplasm is benign, in-situ, malignant, or of uncertain histologic behavior. If malignant, any secondary (metastatic) sites should also be determined.

The neoplasm table in the Alphabetic Index should be referenced first. However, if the histological term is documented, that term should be referenced first, rather than going immediately to the Neoplasm Table, in order to determine which column in the Neoplasm Table is appropriate. For example, if the documentation indicates "adenoma," refer to the term in the Alphabetic Index to review the entries under this term and the instructional note to "see also neoplasm, by site, benign." The table provides the proper code based on the type of neoplasm and the site. It is important to select the proper column in the table that corresponds to the type of neoplasm. The tabular should then be referenced to verify that the correct code has been selected from the table and that a more specific site code does not exist. *See Section I. C. 18.d.4. for information regarding V codes for genetic susceptibility to cancer.*

a. Treatment directed at the malignancy

If the treatment is directed at the malignancy, designate the malignancy as the principal diagnosis.

b. Treatment of secondary site

When a patient is admitted because of a primary neoplasm with metastasis and treatment is directed toward the secondary site only, the secondary neoplasm is designated as the principal diagnosis even though the primary malignancy is still present.

c. Coding and sequencing of complications

Coding and sequencing of complications associated with the malignancies or with the therapy thereof are subject to the following guidelines:

1) Anemia associated with malignancy

When admission/encounter is for management of an anemia associated with the malignancy, and the treatment is only for anemia, the appropriate anemia code (such as code 285.22, Anemia in neoplastic disease) is designated as the principal diagnosis and is followed by the appropriate code(s) for the malignancy.

Code 285.22 may also be used as a secondary code if the patient suffers from anemia and is being treated for the malignancy.

2) Anemia associated with chemotherapy, immunotherapy and radiation therapy

When the admission/encounter is for management of an anemia associated with chemotherapy, immunotherapy or radiotherapy and the only treatment is for the anemia, the anemia is sequenced first followed by code E933.1. The appropriate neoplasm code should be assigned as an additional code.

3) Management of dehydration due to the malignancy

When the admission/encounter is for management of dehydration due to the malignancy or the therapy, or a combination of both, and only the dehydration is being treated (intravenous rehydration), the dehydration is sequenced first, followed by the code(s) for the malignancy.

4) Treatment of a complication resulting from a surgical procedure

When the admission/encounter is for treatment of a complication resulting from a surgical procedure, designate the complication as the principal or first-listed diagnosis if treatment is directed at resolving the complication.

d. Primary malignancy previously excised

When a primary malignancy has been previously excised or eradicated from its site and there is no further treatment directed to that site and there is no evidence of any existing primary malignancy, a code from category V10, Personal history of malignant neoplasm, should be used to indicate the former site of the malignancy. Any mention of extension, invasion, or metastasis to another site is coded as a secondary malignant neoplasm to that site. The secondary site may be the principal or first-listed with the V10 code used as a secondary code.

e. Admissions/Encounters involving chemotherapy, immunotherapy and radiation therapy

1) Episode of care involves surgical removal of neoplasm

When an episode of care involves the surgical removal of a neoplasm, primary or secondary site, followed by adjunct chemotherapy or radiation treatment during the same episode of care, the neoplasm code should be assigned as principal or first-listed diagnosis, using codes in the 140-198 series or where appropriate in the 200-203 series.

2) Patient admission/encounter solely for administration of chemotherapy, immunotherapy and radiation therapy

If a patient admission/encounter is solely for the administration of chemotherapy, immunotherapy or radiation therapy assign code V58.0, Encounter for radiation therapy, or V58.11, Encounter for antineoplastic chemotherapy, or V58.12, Encounter for antineoplastic immunotherapy as the first-listed or principal diagnosis. If a patient receives more than one of these therapies during the same admission more than one of these codes may be assigned, in any sequence.

3) Patient admitted for radiotherapy/chemotherapy and immunotherapy and develops complications

When a patient is admitted for the purpose of radiotherapy, immunotherapy or chemotherapy and develops complications such as uncontrolled nausea and vomiting or dehydration, the principal or first-listed diagnosis is V58.0, Encounter for radiotherapy, or V58.11, Encounter for antineoplastic chemotherapy, or V58.12, Encounter for antineoplastic immunotherapy followed by any codes for the complications.

f. Admission/encounter to determine extent of malignancy

When the reason for admission/encounter is to determine the extent of the malignancy, or for a procedure such as paracentesis or thoracentesis, the primary malignancy or appropriate metastatic site is designated as the principal or first-listed diagnosis, even though chemotherapy or radiotherapy is administered.

g. Symptoms, signs, and ill-defined conditions listed in Chapter 16 <u>associated with neoplasms</u>

Symptoms, signs, and ill-defined conditions listed in Chapter 16 characteristic of, or associated with, an existing primary or secondary site malignancy cannot be used to replace the malignancy as principal or first-listed diagnosis, regardless of the number of admissions or encounters for treatment and care of the neoplasm.
    See section I.C.18.d.14, Encounter for prophylactic organ removal.

h. Admission/encounter for pain control/management

See Section I.C.6.a.5 for information on coding admission/encounter for pain control/management.

3. Chapter 3: Endocrine, Nutritional, and Metabolic Diseases and Immunity Disorders (240-279)

a. Diabetes mellitus

Codes under category 250, Diabetes mellitus, identify complications/manifestations associated with diabetes mellitus. A fifth-digit is required for all category 250 codes to identify the type of diabetes mellitus and whether the diabetes is controlled or uncontrolled.

1) Fifth-digits for category 250:

The following are the fifth-digits for the codes under category 250:
0 type II or unspecified type, not stated as uncontrolled
1 type I, [juvenile type], not stated as uncontrolled
2 type II or unspecified type, uncontrolled
3 type I, [juvenile type], uncontrolled
    The age of a patient is not the sole determining factor, though most type I diabetics develop the condition before reaching puberty. For this reason type I diabetes mellitus is also referred to as juvenile diabetes.

2) Type of diabetes mellitus not documented

If the type of diabetes mellitus is not documented in the medical record the default is type II.

3) Diabetes mellitus and the use of insulin

All type I diabetics must use insulin to replace what their bodies do not produce. However, the use of insulin does not mean that a patient is a type I diabetic. Some patients with type II diabetes mellitus are unable to control their blood sugar through diet and oral medication alone and do require insulin. If the documentation in a medical record does not indicate the type of diabetes but does indicate that the patient uses insulin, the appropriate fifth-digit for type II must be used. For type II patients who routinely use insulin, code V58.67, Long-term (current) use of insulin, should also be assigned to indicate that the patient uses insulin. Code V58.67 should not be assigned if insulin is given temporarily to bring a type II patient's blood sugar under control during an encounter.

4) Assigning and sequencing diabetes codes and associated conditions

When assigning codes for diabetes and its associated conditions, the code(s) from category 250 must be sequenced before the codes for the associated conditions. The diabetes codes and the secondary codes that correspond to them are paired codes that follow the etiology/manifestation convention of the classification *(See Section I.A.6., Etiology/manifestation convention).* Assign as many codes from category 250 as needed to identify all of the associated conditions that the patient has. The corresponding secondary codes are listed under each of the diabetes codes.

(a) Diabetic retinopathy/diabetic macular edema

Diabetic macular edema, code 362.07, is only present with diabetic retinopathy. Another code from subcategory 362.0, Diabetic retinopathy, must be used with code 362.07. Codes under subcategory 362.0 are diabetes manifestation codes, so they must be used following the appropriate diabetes code.

5) Diabetes mellitus in pregnancy and gestational diabetes

(a) For diabetes mellitus complicating pregnancy, see Section I.C.11.f., Diabetes mellitus in pregnancy.

(b) For gestational diabetes, see Section I.C.11, g., Gestational diabetes.

6) Insulin pump malfunction

(a) Underdose of insulin due insulin pump failure

An underdose of insulin due to an insulin pump failure should be assigned 996.57, Mechanical complication due to insulin pump, as the principal or first listed code, followed by the appropriate diabetes mellitus code based on documentation.

(b) Overdose of insulin due to insulin pump failure

The principal or first listed code for an encounter due to an insulin pump malfunction resulting in an overdose of insulin, should also be 996.57, Mechanical complication due to insulin pump, followed by code 962.3, Poisoning by insulins and antidiabetic agents, and the appropriate diabetes mellitus code based on documentation.

4. **Chapter 4: Diseases of Blood and Blood Forming Organs (280-289)**

   a. **Anemia of chronic disease**

   Subcategory 285.2, Anemia in chronic illness, has codes for anemia in chronic kidney disease, code 285.21; anemia in neoplastic disease, code 285.22; and anemia in other chronic illness, code 285.29. These codes can be used as the principal/first listed code if the reason for the encounter is to treat the anemia. They may also be used as secondary codes if treatment of the anemia is a component of an encounter, but not the primary reason for the encounter. When using a code from subcategory 285 it is also necessary to use the code for the chronic condition causing the anemia.

   1) **Anemia in chronic kidney disease**

      When assigning code 285.21, Anemia in chronic kidney disease, it is also necessary to assign a code from category 585, Chronic kidney disease, to indicate the stage of chronic kidney disease.

      See I.C.10.a. Chronic kidney disease (CKD).

   2) **Anemia in neoplastic disease**

      When assigning code 285.22, Anemia in neoplastic disease, it is also necessary to assign the neoplasm code that is responsible for the anemia. Code 285.22 is for use for anemia that is due to the malignancy, not for anemia due to antineoplastic chemotherapy drugs, which is an adverse effect.

      See I.C.2.c.1 Anemia associated with malignancy.

      See I.C.2.c.2 Anemia associated with chemotherapy, immunotherapy and radiation therapy.

      See I.C.17.e.1. Adverse effects.

5. **Chapter 5: Mental Disorders (290-319)**

   Reserved for future guideline expansion

6. **Chapter 6: Diseases of Nervous System and Sense Organs (320-389)**

   a. **Pain - Category 338**

   1) **General coding information**

      Codes in category 338 may be used in conjunction with codes from other categories and chapters to provide more detail about acute or chronic pain and neoplasm-related pain, unless otherwise indicated below.

      If the pain is not specified as acute or chronic, do not assign codes from category 338, except for post-thoracotomy pain, postoperative pain or neoplasm related pain, or central pain syndrome.

      A code from subcategories 338.1 and 338.2 should not be assigned if the underlying (definitive) diagnosis is known, unless the reason for the encounter is pain control/management and not management of the underlying condition.

(a) Category 338 Codes as Principal or First-Listed Diagnosis

Category 338 codes are acceptable as principal diagnosis or the first-listed code:

- When pain control or pain management is the reason for the admission/encounter (e.g., a patient with displaced intervertebral disc, nerve impingement and severe back pain presents for injection of steroid into the spinal canal). The underlying cause of the pain should be reported as an additional diagnosis, if known.

- When an admission or encounter is for a procedure aimed at treating the underlying condition (e.g., spinal fusion, kyphoplasty), a code for the underlying condition (e.g., vertebral fracture, spinal stenosis) should be assigned as the principal diagnosis. No code from category 338 should be assigned.

- When a patient is admitted for the insertion of a neurostimulator for pain control, assign the appropriate pain code as the principal or first listed diagnosis. When an admission or encounter is for a procedure aimed at treating the underlying condition and a neurostimulator is inserted for pain control during the same admission/encounter, a code for the underlying condition should be assigned as the principal diagnosis and the appropriate pain code should be assigned as a secondary diagnosis.

(b) Use of Category 338 Codes in Conjunction with Site Specific Pain Codes

(i) Assigning Category 338 Codes and Site-Specific Pain Codes

Codes from category 338 may be used in conjunction with codes that identify the site of pain (including codes from chapter 16) if the category 338 code provides additional information. For example, if the code describes the site of the pain, but does not fully describe whether the pain is acute or chronic, then both codes should be assigned.

(ii) Sequencing of Category 338 Codes with Site-Specific Pain Codes

The sequencing of category 338 codes with site-specific pain codes (including chapter 16 codes), is dependent on the circumstances of the encounter/admission as follows:

- If the encounter is for pain control or pain management, assign the code from category 338 followed by the code identifying the specific site of pain (e.g., encounter for pain management for acute neck pain from trauma is assigned code 338.11, Acute pain due to trauma, followed by code 723.1, Cervicalgia, to identify the site of pain).

- If the encounter is for any other reason except pain control or pain management, and a related definitive diagnosis has not been established (confirmed) by the provider, assign the code for the specific site of pain first, followed by the appropriate code from category 338.

2) Pain due to devices, <u>implants and grafts</u>

Pain associated with devices, **implants and grafts** left in a surgical site **(for example painful hip prosthesis)** is assigned to the appropriate code(s) found in Chapter 17, Injury and Poisoning. Use additional code(s) from category 338 to identify acute or chronic pain due to presence of the device, implant or graft (338.18-338.19 or 338.28-338.29).

3) Postoperative Pain

Post-thoracotomy pain and other postoperative pain are classified to subcategories 338.1 and 338.2, depending on whether the pain is acute or chronic. The default for post-thoracotomy and other postoperative pain not specified as acute or chronic is the code for the acute form.

<u>Routine or expected postoperative pain immediately after surgery should not be coded.</u>

(a) Postoperative pain not associated with specific postoperative complication

Postoperative pain not associated with a specific postoperative complication is assigned to the appropriate postoperative pain code in category 338.

(b) Postoperative pain associated with specific postoperative complication

Postoperative pain associated with a specific postoperative complication (such as **painful suture wires**) is assigned to the appropriate code(s) found in Chapter 17, Injury and Poisoning. **If appropriate, use additional code(s) from category 338 to identify acute or chronic pain (338.18 or 338.28).** If pain control/management is the reason for the encounter, a code from category 338 should be assigned as the principal or first-listed diagnosis in accordance with *Section I.C.6.a.1.a above.*

(c) Postoperative pain as principal or first-listed diagnosis

Postoperative pain may be reported as the principal or first-listed diagnosis when the stated reason for the admission/encounter is documented as postoperative pain control/management.

(d) Postoperative pain as secondary diagnosis

Postoperative pain may be reported as a secondary diagnosis code when a patient presents for outpatient surgery and develops an unusual or inordinate amount of postoperative pain.

Routine or expected postoperative pain immediately after surgery should not be coded.

The provider's documentation should be used to guide the coding of postoperative pain, as well as *Section III. Reporting Additional Diagnoses and Section IV. Diagnostic Coding and Reporting in the Outpatient Setting.*

See Section II.I.2 for information on sequencing of diagnoses for patients admitted to hospital inpatient care following post-operative observation.

See Section II.J for information on sequencing of diagnoses for patients admitted to hospital inpatient care from outpatient surgery.

See Section IV.A.2 for information on sequencing of diagnoses for patients admitted for observation.

4) Chronic pain

Chronic pain is classified to subcategory 338.2. There is no time frame defining when pain becomes chronic pain. The provider's documentation should be used to guide use of these codes.

5) Neoplasm Related Pain

Code 338.3 is assigned to pain documented as being related, associated or due to cancer, primary or secondary malignancy, or tumor. This code is assigned regardless of whether the pain is acute or chronic.

This code may be assigned as the principal or first-listed code when the stated reason for the admission/encounter is documented as pain control/pain management. The underlying neoplasm should be reported as an additional diagnosis.

When the reason for the admission/encounter is management of the neoplasm and the pain associated with the neoplasm is also documented, code 338.3 may be assigned as an additional diagnosis.

See Section I.C.2 for instructions on the sequencing of neoplasms for all other stated reasons for the admission/encounter (except for pain control/pain management).

6) Chronic pain syndrome

This condition is different than the term "chronic pain," and therefore this code should only be used when the provider has specifically documented this condition.

7. Chapter 7: Diseases of Circulatory System (390-459)

a. Hypertension

Hypertension Table

The Hypertension Table, found under the main term, "Hypertension", in the Alphabetic Index, contains a complete listing of all conditions due to or associated with hypertension and classifies them according to malignant, benign, and unspecified.

1) Hypertension, Essential, or NOS

Assign hypertension (arterial) (essential) (primary) (systemic) (NOS) to category code 401 with the appropriate fourth digit to indicate malignant (.0), benign (.1), or unspecified (.9). Do not use either .0 malignant or .1 benign unless medical record documentation supports such a designation.

2) Hypertension with Heart Disease

Heart conditions (425.8, 429.0-429.3, 429.8, 429.9) are assigned to a code from category 402 when a causal relationship is stated (due to hypertension) or implied (hypertensive). Use an additional code from category 428 to identify the type of heart failure in those patients with heart failure. More than one code from category 428 may be assigned if the patient has systolic or diastolic failure and congestive heart failure.

The same heart conditions (425.8, 429.0-429.3, 429.8, 429.9) with hypertension, but without a stated causal relationship, are coded separately. Sequence according to the circumstances of the admission/encounter.

3) Hypertensive Chronic Kidney Disease

Assign codes from category 403, Hypertensive chronic kidney disease, when conditions classified to categories 585-587 are present. Unlike hypertension with heart disease, ICD-9-CM presumes a cause-and-effect relationship and classifies chronic kidney disease (CKD) with hypertension as hypertensive chronic kidney disease.

Fifth digits for category 403 should be assigned as follows:

- 0 with CKD stage I through stage IV, or unspecified.

- 1 with CKD stage V or end stage renal disease. The appropriate code from category 585, Chronic kidney disease, should be used as a secondary code with a code from category 403 to identify the stage of chronic kidney disease.

See Section I.C.10.a for information on the coding of chronic kidney disease.

4) Hypertensive Heart and Chronic Kidney Disease

Assign codes from combination category 404, Hypertensive heart and chronic kidney disease, when both hypertensive kidney disease and hypertensive heart disease are stated in the diagnosis. Assume a relationship between the hypertension and the chronic kidney disease, whether or not the condition is so designated. Assign an additional code from category 428, to identify the type of heart failure. More than one code from category 428 may be assigned if the patient has systolic or diastolic failure and congestive heart failure.

Fifth digits for category 404 should be assigned as follows:

- 0 without heart failure and with chronic kidney disease (CKD) stage I through stage IV, or unspecified

- 1 with heart failure and with CKD stage I through stage IV, or unspecified

- 2 without heart failure and with CKD stage V or end stage renal disease

- 3 with heart failure and with CKD stage V or end stage renal disease

The appropriate code from category 585, Chronic kidney disease, should be used as a secondary code with a code from category 404 to identify the stage of kidney disease. *See Section I.C.10.a for information on the coding of chronic kidney disease.*

5) Hypertensive Cerebrovascular Disease

First assign codes from 430-438, Cerebrovascular disease, then the appropriate hypertension code from categories 401-405.

6) Hypertensive Retinopathy

Two codes are necessary to identify the condition. First assign the code from subcategory 362.11, Hypertensive retinopathy, then the appropriate code from categories 401-405 to indicate the type of hypertension.

7) Hypertension, Secondary

Two codes are required: one to identify the underlying etiology and one from category 405 to identify the hypertension. Sequencing of codes is determined by the reason for admission/encounter.

8) Hypertension, Transient

Assign code 796.2, Elevated blood pressure reading without diagnosis of hypertension, unless patient has an established diagnosis of hypertension. Assign code 642.3x for transient hypertension of pregnancy.

9) Hypertension, Controlled

Assign appropriate code from categories 401-405. This diagnostic statement usually refers to an existing state of hypertension under control by therapy.

10) Hypertension, Uncontrolled

Uncontrolled hypertension may refer to untreated hypertension or hypertension not responding to current therapeutic regimen. In either case, assign the appropriate code from categories 401-405 to designate the stage and type of hypertension. Code to the type of hypertension.

11) Elevated Blood Pressure

For a statement of elevated blood pressure without further specificity, assign code 796.2, Elevated blood pressure reading without diagnosis of hypertension, rather than a code from category 401.

b. Cerebral infarction/stroke/cerebrovascular accident (CVA)

The terms stroke and CVA are often used interchangeably to refer to a cerebral infarction. The terms stroke, CVA, and cerebral infarction NOS are all indexed to the default code 434.91, Cerebral artery occlusion, unspecified, with infarction. Code 436, Acute, but ill-defined, cerebrovascular disease, should not be used when the documentation states stroke or CVA.

c. Postoperative cerebrovascular accident

A cerebrovascular hemorrhage or infarction that occurs as a result of medical intervention is coded to 997.02, Iatrogenic cerebrovascular infarction or hemorrhage. Medical record documentation should clearly specify the cause- and-effect relationship between the medical intervention and the cerebrovascular accident in order to assign this code. A secondary code from the code range 430-432 or from a code from subcategories 433 or 434 with a fifth digit of "1" should also be used to identify the type of hemorrhage or infarct.

This guideline conforms to the use additional code note instruction at category 997. Code 436, Acute, but ill-defined, cerebrovascular disease, should not be used as a secondary code with code 997.02.

d. Late Effects of Cerebrovascular Disease

1) Category 438, Late Effects of Cerebrovascular disease

Category 438 is used to indicate conditions classifiable to categories 430-437 as the causes of late effects (neurologic deficits), themselves classified elsewhere. These "late effects" include neurologic deficits that persist after initial onset of conditions classifiable to 430-437. The neurologic deficits caused by cerebrovascular disease may be present from the onset or may arise at any time after the onset of the condition classifiable to 430-437.

2) Codes from category 438 with codes from 430-437

Codes from category 438 may be assigned on a health care record with codes from 430-437, if the patient has a current cerebrovascular accident (CVA) and deficits from an old CVA.

3) Code V12.54

Assign code V12.**54, Transient ischemic attack (TIA), and cerebral infarction without residual deficits** (and not a code from category 438) as an additional code for history of cerebrovascular disease when no neurologic deficits are present.

e. Acute myocardial infarction (AMI)

1) ST elevation myocardial infarction (STEMI) and non ST elevation myocardial infarction (NSTEMI)

The ICD-9-CM codes for acute myocardial infarction (AMI) identify the site, such as anterolateral wall or true posterior wall. Subcategories 410.0-410.6 and 410.8 are used for ST elevation myocardial infarction (STEMI). Subcategory 410.7, Subendocardial infarction, is used for non ST elevation myocardial infarction (NSTEMI) and nontransmural MIs.

2) Acute myocardial infarction, unspecified

Subcategory 410.9 is the default for the unspecified term acute myocardial infarction. If only STEMI or transmural MI without the site is documented, query the provider as to the site, or assign a code from subcategory 410.9.

3) AMI documented as nontransmural or subendocardial but site provided

If an AMI is documented as nontransmural or subendocardial, but the site is provided, it is still coded as a subendocardial AMI. If NSTEMI evolves to STEMI, assign the STEMI code. If STEMI converts to NSTEMI due to thrombolytic therapy, it is still coded as STEMI.

8. **Chapter 8: Diseases of Respiratory System (460-519)**

   a. **Chronic Obstructive Pulmonary Disease [COPD] and Asthma**

      1) **Conditions that comprise COPD and Asthma**

      The conditions that comprise COPD are obstructive chronic bronchitis, subcategory 491.2, and emphysema, category 492. All asthma codes are under category 493, Asthma. Code 496, Chronic airway obstruction, not elsewhere classified, is a nonspecific code that should only be used when the documentation in a medical record does not specify the type of COPD being treated.

      2) **Acute exacerbation of chronic obstructive bronchitis and asthma**

      The codes for chronic obstructive bronchitis and asthma distinguish between uncomplicated cases and those in acute exacerbation. An acute exacerbation is a worsening or a decompensation of a chronic condition. An acute exacerbation is not equivalent to an infection superimposed on a chronic condition, though an exacerbation may be triggered by an infection.

      3) **Overlapping nature of the conditions that comprise COPD and asthma**

      Due to the overlapping nature of the conditions that make up COPD and asthma, there are many variations in the way these conditions are documented. Code selection must be based on the terms as documented. When selecting the correct code for the documented type of COPD and asthma, it is essential to first review the index, and then verify the code in the tabular list. There are many instructional notes under the different COPD subcategories and codes. It is important that all such notes be reviewed to assure correct code assignment.

      4) **Acute exacerbation of asthma and status asthmaticus**

      An acute exacerbation of asthma is an increased severity of the asthma symptoms, such as wheezing and shortness of breath. Status asthmaticus refers to a patient's failure to respond to therapy administered during an asthmatic episode and is a life threatening complication that requires emergency care. If status asthmaticus is documented by the provider with any type of COPD or with acute bronchitis, the status asthmaticus should be sequenced first. It supersedes any type of COPD including that with acute exacerbation or acute bronchitis. It is inappropriate to assign an asthma code with 5th digit 2, with acute exacerbation, together with an asthma code with 5th digit 1, with status asthmatics. Only the 5th digit 1 should be assigned.

   b. **Chronic Obstructive Pulmonary Disease [COPD] and Bronchitis**

      1) **Acute bronchitis with COPD**

      Acute bronchitis, code 466.0, is due to an infectious organism. When acute bronchitis is documented with COPD, code 491.22, Obstructive chronic bronchitis with acute bronchitis, should be assigned. It is not necessary to also assign code 466.0. If a medical record documents acute bronchitis with COPD with acute exacerbation, only code 491.22 should be assigned. The acute bronchitis included in code 491.22 supersedes the acute exacerbation. If a medical record documents COPD with acute exacerbation without mention of acute bronchitis, only code 491.21 should be assigned.

c. **Acute Respiratory Failure**

1) **Acute respiratory failure as principal diagnosis**

Code 518.81, Acute respiratory failure, may be assigned as a principal diagnosis when it is the condition established after study to be chiefly responsible for occasioning the admission to the hospital, and the selection is supported by the Alphabetic Index and Tabular List. However, chapter-specific coding guidelines (such as obstetrics, poisoning, HIV, newborn) that provide sequencing direction take precedence.

2) **Acute respiratory failure as secondary diagnosis**

Respiratory failure may be listed as a secondary diagnosis if it occurs after admission, or if it is present on admission, but does not meet the definition of principal diagnosis.

3) **Sequencing of acute respiratory failure and another acute condition**

When a patient is admitted with respiratory failure and another acute condition, (e.g., myocardial infarction, cerebrovascular accident), the principal diagnosis will not be the same in every situation. Selection of the principal diagnosis will be dependent on the circumstances of admission. If both the respiratory failure and the other acute condition are equally responsible for occasioning the admission to the hospital, and there are no chapter-specific sequencing rules, the guideline regarding two or more diagnoses that equally meet the definition for principal diagnosis *(Section II, C.)* may be applied in these situations.

If the documentation is not clear as to whether acute respiratory failure and another condition are equally responsible for occasioning the admission, query the provider for clarification.

d. **Influenza due to identified avian influenza virus (avian influenza)**

Code only confirmed cases of avian influenza. This is an exception to the hospital inpatient guideline Section II, H. (Uncertain Diagnosis).

In this context, "confirmation" does not require documentation of positive laboratory testing specific for avian influenza. However, coding should be based on the provider's diagnostic statement that the patient has avian influenza.

If the provider records "suspected or possible or probable avian influenza," the appropriate influenza code from category 487 should be assigned. Code 488, Influenza due to identified avian influenza virus, should not be assigned.

9. **Chapter 9: Diseases of Digestive System (520-579)**

Reserved for future guideline expansion

10. **Chapter 10: Diseases of Genitourinary System (580-629)**

a. **Chronic kidney disease**

1) **Stages of chronic kidney disease (CKD)**

The ICD-9-CM classifies CKD based on severity. The severity of CKD is designated by stages I-V. Stage II, code 585.2, equates to mild CKD; stage III, code 585.3, equates to moderate CKD; and stage IV, code 585.4, equates to severe CKD. Code 585.6, End stage renal disease (ESRD), is assigned when the provider has documented end-stage-renal disease (ESRD).

If both a stage of CKD and ESRD are documented, assign code 585.6 only.

2) **Chronic kidney disease and kidney transplant status**

Patients who have undergone kidney transplant may still have some form of CKD, because the kidney transplant may not fully restore kidney function. Therefore, the presence of CKD alone does not constitute a transplant complication. Assign the appropriate 585 code for the patient's stage of CKD and code V42.0. If a transplant complication such as failure or rejection is documented, see section I.C.17.f.1.b for information on coding complications of a kidney transplant. If the documentation is unclear as to whether the patient has a complication of the transplant, query the provider.

3) **Chronic kidney disease with other conditions**

Patients with CKD may also suffer from other serious conditions, most commonly diabetes mellitus and hypertension. The sequencing of the CKD code in relationship to codes for other contributing conditions is based on the conventions in the tabular list.

See I.C.3.a.4 for sequencing instructions for diabetes.

See I.C.4.a.1 for anemia in CKD.

See I.C.7.a.3 for hypertensive chronic kidney disease.

See I.C.17.f.1.b, Kidney transplant complications, for instructions on coding of documented rejection or failure.

11. **Chapter 11: Complications of Pregnancy, Childbirth, and the Puerperium (630-677)**

a. **General Rules for Obstetric Cases**

1) **Codes from chapter 11 and sequencing priority**

Obstetric cases require codes from chapter 11, codes in the range 630-677, Complications of Pregnancy, Childbirth, and the Puerperium. Chapter 11 codes have sequencing priority over codes from other chapters. Additional codes from other chapters may be used in conjunction with chapter 11 codes to further specify conditions. Should the provider document that the pregnancy is incidental to the encounter, then code V22.2 should be used in place of any chapter 11 codes. It is the provider's responsibility to state that the condition being treated is not affecting the pregnancy.

2) Chapter 11 codes used only on the maternal record

Chapter 11 codes are to be used only on the maternal record, never on the record of the newborn.

3) Chapter 11 fifth-digits

Categories 640-648, 651-676 have required fifth-digits, which indicate whether the encounter is antepartum, postpartum and whether a delivery has also occurred.

4) Fifth-digits, appropriate for each code

The fifth-digits, which are appropriate for each code number, are listed in brackets under each code. The fifth-digits on each code should all be consistent with each other. That is, should a delivery occur all of the fifth-digits should indicate the delivery.

b. Selection of OB Principal or First-listed Diagnosis

1) Routine outpatient prenatal visits

For routine outpatient prenatal visits when no complications are present codes V22.0, Supervision of normal first pregnancy, and V22.1, Supervision of other normal pregnancy, should be used as the first-listed diagnoses. These codes should not be used in conjunction with chapter 11 codes.

2) Prenatal outpatient visits for high-risk patients

For prenatal outpatient visits for patients with high-risk pregnancies, a code from category V23, Supervision of high-risk pregnancy, should be used as the principal or first-listed diagnosis. Secondary chapter 11 codes may be used in conjunction with these codes if appropriate.

3) Episodes when no delivery occurs

In episodes when no delivery occurs, the principal diagnosis should correspond to the principal complication of the pregnancy, which necessitated the encounter. Should more than one complication exist, all of which are treated or monitored, any of the complications codes may be sequenced first.

4) When a delivery occurs

When a delivery occurs, the principal diagnosis should correspond to the main circumstances or complication of the delivery. In cases of cesarean delivery, the selection of the principal diagnosis should correspond to the reason the cesarean delivery was performed unless the reason for admission/encounter was unrelated to the condition resulting in the cesarean delivery.

5) Outcome of delivery

An outcome of delivery code, V27.0-V27.9, should be included on every maternal record when a delivery has occurred. These codes are not to be used on subsequent records or on the newborn record.

c. Fetal Conditions Affecting the Management of the Mother

1) Codes from category 655

Known or suspected fetal abnormality affecting management of the mother, and category 656, Other fetal and placental problems affecting the management of the mother, are assigned only when the fetal condition is actually responsible for modifying the management of the mother, i.e., by requiring diagnostic studies, additional observation, special care, or termination of pregnancy. The fact that the fetal condition exists does not justify assigning a code from this series to the mother's record.

2) In utero surgery

In cases when surgery is performed on the fetus, a diagnosis code from category 655, Known or suspected fetal abnormalities affecting management of the mother, should be assigned identifying the fetal condition. Procedure code 75.36, Correction of fetal defect, should be assigned on the hospital inpatient record.

No code from Chapter 15, the perinatal codes, should be used on the mother's record to identify fetal conditions. Surgery performed in utero on a fetus is still to be coded as an obstetric encounter.

d. HIV Infection in Pregnancy, Childbirth and the Puerperium

During pregnancy, childbirth or the puerperium, a patient admitted because of an HIV-related illness should receive a principal diagnosis of 647.6X, Other specified infectious and parasitic diseases in the mother classifiable elsewhere, but complicating the pregnancy, childbirth or the puerperium, followed by 042 and the code(s) for the HIV-related illness(es).

Patients with asymptomatic HIV infection status admitted during pregnancy, childbirth, or the puerperium should receive codes of 647.6X and V08.

e. Current Conditions Complicating Pregnancy

Assign a code from subcategory 648.x for patients that have current conditions when the condition affects the management of the pregnancy, childbirth, or the puerperium. Use additional secondary codes from other chapters to identify the conditions, as appropriate.

f. Diabetes mellitus in pregnancy

Diabetes mellitus is a significant complicating factor in pregnancy. Pregnant women who are diabetic should be assigned code 648.0x, Diabetes mellitus complicating pregnancy, and a secondary code from category 250, Diabetes mellitus, to identify the type of diabetes.

Code V58.67, Long-term (current) use of insulin, should also be assigned if the diabetes mellitus is being treated with insulin.

g. Gestational diabetes

Gestational diabetes can occur during the second and third trimester of pregnancy in women who were not diabetic prior to pregnancy. Gestational diabetes can cause complications in the pregnancy similar to those of pre-existing diabetes mellitus. It also puts the woman at greater risk of developing diabetes after the pregnancy.

Gestational diabetes is coded to 648.8x, Abnormal glucose tolerance. Codes 648.0x and 648.8x should never be used together on the same record.

Code V58.67, Long-term (current) use of insulin, should also be assigned if the gestational diabetes is being treated with insulin.

h. Normal Delivery, Code 650

1) Normal delivery

Code 650 is for use in cases when a woman is admitted for a full-term normal delivery and delivers a single, healthy infant without any complications antepartum, during the delivery, or postpartum during the delivery episode. Code 650 is always a principal diagnosis. It is not to be used if any other code from chapter 11 is needed to describe a current complication of the antenatal, delivery, or perinatal period. Additional codes from other chapters may be used with code 650 if they are not related to or are in any way complicating the pregnancy.

2) Normal delivery with resolved antepartum complication

Code 650 may be used if the patient had a complication at some point during her pregnancy, but the complication is not present at the time of the admission for delivery.

3) V27.0, Single liveborn, outcome of delivery

V27.0, Single liveborn, is the only outcome of delivery code appropriate for use with 650.

i. The Postpartum and Peripartum Periods

1) Postpartum and peripartum periods

The postpartum period begins immediately after delivery and continues for six weeks following delivery. The peripartum period is defined as the last month of pregnancy to five months postpartum.

2) Postpartum complication

A postpartum complication is any complication occurring within the six-week period.

3) Pregnancy-related complications after 6 week period

Chapter 11 codes may also be used to describe pregnancy-related complications after the six-week period should the provider document that a condition is pregnancy related.

4) Postpartum complications occurring during the same admission as delivery

Postpartum complications that occur during the same admission as the delivery are identified with a fifth digit of "2." Subsequent admissions/encounters for postpartum complications should be identified with a fifth digit of "4."

5) Admission for routine postpartum care following delivery outside hospital

When the mother delivers outside the hospital prior to admission and is admitted for routine postpartum care and no complications are noted, code V24.0, Postpartum care and examination immediately after delivery, should be assigned as the principal diagnosis.

6) Admission following delivery outside hospital with postpartum conditions

A delivery diagnosis code should not be used for a woman who has delivered prior to admission to the hospital. Any postpartum conditions and/or postpartum procedures should be coded.

j. Code 677, Late effect of complication of pregnancy

1) Code 677

Code 677, Late effect of complication of pregnancy, childbirth, and the puerperium is for use in those cases when an initial complication of a pregnancy develops a sequelae requiring care or treatment at a future date.

2) After the initial postpartum period

This code may be used at any time after the initial postpartum period.

3) Sequencing of Code 677

This code, like all late effect codes, is to be sequenced following the code describing the sequelae of the complication.

k. Abortions

1) Fifth-digits required for abortion categories

Fifth-digits are required for abortion categories 634-637. Fifth-digit 1, incomplete, indicates that all of the products of conception have not been expelled from the uterus. Fifth-digit 2, complete, indicates that all products of conception have been expelled from the uterus prior to the episode of care.

2) Code from categories 640-648 and 651-659

A code from categories 640-648 and 651-659 may be used as additional codes with an abortion code to indicate the complication leading to the abortion.

Fifth digit 3 is assigned with codes from these categories when used with an abortion code because the other fifth digits will not apply. Codes from the 660-669 series are not to be used for complications of abortion.

3) Code 639 for complications

Code 639 is to be used for all complications following abortion. Code 639 cannot be assigned with codes from categories 634-638.

4) Abortion with Liveborn Fetus

When an attempted termination of pregnancy results in a liveborn fetus assign code 644.21, Early onset of delivery, with an appropriate code from category V27, Outcome of Delivery. The procedure code for the attempted termination of pregnancy should also be assigned.

5) Retained Products of Conception following an abortion

Subsequent admissions for retained products of conception following a spontaneous or legally induced abortion are assigned the appropriate code from category 634, Spontaneous abortion, or 635 Legally induced abortion, with a fifth digit of "1" (incomplete). This advice is appropriate even when the patient was discharged previously with a discharge diagnosis of complete abortion.

12. Chapter 12: Diseases Skin and Subcutaneous Tissue (680-709)

Reserved for future guideline expansion

13. Chapter 13: Diseases of Musculoskeletal and Connective Tissue (710-739)

a. Coding of Pathologic Fractures

1) Acute Fractures vs. Aftercare

Pathologic fractures are reported using subcategory 733.1, when the fracture is newly diagnosed. Subcategory 733.1 may be used while the patient is receiving active treatment for the fracture. Examples of active treatment are: surgical treatment, emergency department encounter, evaluation and treatment by a new physician.

Fractures are coded using the aftercare codes (subcategories V54.0, V54.2, V54.8 or V54.9) for encounters after the patient has completed active treatment of the fracture and is receiving routine care for the fracture during the healing or recovery phase. Examples of fracture aftercare are: cast change or removal, removal of external or internal fixation device, medication adjustment, and follow up visits following fracture treatment.

Care for complications of surgical treatment for fracture repairs during the healing or recovery phase should be coded with the appropriate complication codes.

Care of complications of fractures, such as malunion and nonunion, should be reported with the appropriate codes.

See Section I. C. 17.b for information on the coding of traumatic fractures.

14. Chapter 14: Congenital Anomalies (740-759)

a. Codes in categories 740-759, Congenital Anomalies

Assign an appropriate code(s) from categories 740-759, Congenital Anomalies, when an anomaly is documented. A congenital anomaly may be the principal/first listed diagnosis on a record or a secondary diagnosis.

When a congenital anomaly does not have a unique code assignment, assign additional code(s) for any manifestations that may be present. When the code assignment specifically identifies the congenital anomaly, manifestations that are an inherent component of the anomaly should not be coded separately. Additional codes should be assigned for manifestations that are not an inherent component.

Codes from Chapter 14 may be used throughout the life of the patient. If a congenital anomaly has been corrected, a personal history code should be used to identify the history of the anomaly.

Although present at birth, a congenital anomaly may not be identified until later in life. Whenever the condition is diagnosed by the physician, it is appropriate to assign a code from codes 740-759.

For the birth admission, the appropriate code from category V30, Liveborn infants, according to type of birth should be sequenced as the principal diagnosis, followed by any congenital anomaly codes, 740759.

15. Chapter 15: Newborn (Perinatal) Guidelines (760-779)

For coding and reporting purposes the perinatal period is defined as **before** birth through the 28th day following birth. The following guidelines are provided for reporting purposes. Hospitals may record other diagnoses as needed for internal data use.

a. General Perinatal Rules

1) Chapter 15 Codes

They are <u>never</u> for use on the maternal record. Codes from Chapter 11, the obstetric chapter, are never permitted on the newborn record. Chapter 15 code may be used throughout the life of the patient if the condition is still present.

2) Sequencing of perinatal codes

Generally, codes from Chapter 15 should be sequenced as the principal/first-listed diagnosis on the newborn record, with the exception of the appropriate V30 code for the birth episode, followed by codes from any other chapter that provide additional detail. The "use additional code" note at the beginning of the chapter supports this guideline. If the index does not provide a specific code for a perinatal condition, assign code 779.89, Other specified conditions originating in the perinatal period, followed by the code from another chapter that specifies the condition. Codes for signs and symptoms may be assigned when a definitive diagnosis has not been established.

3) Birth process or community acquired conditions

If a newborn has a condition that may be either due to the birth process or community acquired and the documentation does not indicate which it is, the default is due to the birth process and the code from Chapter 15 should be used. If the condition is community-acquired, a code from Chapter 15 should not be assigned.

4) Code all clinically significant conditions

All clinically significant conditions noted on routine newborn examination should be coded. A condition is clinically significant if it requires:

- clinical evaluation; or
- therapeutic treatment; or
- diagnostic procedures; or
- extended length of hospital stay; or
- increased nursing care and/or monitoring; or
- has implications for future health care needs

Note: The perinatal guidelines listed above are the same as the general coding guidelines for "additional diagnoses", except for the final point regarding implications for future health care needs. Codes should be assigned for conditions that have been specified by the provider as having implications for future health care needs. Codes from the perinatal chapter should not be assigned unless the provider has established a definitive diagnosis.

b. Use of codes V30-V39

When coding the birth of an infant, assign a code from categories V30-V39, according to the type of birth. A code from this series is assigned as a principal diagnosis, and assigned only once to a newborn at the time of birth.

c. Newborn transfers

If the newborn is transferred to another institution, the V30 series is not used at the receiving hospital.

d. Use of category V29

1) Assigning a code from category V29

Assign a code from category V29, Observation and evaluation of newborns and infants for suspected conditions not found, to identify those instances when a healthy newborn is evaluated for a suspected condition that is determined after study not to be present. Do not use a code from category V29 when the patient has identified signs or symptoms of a suspected problem; in such cases, code the sign or symptom.

A code from category V29 may also be assigned as a principal code for readmissions or encounters when the V30 code no longer applies. Codes from category V29 are for use only for healthy newborns and infants for which no condition after study is found to be present.

2) V29 code on a birth record

A V29 code is to be used as a secondary code after the V30, Outcome of delivery, code.

e. Use of other V codes on perinatal records

V codes other than V30 and V29 may be assigned on a perinatal or newborn record code. The codes may be used as a principal or first-listed diagnosis for specific types of encounters or for readmissions or encounters when the V30 code no longer applies.

See Section I.C.18 for information regarding the assignment of V codes.

f. Maternal Causes of Perinatal Morbidity

Codes from categories 760-763, Maternal causes of perinatal morbidity and mortality, are assigned only when the maternal condition has actually affected the fetus or newborn. The fact that the mother has an associated medical condition or experiences some complication of pregnancy, labor or delivery does not justify the routine assignment of codes from these categories to the newborn record.

g. Congenital Anomalies in Newborns

For the birth admission, the appropriate code from category V30, Liveborn infants according to type of birth, should be used, followed by any congenital anomaly codes, categories 740-759. Use additional secondary codes from other chapters to specify conditions associated with the anomaly, if applicable.

Also, see Section I.C.14 for information on the coding of congenital anomalies.

h. Coding Additional Perinatal Diagnoses

1) Assigning codes for conditions that require treatment

Assign codes for conditions that require treatment or further investigation, prolong the length of stay, or require resource utilization.

2) Codes for conditions specified as having implications for future health care needs

Assign codes for conditions that have been specified by the provider as having implications for future health care needs.

Note: This guideline should not be used for adult patients.

3) Codes for newborn conditions originating in the perinatal period

Assign a code for newborn conditions originating in the perinatal period (categories 760-779), as well as complications arising during the current episode of care classified in other chapters, only if the diagnoses have been documented by the responsible provider at the time of transfer or discharge as having affected the fetus or newborn.

i. Prematurity and Fetal Growth Retardation

Providers utilize different criteria in determining prematurity. A code for prematurity should not be assigned unless it is documented. The 5th digit assignment for codes from category 764 and subcategories 765.0 and 765.1 should be based on the recorded birth weight and estimated gestational age.

A code from subcategory 765.2, Weeks of gestation, should be assigned as an additional code with category 764 and codes from 765.0 and 765.1 to specify weeks of gestation as documented by the provider in the record.

j. Newborn sepsis

Code 771.81, Septicemia [sepsis] of newborn, should be assigned with a secondary code from category 041, Bacterial infections in conditions classified elsewhere and of unspecified site, to identify the organism. It is not necessary to use a code from subcategory 995.9, Systemic inflammatory response syndrome (SIRS), on a newborn record. A code from category 038, Septicemia, should not be used on a newborn record. Code 771.81 describes the sepsis.

16. Chapter 16: Signs, Symptoms and Ill-Defined Conditions (780-799)

Reserved for future guideline expansion

17. Chapter 17: Injury and Poisoning (800-999)

a. Coding of Injuries

When coding injuries, assign separate codes for each injury unless a combination code is provided, in which case the combination code is assigned. Multiple injury codes are provided in ICD-9-CM, but should not be assigned unless information for a more specific code is not available. These codes are not to be used for normal, healing surgical wounds or to identify complications of surgical wounds.

The code for the most serious injury, as determined by the provider and the focus of treatment, is sequenced first.

1) Superficial injuries

Superficial injuries such as abrasions or contusions are not coded when associated with more severe injuries of the same site.

2) Primary injury with damage to nerves/blood vessels

When a primary injury results in minor damage to peripheral nerves or blood vessels, the primary injury is sequenced first with additional code(s) from categories 950-957, Injury to nerves and spinal cord, and/or 900-904, Injury to blood vessels. When the primary injury is to the blood vessels or nerves, that injury should be sequenced first.

b. Coding of Traumatic Fractures

The principles of multiple coding of injuries should be followed in coding fractures. Fractures of specified sites are coded individually by site in accordance with both the provisions within categories 800-829 and the level of detail furnished by medical record content. Combination categories for multiple fractures are provided for use when there is insufficient detail in the medical record (such as trauma cases transferred to another hospital), when the reporting form limits the number of codes that can be used in reporting pertinent clinical data, or when there is insufficient specificity at the fourth-digit or fifth-digit level. More specific guidelines are as follows:

1) Acute Fractures vs. Aftercare

Traumatic fractures are coded using the acute fracture codes (800-829) while the patient is receiving active treatment for the fracture. Examples of active treatment are: surgical treatment, emergency department encounter, and evaluation and treatment by a new physician.

Fractures are coded using the aftercare codes (subcategories V54.0, V54.1, V54.8, or V54.9) for encounters after the patient has completed active treatment of the fracture and is receiving routine care for the fracture during the healing or recovery phase. Examples of fracture aftercare are: cast change or removal, removal of external or internal fixation device, medication adjustment, and follow up visits following fracture treatment.

Care for complications of surgical treatment for fracture repairs during the healing or recovery phase should be coded with the appropriate complication codes.

Care of complications of fractures, such as malunion and nonunion, should be reported with the appropriate codes.

Pathologic fractures are not coded in the 800-829 range, but instead are assigned to subcategory 733.1. *See Section I.C.13.a for additional information.*

2) Multiple fractures of same limb

Multiple fractures of same limb classifiable to the same three-digit or four-digit category are coded to that category.

3) Multiple unilateral or bilateral fractures of same bone

Multiple unilateral or bilateral fractures of same bone(s) but classified to different fourth-digit subdivisions (bone part) within the same three-digit category are coded individually by site.

4) Multiple fracture categories 819 and 828

Multiple fracture categories 819 and 828 classify bilateral fractures of both upper limbs (819) and both lower limbs (828), but without any detail at the fourth-digit level other than open and closed type of fractures.

5) Multiple fractures sequencing

Multiple fractures are sequenced in accordance with the severity of the fracture. The provider should be asked to list the fracture diagnoses in the order of severity.

c. Coding of Burns

Current burns (940-948) are classified by depth, extent and by agent (E code). Burns are classified by depth as first degree (erythema), second degree (blistering), and third degree (full-thickness involvement).

1) Sequencing of burn and related condition codes

Sequence first the code that reflects the highest degree of burn when more than one burn is present.

a. When the reason for the admission or encounter is for treatment of external multiple burns, sequence first the code that reflects the burn of the highest degree.

b. When a patient has both internal and external burns, the circumstances of admission govern the selection of the principal diagnosis or first-listed diagnosis.

c. When a patient is admitted for burn injuries and other related conditions such as smoke inhalation and/or respiratory failure, the circumstances of admission govern the selection of the principal or first-listed diagnosis.

2) Burns of the same local site

Classify burns of the same local site (three-digit category level, 940-947) but of different degrees to the subcategory identifying the highest degree recorded in the diagnosis.

3) Non-healing burns

Non-healing burns are coded as acute burns.

Necrosis of burned skin should be coded as a non-healed burn.

4) Code 958.3, Posttraumatic wound infection

Assign code 958.3, Posttraumatic wound infection, not elsewhere classified, as an additional code for any documented infected burn site.

5) Assign separate codes for each burn site

When coding burns, assign separate codes for each burn site. Category 946 Burns of Multiple specified sites, should only be used if the location of the burns are not documented. Category 949, Burn, unspecified, is extremely vague and should rarely be used.

6) Assign codes from category 948, Burns

Burns classified according to extent of body surface involved, when the site of the burn is not specified or when there is a need for additional data. It is advisable to use category 948 as additional coding when needed to provide data for evaluating burn mortality, such as that needed by burn units. It is also advisable to use category 948 as an additional code for reporting purposes when there is mention of a third-degree burn involving 20 percent or more of the body surface.

In assigning a code from category 948:

Fourth-digit codes are used to identify the percentage of total body surface involved in a burn (all degree).

Fifth-digits are assigned to identify the percentage of body surface involved in third-degree burn.

Fifth-digit zero (0) is assigned when less than 10 percent or when no body surface is involved in a third-degree burn.

Category 948 is based on the classic "rule of nines" in estimating body surface involved: head and neck are assigned nine percent, each arm nine percent, each leg 18 percent, the anterior trunk 18 percent, posterior trunk 18 percent, and genitalia one percent. Providers may change these percentage assignments where necessary to accommodate infants and children who have proportionately larger heads than adults and patients who have large buttocks, thighs, or abdomen that involve burns.

7) Encounters for treatment of late effects of burns

Encounters for the treatment of the late effects of burns (i.e., scars or joint contractures) should be coded to the residual condition (sequelae) followed by the appropriate late effect code (906.5-906.9). A late effect E code may also be used, if desired.

8) Sequelae with a late effect code and current burn

When appropriate, both a sequelae with a late effect code, and a current burn code may be assigned on the same record (when both a current burn and sequelae of an old burn exist).

d. Coding of Debridement of Wound, Infection, or Burn

Excisional debridement involves surgical removal or cutting away, as opposed to a mechanical (brushing, scrubbing, washing) debridement.

For coding purposes, excisional debridement is assigned to code 86.22.

Nonexcisional debridement is assigned to code 86.28.

e. Adverse Effects, Poisoning and Toxic Effects

The properties of certain drugs, medicinal and biological substances or combinations of such substances, may cause toxic reactions. The occurrence of drug toxicity is classified in ICD-9-CM as follows:

1) Adverse Effect

When the drug was correctly prescribed and properly administered, code the reaction plus the appropriate code from the E930-E949 series. Codes from the E930-E949 series must be used to identify the causative substance for an adverse effect of drug, medicinal and biological substances, correctly prescribed and properly administered. The effect, such as tachycardia, delirium, gastrointestinal hemorrhaging, vomiting, hypokalemia, hepatitis, renal failure, or respiratory failure, is coded and followed by the appropriate code from the E930-E949 series.

Adverse effects of therapeutic substances correctly prescribed and properly administered (toxicity, synergistic reaction, side effect, and idiosyncratic reaction) may be due to (1) differences among patients, such as age, sex, disease, and genetic factors, and (2) drug-related factors, such as type of drug, route of administration, duration of therapy, dosage, and bioavailability.

2) Poisoning

(a) Error was made in drug prescription

Errors made in drug prescription or in the administration of the drug by provider, nurse, patient, or other person, use the appropriate poisoning code from the 960-979 series.

(b) Overdose of a drug intentionally taken

If an overdose of a drug was intentionally taken or administered and resulted in drug toxicity, it would be coded as a poisoning (960-979 series).

(c) Nonprescribed drug taken with correctly prescribed and properly administered drug

If a nonprescribed drug or medicinal agent was taken in combination with a correctly prescribed and properly administered drug, any drug toxicity or other reaction resulting from the interaction of the two drugs would be classified as a poisoning.

(d) Sequencing of poisoning

When coding a poisoning or reaction to the improper use of a medication (e.g., wrong dose, wrong substance, wrong route of administration) the poisoning code is sequenced first, followed by a code for the manifestation. If there is also a diagnosis of drug abuse or dependence to the substance, the abuse or dependence is coded as an additional code.

See Section I.C.3.a.6.b. if poisoning is the result of insulin pump malfunctions and Section I.C.19 for general use of E-codes.

3) Toxic Effects

(a) Toxic effect codes

When a harmful substance is ingested or comes in contact with a person, this is classified as a toxic effect. The toxic effect codes are in categories 980-989.

(b) Sequencing toxic effect codes

A toxic effect code should be sequenced first, followed by the code(s) that identify the result of the toxic effect.

(c) External cause codes for toxic effects

An external cause code from categories E860-E869 for accidental exposure, codes E950.6 or E950.7 for intentional self-harm, category E962 for assault, or categories E980-E982, for undetermined, should also be assigned to indicate intent.

f. Complications of care

1) Transplant complications

(a) Transplant complications other than kidney

Codes under subcategory 996.8, Complications of transplanted organ, are for use for both complications and rejection of transplanted organs. A transplant complication code is only assigned if the complication affects the function of the transplanted organ. Two codes are required to fully describe a transplant complication, the appropriate code from subcategory 996.8 and a secondary code that identifies the complication.

Pre-existing conditions or conditions that develop after the transplant are not coded as complications unless they affect the function of the transplanted organs.

(b) Kidney transplant complications

Code 996.81 should be assigned for documented complications of a kidney transplant, such as transplant failure or rejection. Code 996.81 should not be assigned for post kidney transplant patients who have chronic kidney (CKD) unless a transplant complication such as transplant failure or rejection is documented. If the documentation is unclear as to whether the patient has a complication of the transplant, query the provider.

For patients with CKD following a kidney transplant, but who do not have a complication such as failure or rejection, *see section I.C.10.a.2, Chronic kidney disease and kidney transplant status.*

g. SIRS due to Non-infectious Process

The systemic inflammatory response syndrome (SIRS) can develop as a result of certain non-infectious disease processes, such as trauma, malignant neoplasm, or pancreatitis. When SIRS is documented with a noninfectious condition, and no subsequent infection is documented, the code for the underlying condition, such as an injury, should be assigned, followed by code 995.93, Systemic inflammatory response syndrome due to noninfectious process without acute organ dysfunction, or 995.94, Systemic inflammatory response syndrome due to non-infectious process with acute organ dysfunction. If an acute organ dysfunction is documented, the appropriate code(s) for the associated acute organ dysfunction(s) should be assigned in addition to code 995.94. If acute organ dysfunction is documented, but it cannot be determined if the acute organ dysfunction is associated with SIRS or due to another condition (e.g., directly due to the trauma), the provider should be queried.

When the non-infectious condition has led to an infection that results in SIRS, *see Section I.C.1.b.11 for the guideline for sepsis and severe sepsis associated with a non-infectious process.*

18. **Classification of Factors Influencing Health Status and Contact with Health Service (Supplemental V01-V84)**

Note: The chapter specific guidelines provide additional information about the use of V codes for specified encounters.

a. **Introduction**

ICD-9-CM provides codes to deal with encounters for circumstances other than a disease or injury. The Supplementary Classification of Factors Influencing Health Status and Contact with Health Services (V01.0-V84.8) is provided to deal with occasions when circumstances other than a disease or injury (codes 001-999) are recorded as a diagnosis or problem.

There are four primary circumstances for the use of V codes:

1) A person who is not currently sick encounters the health services for some specific reason, such as to act as an organ donor, to receive prophylactic care, such as inoculations or health screenings, or to receive counseling on health related issues.

2) A person with a resolving disease or injury, or a chronic, long-term condition requiring continuous care, encounters the health care system for specific aftercare of that disease or injury (e.g., dialysis for renal disease; chemotherapy for malignancy; cast change). A diagnosis/symptom code should be used whenever a current, acute, diagnosis is being treated or a sign or symptom is being studied.

3) Circumstances or problems influence a person's health status but are not in themselves a current illness or injury.

4) Newborns, to indicate birth status

b. **V codes use in any healthcare setting**

V codes are for use in any healthcare setting. V codes may be used as either a first listed (principal diagnosis code in the inpatient setting) or secondary code, depending on the circumstances of the encounter. Certain V codes may only be used as first listed, others only as secondary codes.

See Section I.C.18.e, V Code Table.

c. V Codes indicate a reason for an encounter

They are not procedure codes. A corresponding procedure code must accompany a V code to describe the procedure performed.

d. Categories of V Codes

1) Contact/Exposure

Category V01 indicates contact with or exposure to communicable diseases. These codes are for patients who do not show any sign or symptom of a disease but have been exposed to it by close personal contact with an infected individual or are in an area where a disease is epidemic. These codes may be used as a first listed code to explain an encounter for testing, or, more commonly, as a secondary code to identify a potential risk.

2) Inoculations and vaccinations

Categories V03-V06 are for encounters for inoculations and vaccinations. They indicate that a patient is being seen to receive a prophylactic inoculation against a disease. The injection itself must be represented by the appropriate procedure code. A code from V03-V06 may be used as a secondary code if the inoculation is given as a routine part of preventive health care, such as a well-baby visit.

3) Status

Status codes indicate that a patient is either a carrier of a disease or has the sequelae or residual of a past disease or condition. This includes such things as the presence of prosthetic or mechanical devices resulting from past treatment. A status code is informative, because the status may affect the course of treatment and its outcome. A status code is distinct from a history code. The history code indicates that the patient no longer has the condition.

A status code should not be used with a diagnosis code from one of the body system chapters, if the diagnosis code includes the information provided by the status code. For example, code V42.1, Heart transplant status, should not be used with code 996.83, Complications of transplanted heart. The status code does not provide additional information. The complication code indicates that the patient is a heart transplant patient.

The status V codes/categories are:

V02   Carrier or suspected carrier of infectious diseases

Carrier status indicates that a person harbors the specific organisms of a disease without manifest symptoms and is capable of transmitting the infection.

V08   Asymptomatic HIV infection status

This code indicates that a patient has tested positive for HIV but has manifested no signs or symptoms of the disease.

V09   Infection with drug-resistant microorganisms

This category indicates that a patient has an infection that is resistant to drug treatment.

Sequence the infection code first.

V21   Constitutional states in development

V22.2   Pregnant state, incidental This code is a secondary code only for use when the pregnancy is in no way complicating the reason for visit. Otherwise, a code from the obstetric chapter is required.

V26.5x Sterilization status

V42   Organ or tissue replaced by transplant

V43   Organ or tissue replaced by other means

V44   Artificial opening status

V45   Other postsurgical states

V46   Other dependence on machines

V49.6   Upper limb amputation status

V49.7   Lower limb amputation status

> **Note:** Categories V42-V46, and subcategories V49.6, V49.7 are for use only if there are no complications or malfunctions of the organ or tissue replaced, the amputation site or the equipment on which the patient is dependent.

V49.81 Postmenopausal status

V49.82 Dental sealant status

V49.83 Awaiting organ transplant status

V58.6x Long-term (current) drug use

> **Codes from** this subcategory indicate a patient's continuous use of a prescribed drug (including such things as aspirin therapy) for the long-term treatment of a condition or for prophylactic use. It is not for use for patients who have addictions to drugs.
>
> Assign a code from subcategory V58.6, Long-term (current) drug use, if the patient is receiving a medication for an extended period as a prophylactic measure (such as for the prevention of deep vein thrombosis) or as treatment of a chronic condition (such as arthritis) or a disease requiring a lengthy course of treatment (such as cancer). Do not assign a code from subcategory V58.6 for medication being administered for a brief period of time to treat an acute illness or injury (such as a course of antibiotics to treat acute bronchitis).

V83   Genetic carrier status

> Genetic carrier status indicates that a person carries a gene, associated with a particular disease, which may be passed to offspring who may develop that disease. The person does not have the disease and is not at risk of developing the disease.

V84   Genetic susceptibility status

> Genetic susceptibility indicates that a person has a gene that increases the risk of that person developing the disease.

Codes from category V84, Genetic susceptibility to disease, should not be used as principal or first-listed codes. If the patient has the condition to which he/she is susceptible, and that condition is the reason for the encounter, the code for the current condition should be sequenced first. If the patient is being seen for follow-up after completed treatment for this condition, and the condition no longer exists, a follow-up code should be sequenced first, followed by the appropriate personal history and genetic susceptibility codes. If the purpose of the encounter is genetic counseling associated with procreative management, a code from subcategory V26.3, Genetic counseling and testing, should be assigned as the first-listed code, followed by a code from category V84. Additional codes should be assigned for any applicable family or personal history.

See Section I.C. 18.d.14 for information on prophylactic organ removal due to a genetic susceptibility.

V86   Estrogen receptor status

4) History (of)

There are two types of history V codes, personal and family. Personal history codes explain a patient's past medical condition that no longer exists and is not receiving any treatment, but that has the potential for recurrence, and therefore may require continued monitoring. The exceptions to this general rule are category V14, Personal history of allergy to medicinal agents, and subcategory V15.0, Allergy, other than to medicinal agents. A person who has had an allergic episode to a substance or food in the past should always be considered allergic to the substance.

Family history codes are for use when a patient has a family member(s) who has had a particular disease that causes the patient to be at higher risk of also contracting the disease.

Personal history codes may be used in conjunction with follow-up codes and family history codes may be used in conjunction with screening codes to explain the need for a test or procedure. History codes are also acceptable on any medical record regardless of the reason for visit. A history of an illness, even if no longer present, is important information that may alter the type of treatment ordered.

The history V code categories are:

V10   Personal history of malignant neoplasm

V12   Personal history of certain other diseases

V13   Personal history of other diseases

Except: V13.4, Personal history of arthritis, and V13.6, Personal history of congenital malformations. These conditions are life-long so are not true history codes.

V14   Personal history of allergy to medicinal agents

V15   Other personal history presenting hazards to health

Except: V15.7, Personal history of contraception.

V16   Family history of malignant neoplasm

V17   Family history of certain chronic disabling diseases

V18   Family history of certain other specific diseases

V19   Family history of other conditions

5) Screening

Screening is the testing for disease or disease precursors in seemingly well individuals so that early detection and treatment can be provided for those who test positive for the disease. Screenings that are recommended for many subgroups in a population include: routine mammograms for women over 40, a fecal occult blood test for everyone over 50, an amniocentesis to rule out a fetal anomaly for pregnant women over 35, because the incidence of breast cancer and colon cancer in these subgroups is higher than in the general population, as is the incidence of Down's syndrome in older mothers.

The testing of a person to rule out or confirm a suspected diagnosis because the patient has some sign or symptom is a diagnostic examination, not a screening. In these cases, the sign or symptom is used to explain the reason for the test.

A screening code may be a first listed code if the reason for the visit is specifically the screening exam. It may also be used as an additional code if the screening is done during an office visit for other health problems. A screening code is not necessary if the screening is inherent to a routine examination, such as a pap smear done during a routine pelvic examination.

Should a condition be discovered during the screening then the code for the condition may be assigned as an additional diagnosis.

The V code indicates that a screening exam is planned. A procedure code is required to confirm that the screening was performed.

The screening V code categories:

V28   Antenatal screening

V73-V82 Special screening examinations

6) Observation

There are two observation V code categories. They are for use in very limited circumstances when a person is being observed for a suspected condition that is ruled out. The observation codes are not for use if an injury or illness or any signs or symptoms related to the suspected condition are present. In such cases the diagnosis/symptom code is used with the corresponding E code to identify any external cause.

The observation codes are to be used as principal diagnosis only. The only exception to this is when the principal diagnosis is required to be a code from the V30, Live born infant, category. Then the V29 observation code is sequenced after the V30 code. Additional codes may be used in addition to the observation code but only if they are unrelated to the suspected condition being observed.

The observation V code categories:

V29   Observation and evaluation of newborns for suspected condition not found
For the birth encounter, a code from category V30 should be sequenced before the V29 code.

V71   Observation and evaluation for suspected condition not found

7) Aftercare

Aftercare visit codes cover situations when the initial treatment of a disease or injury has been performed and the patient requires continued care during the healing or recovery phase, or for the long-term consequences of the disease. The aftercare V code should not be used if treatment is directed at a current, acute disease or injury. The diagnosis code is to be used in these cases. Exceptions to this rule are codes V58.0, Radiotherapy, and codes from subcategory V58.1, Encounter for chemotherapy and immunotherapy for neoplastic conditions. These codes are to be first listed, followed by the diagnosis code when a patient's encounter is solely to receive radiation therapy or chemotherapy for the treatment of a neoplasm. Should a patient receive both chemotherapy and radiation therapy during the same encounter code V58.0 and V58.1 may be used together on a record with either one being sequenced first.

The aftercare codes are generally first listed to explain the specific reason for the encounter. An aftercare code may be used as an additional code when some type of aftercare is provided in addition to the reason for admission and no diagnosis code is applicable. An example of this would be the closure of a colostomy during an encounter for treatment of another condition.

Certain aftercare V code categories need a secondary diagnosis code to describe the resolving condition or sequelae, for others, the condition is inherent in the code title.

Additional V code aftercare category terms include, fitting and adjustment, and attention to artificial openings.

Status V codes may be used with aftercare V codes to indicate the nature of the aftercare. For example code V45.81, Aortocoronary bypass status, may be used with code V58.73, Aftercare following surgery of the circulatory system, NEC, to indicate the surgery for which the aftercare is being performed. Also, a transplant status code may be used following code V58.44, Aftercare following organ transplant, to identify the organ transplanted. A status code should not be used when the aftercare code indicates the type of status, such as using V55.0, Attention to tracheostomy with V44.0, Tracheostomy status.

The aftercare V category/codes:

V52   Fitting and adjustment of prosthetic device and implant

V53   Fitting and adjustment of other device

V54   Other orthopedic aftercare

V55   Attention to artificial openings

V56   Encounter for dialysis and dialysis catheter care

V57   Care involving the use of rehabilitation procedures

V58.0   Radiotherapy

V58.11   Encounter for antineoplastic chemotherapy

V58.12   Encounter for antineoplastic immunotherapy

V58.3x   Attention to dressings and sutures

V58.41   Encounter for planned post-operative wound closure

V58.42   Aftercare, surgery, neoplasm

V58.43   Aftercare, surgery, trauma

V58.44   Aftercare involving organ transplant

V58.49   Other specified aftercare following surgery

V58.7x   Aftercare following surgery

V58.81   Fitting and adjustment of vascular catheter

V58.82   Fitting and adjustment of non-vascular catheter

V58.83   Monitoring therapeutic drug

V58.89   Other specified aftercare

8) Follow-up

The follow-up codes are used to explain continuing surveillance following completed treatment of a disease, condition, or injury. They imply that the condition has been fully treated and no longer exists. They should not be confused with aftercare codes that explain current treatment for a healing condition or its sequelae. Follow-up codes may be used in conjunction with history codes to provide the full picture of the healed condition and its treatment. The follow-up code is sequenced first, followed by the history code.

A follow-up code may be used to explain repeated visits. Should a condition be found to have recurred on the follow-up visit, then the diagnosis code should be used in place of the follow-up code.

The follow-up V code categories:

V24   Postpartum care and evaluation

V67   Follow-up examination

9) Donor

Category V59 is the donor codes. They are used for living individuals who are donating blood or other body tissue. These codes are only for individuals donating for others, not for self donations. They are not for use to identify cadaveric donations.

10) Counseling

Counseling V codes are used when a patient or family member receives assistance in the aftermath of an illness or injury, or when support is required in coping with family or social problems. They are not necessary for use in conjunction with a diagnosis code when the counseling component of care is considered integral to standard treatment.

The counseling V categories/codes:

V25.0   General counseling and advice for contraceptive management

V26.3   Genetic counseling

V26.4   General counseling and advice for procreative management

V61   Other family circumstances

V65.1   Person consulted on behalf of another person

V65.3   Dietary surveillance and counseling

V65.4   Other counseling, not elsewhere classified

11) Obstetrics and related conditions

See Section I.C.11., the Obstetrics guidelines for further instruction on the use of these codes.

V codes for pregnancy are for use in those circumstances when none of the problems or complications included in the codes from the Obstetrics chapter exist (a routine prenatal visit or postpartum care). Codes V22.0, Supervision of normal first pregnancy, and V22.1, Supervision of other normal pregnancy, are always first listed and are not to be used with any other code from the OB chapter.

The outcome of delivery, category V27, should be included on all maternal delivery records. It is always a secondary code.

V codes for family planning (contraceptive) or procreative management and counseling should be included on an obstetric record either during the pregnancy or the postpartum stage, if applicable.

Obstetrics and related conditions V code categories:

V22   Normal pregnancy

V23   Supervision of high-risk pregnancy

Except: V23.2, Pregnancy with history of abortion. Code 646.3, Habitual aborter, from the OB chapter is required to indicate a history of abortion during a pregnancy.

V24 Postpartum care and evaluation

V25 Encounter for contraceptive management

Except V25.0x
(See Section I.C.18.d.11, Counseling)

V26 Procreative management Except V26.5x, Sterilization status, V26.3 and V26.4
(See Section I.C.18.d.11., Counseling)

V27 Outcome of delivery

V28 Antenatal screening
(See Section I.C.18.d.6., Screening)

12) Newborn, infant and child

See Section I.C.15, the Newborn guidelines for further instruction on the use of these codes.

Newborn   V code categories:

V20   Health supervision of infant or child

V29   Observation and evaluation of newborns for suspected condition not found

(See Section I.C.18.d.7, Observation)

V30-V39   Liveborn infant according to type of birth

13) Routine and administrative examinations

The V codes allow for the description of encounters for routine examinations, such as, a general check-up, or, examinations for administrative purposes, such as, a pre-employment physical. The codes are not to be used if the examination is for diagnosis of a suspected condition or for treatment purposes. In such cases the diagnosis code is used. During a routine exam, should a diagnosis or condition be discovered, it should be coded as an additional code. Pre-existing and chronic conditions and history codes may also be included as additional codes as long as the examination is for administrative purposes and not focused on any particular condition.

Pre-operative examination V codes are for use only in those situations when a patient is being cleared for surgery and no treatment is given.

The V codes categories/code for routine and administrative examinations:

V20.2   Routine infant or child health check

Any injections given should have a corresponding procedure code.

V70   General medical examination

V72   Special investigations and examinations

Codes V72.5 and V72.6 may be used if the reason for the patient encounter is for routine laboratory/radiology testing in the absence of any signs, symptoms, or associated diagnosis. If routine testing is performed during the same encounter as a test to evaluate a sign, symptom, or diagnosis, it is appropriate to assign both the V code and the code describing the reason for the non-routine test.

14) Miscellaneous V codes

The miscellaneous V codes capture a number of other health care encounters that do not fall into one of the other categories. Certain of these codes identify the reason for the encounter, others are for use as additional codes that provide useful information on circumstances that may affect a patient's care and treatment.

Prophylactic Organ Removal

For encounters specifically for prophylactic removal of breasts, ovaries, or another organ due to a genetic susceptibility to cancer or a family history of cancer, the principal or first listed code should be a code from subcategory V50.4, Prophylactic organ removal, followed by the appropriate genetic susceptibility code and the appropriate family history code.

If the patient has a malignancy of one site and is having prophylactic removal at another site to prevent either a new primary malignancy or metastatic disease, a code for the malignancy should also be assigned in addition to a code from subcategory V50.4. A V50.4 code should not be assigned if the patient is having organ removal for treatment of a malignancy, such as the removal of the testes for the treatment of prostate cancer.

Miscellaneous V code categories/codes:

V07   Need for isolation and other prophylactic measures

V50   Elective surgery for purposes other than remedying health states

V58.5 Orthodontics

V60   Housing, household, and economic circumstances

V62   Other psychosocial circumstances

V63   Unavailability of other medical facilities for care

V64   Persons encountering health services for specific procedures, not carried out

V66   Convalescence and Palliative Care

V68   Encounters for administrative purposes

V69   Problems related to lifestyle

V85   Body Mass Index

15) Nonspecific V codes

Certain V codes are so non-specific, or potentially redundant with other codes in the classification, that there can be little justification for their use in the inpatient setting. Their use in the outpatient setting should be limited to those instances when there is no further documentation to permit more precise coding. Otherwise, any sign or symptom or any other reason for visit that is captured in another code should be used.

Nonspecific V code categories/codes:

V11   Personal history of mental disorder A code from the mental disorders chapter, with an in remission fifth-digit, should be used.

V13.4 Personal history of arthritis

V13.6 Personal history of congenital malformations

V15.7 Personal history of contraception

V23.2 Pregnancy with history of abortion

V40   Mental and behavioral problems

V41   Problems with special senses and other special functions

V47   Other problems with internal organs

V48   Problems with head, neck, and trunk

V49   Problems with limbs and other problems

Exceptions:

V49.6   Upper limb amputation status

V49.7   Lower limb amputation status

V49.81   Postmenopausal status

V49.82   Dental sealant status

V49.83   Awaiting organ transplant status

V51   Aftercare involving the use of plastic surgery

V58.2   Blood transfusion, without reported diagnosis

V58.9   Unspecified aftercare

See Section IV.K. and Section IV.L. of the Outpatient guidelines.

V CODE TABLE
October 1, 2007 (FY2008)
Items in bold indicate a new entry or change from the November 2006 table
Items underlined have been moved within the table since November 2006

The V code table below contains columns for 1st listed, 1st or additional, additional only, and non-specific. Each code or category is listed on the left hand column and the allowable sequencing of the code or codes within the category is noted under the appropriate column.

Code(s)	Description	1st Dx Only[1]	1st or Add'l Dx[2]	Add'l Dx Only[3]	Non-Specific Diagnosis[4]
V01.X	Contact with or exposure to communicable diseases		X		
V02.X	Carrier or suspected carrier of infectious diseases		X		
V03.X	Need for prophylactic vaccination and inoculation against bacterial diseases		X		
V04.X	Need for prophylactic vaccination and inoculation against certain diseases		X		
V05.X	Need for prophylactic vaccination and inoculation against single diseases		X		
V06.X	Need for prophylactic vaccination and inoculation against combinations of diseases		X		
V07.X	Need for isolation and other prophylactic measures		X		
V08	Asymptomatic HIV infection status		X		
V09.X	Infection with drug resistant organisms			X	
V10.X	Personal history of malignant neoplasm		X		
V11.X	Personal history of mental disorder				X
V12.X	Personal history of certain other diseases		X		
V13.0X	Personal history of other disorders of urinary system		X		
V13.1	Personal history of trophoblastic disease		X		
V13.2X	Personal history of other genital system and obstetric disorders		X		

[1]Generally for use as first listed only but may be used as additional if patient has more than one encounter on one day **or there is more than one reason for the encounter**
[2]These codes may be used as first listed or additional codes
[3]These codes are only for use as additional codes
[4]These codes are primarily for use in the nonacute setting and should be limited to encounters for which no sign or symptom or reason for visit is documented in the record. Their use may be as either a first listed or additional code.

Code(s)	Description	1st Dx Only[1]	1st or Add'l Dx[2]	Add'l Dx Only[3]	Non-Specific Diagnosis[4]
V13.3	Personal history of diseases of skin and subcutaneous tissue		X		
V13.4	Personal history of arthritis				X
V13.5	Personal history of other musculoskeletal disorders		X		
V13.61	Personal history of hypospadias			X	
V13.69	Personal history of congenital malformations				X
V13.7	Personal history of perinatal problems		X		
V13.8	Personal history of other specified diseases		X		
V13.9	Personal history of unspecified disease				X
V14.X	Personal history of allergy to medicinal agents			X	
V15.0X	Personal history of allergy, other than to medicinal agents			X	
V15.1	Personal history of surgery to heart and great vessels			X	
V15.2	Personal history of surgery to other major organs			X	
V15.3	Personal history of irradiation			X	
V15.4X	Personal history of psychological trauma			X	
V15.5	Personal history of injury			X	
V15.6	Personal history of poisoning			X	
V15.7	Personal history of contraception				X
V15.81	Personal history of noncompliance with medical treatment			X	
V15.82	Personal history of tobacco use			X	
V15.84	Personal history of exposure to asbestos			X	
V15.85	Personal history of exposure to potentially hazardous body fluids			X	
V15.86	Personal history of exposure to lead			X	
V15.87	Personal history of extracorporeal membrane oxygenation [ECMO]			X	
V15.88	History of fall		X		
V15.89	Other specified personal history presenting hazards to health			X	
V16.X	Family history of malignant neoplasm		X		

[1]Generally for use as first listed only but may be used as additional if patient has more than one encounter on one day **or there is more than one reason for the encounter**

[2]These codes may be used as first listed or additional codes

[3]These codes are only for use as additional codes

[4]These codes are primarily for use in the nonacute setting and should be limited to encounters for which no sign or symptom or reason for visit is documented in the record. Their use may be as either a first listed or additional code.

Code(s)	Description	1st Dx Only[1]	1st or Add'l Dx[2]	Add'l Dx Only[3]	Non-Specific Diagnosis[4]
V17.X	Family history of certain chronic disabling diseases		X		
V18.X	Family history of certain other specific conditions		X		
V19.X	Family history of other conditions		X		
V20.X	Health supervision of infant or child	X			
V21.X	Constitutional states in development			X	
V22.0	Supervision of normal first pregnancy	X			
V22.1	Supervision of other normal pregnancy	X			
V22.2	Pregnancy state, incidental			X	
V23.X	Supervision of high-risk pregnancy		X		
V24.X	Postpartum care and examination	X			
V25.X	Encounter for contraceptive management		X		
V26.0	Tuboplasty or vasoplasty after previous sterilization		X		
V26.1	Artificial insemination		X		
V26.2X	Procreative management investigation and testing		X		
V26.3X	Procreative management, genetic counseling and testing		X		
V26.4X	Procreative management, genetic counseling and advice		X		
V26.5X	Procreative management, sterilization status			X	
V26.81	**Encounter for assisted reproductive fertility procedure cycle**	**X**			
V26.89	Other specified procreative management		X		
V26.9	Unspecified procreative management		X		
V27.X	Outcome of delivery			X	
V28.X	Encounter for antenatal screening of mother		X		
V29.X	Observation and evaluation of newborns for suspected condition not found		X		
V30.X	Single liveborn	X			
V31.X	Twin, mate liveborn	X			
V32.X	Twin, mate stillborn	X			
V33.X	Twin, unspecified	X			
V34.X	Other multiple, mates all liveborn	X			
V35.X	Other multiple, mates all stillborn	X			

[1]Generally for use as first listed only but may be used as additional if patient has more than one encounter on one day **or there is more than one reason for the encounter**

[2]These codes may be used as first listed or additional codes

[3]These codes are only for use as additional codes

[4]These codes are primarily for use in the nonacute setting and should be limited to encounters for which no sign or symptom or reason for visit is documented in the record. Their use may be as either a first listed or additional code.

Code(s)	Description	1st Dx Only[1]	1st or Add'l Dx[2]	Add'l Dx Only[3]	Non-Specific Diagnosis[4]
V36.X	Other multiple, mates live- and stillborn	X			
V37.X	Other multiple, unspecified	X			
V39.X	Unspecified	X			
V40.X	Mental and behavioral problems				X
V41.X	Problems with special senses and other special functions				X
V42.X	Organ or tissue replaced by transplant			X	
V43.0	Organ or tissue replaced by other means, eye globe			X	
V43.1	Organ or tissue replaced by other means, lens			X	
V43.21	Organ or tissue replaced by other means, heart assist device			X	
V43.22	Fully implantable artificial heart status		X		
V43.3	Organ or tissue replaced by other means, heart valve			X	
V43.4	Organ or tissue replaced by other means, blood vessel			X	
V43.5	Organ or tissue replaced by other means, bladder			X	
V43.6X	Organ or tissue replaced by other means, joint			X	
V43.7	Organ or tissue replaced by other means, limb			X	
V43.8X	Other organ or tissue replaced by other means			X	
V44.X	Artificial opening status			X	
V45.0X	Cardiac device in situ			X	
V45.1	Renal dialysis status			X	
V45.2	Presence of cerebrospinal fluid drainage device			X	
V45.3	Intestinal bypass or anastomosis status			X	
V45.4	Arthrodesis status			X	
V45.5X	Presence of contraceptive device			X	
V45.6X	States following surgery of eye and adnexa			X	
V45.7X	Acquired absence of organ		X		
V45.8X	Other postprocedural status			X	

[1]Generally for use as first listed only but may be used as additional if patient has more than one encounter on one day **or there is more than one reason for the encounter**

[2]These codes may be used as first listed or additional codes

[3]These codes are only for use as additional codes

[4]These codes are primarily for use in the nonacute setting and should be limited to encounters for which no sign or symptom or reason for visit is documented in the record. Their use may be as either a first listed or additional code.

Code(s)	Description	1st Dx Only[1]	1st or Add'l Dx[2]	Add'l Dx Only[3]	Non-Specific Diagnosis[4]
V46.0	Other dependence on machines, aspirator			X	
V46.11	Dependence on respiratory, status			X	
V46.12	Encounter for respirator dependence during power failure	X			
V46.13	Encounter for weaning from respirator [ventilator]	X			
V46.14	Mechanical complication of respirator [ventilator]		X		
V46.2	Other dependence on machines, supplemental oxygen			X	
V46.8	Other dependence on other enabling machines			X	
V46.9	Unspecified machine dependence				X
V47.X	Other problems with internal organs				X
V48.X	Problems with head, neck and trunk				X
V49.0	Deficiencies of limbs				X
V49.1	Mechanical problems with limbs				X
V49.2	Motor problems with limbs				X
V49.3	Sensory problems with limbs				X
V49.4	Disfigurements of limbs				X
V49.5	Other problems with limbs				X
V49.6X	Upper limb amputation status		X		
V49.7X	Lower limb amputation status		X		
V49.81	Asymptomatic postmenopausal status (age-related) (natural)		X		
V49.82	Dental sealant status			X	
V49.83	Awaiting organ transplant status			X	
V49.84	Bed confinement status		X		
V49.85	**Dual sensory impairment**			**X**	
V49.89	Other specified conditions influencing health status		X		
V49.9	Unspecified condition influencing health status				X
V50.X	Elective surgery for purposes other than remedying health states		X		
V51	Aftercare involving the use of plastic surgery				X

[1]Generally for use as first listed only but may be used as additional if patient has more than one encounter on one day **or there is more than one reason for the encounter**

[2]These codes may be used as first listed or additional codes

[3]These codes are only for use as additional codes

[4]These codes are primarily for use in the nonacute setting and should be limited to encounters for which no sign or symptom or reason for visit is documented in the record. Their use may be as either a first listed or additional code.

Code(s)	Description	1st Dx Only[1]	1st or Add'l Dx[2]	Add'l Dx Only[3]	Non-Specific Diagnosis[4]
V52.X	Fitting and adjustment of prosthetic device and implant		X		
V53.X	Fitting and adjustment of other device		X		
V54.X	Other orthopedic aftercare		X		
V55.X	Attention to artificial openings		X		
V56.0	Extracorporeal dialysis	X			
V56.1	Encounter for fitting and adjustment of extracorporeal dialysis catheter		X		
V56.2	Encounter for fitting and adjustment of peritoneal dialysis catheter		X		
V56.3X	Encounter for adequacy testing for dialysis		X		
V56.8	Encounter for other dialysis and dialysis catheter care		X		
V57.X	Care involving use of rehabilitation procedures	X			
V58.0	Radiotherapy	X			
V58.11	Encounter for antineoplastic chemotherapy	X			
V58.12	Encounter for antineoplastic immunotherapy	X			
V58.2	Blood transfusion without reported diagnosis				X
V58.3X	Attention to dressings and sutures		X		
V58.4X	Other aftercare following surgery		X		
V58.5	Encounter for orthodontics				X
V58.6X	Long term (current) drug use			X	
V58.7X	Aftercare following surgery to specified body systems, not elsewhere classified		X		
V58.8X	Other specified procedures and aftercare		X		
V58.9	Unspecified aftercare				X
V59.X	Donors	X			
V60.X	Housing, household, and economic circumstances			X	
V61.X	Other family circumstances		X		
V62.X	Other psychosocial circumstances			X	
V63.X	Unavailability of other medical facilities for care		X		
V64.X	Persons encountering health services for specified procedure, not carried out			X	

[1]Generally for use as first listed only but may be used as additional if patient has more than one encounter on one day **or there is more than one reason for the encounter**

[2]These codes may be used as first listed or additional codes

[3]These codes are only for use as additional codes

[4]These codes are primarily for use in the nonacute setting and should be limited to encounters for which no sign or symptom or reason for visit is documented in the record. Their use may be as either a first listed or additional code.

Code(s)	Description	1st Dx Only[1]	1st or Add'l Dx[2]	Add'l Dx Only[3]	Non-Specific Diagnosis[4]
V65.X	Other persons seeking consultation without complaint or sickness		X		
V66.0	Convalescence and palliative care following surgery	X			
V66.1	Convalescence and palliative care following radiotherapy	X			
V66.2	Convalescence and palliative care following chemotherapy	X			
V66.3	Convalescence and palliative care following psychotherapy and other treatment for mental disorder	X			
V66.4	Convalescence and palliative care following treatment of fracture	X			
V66.5	Convalescence and palliative care following other treatment	X			
V66.6	Convalescence and palliative care following combined treatment	X			
V66.7	Encounter for palliative care			X	
V66.9	Unspecified convalescence	X			
V67.X	Follow-up examination		X		
V68.X	Encounters for administrative purposes	X			
V69.X	Problems related to lifestyle		X		
V70.0	Routine general medical examination at a health care facility	X			
V70.1	General psychiatric examination, requested by the authority	X			
V70.2	General psychiatric examination, other and unspecified	X			
V70.3	Other medical examination for administrative purposes	X			
V70.4	Examination for medicolegal reasons	X			
V70.5	Health examination of defined subpopulations	X			
V70.6	Health examination in population surveys	X			
V70.7	Examination of participant in clinical trial		X		

[1]Generally for use as first listed only but may be used as additional if patient has more than one encounter on one day **or there is more than one reason for the encounter**

[2]These codes may be used as first listed or additional codes

[3]These codes are only for use as additional codes

[4]These codes are primarily for use in the nonacute setting and should be limited to encounters for which no sign or symptom or reason for visit is documented in the record. Their use may be as either a first listed or additional code.

Code(s)	Description	1st Dx Only[1]	1st or Add'l Dx[2]	Add'l Dx Only[3]	Non-Specific Diagnosis[4]
V70.8	Other specified general medical examinations	X			
V70.9	Unspecified general medical examination	X			
V71.X	Observation and evaluation for suspected conditions not found	X			
V72.0	Examination of eyes and vision		X		
V72.1X	Examination of ears and hearing		X		
V72.2	Dental examination		X		
V72.3X	Gynecological examination		X		
V72.4X	Pregnancy examination or test		X		
V72.5	Radiological examination, NEC		X		
V72.6	Laboratory examination		X		
V72.7	Diagnostic skin and sensitization tests		X		
V72.81	Preoperative cardiovascular examination		X		
V72.82	Preoperative respiratory examination		X		
V72.83	Other specified preoperative examination		X		
V72.84	Preoperative examination, unspecified		X		
V72.85	Other specified examination		X		
V72.86	Encounter for blood typing		X		
V72.9	Unspecified examination				X
V73.X	Special screening examination for viral and chlamydial diseases		X		
V74.X	Special screening examination for bacterial and spirochetal diseases		X		
V75.X	Special screening examination for other infectious diseases		X		
V76.X	Special screening examination for malignant neoplasms		X		
V77.X	Special screening examination for endocrine, nutritional, metabolic and immunity disorders		X		
V78.X	Special screening examination for disorders of blood and blood-forming organs		X		
V79.X	Special screening examination for mental disorders and developmental handicaps		X		

[1]Generally for use as first listed only but may be used as additional if patient has more than one encounter on one day **or there is more than one reason for the encounter**
[2]These codes may be used as first listed or additional codes
[3]These codes are only for use as additional codes
[4]These codes are primarily for use in the nonacute setting and should be limited to encounters for which no sign or symptom or reason for visit is documented in the record. Their use may be as either a first listed or additional code.

Code(s)	Description	1st Dx Only[1]	1st or Add'l Dx[2]	Add'l Dx Only[3]	Non-Specific Diagnosis[4]
V80.X	Special screening examination for neurological, eye, and ear diseases		X		
V81.X	Special screening examination for cardiovascular, respiratory, and genitourinary diseases		X		
V82.X	Special screening examination for other conditions		X		
V83.X	Genetic carrier status		X		
V84.X	Genetic susceptibility to disease			X	
V85	Body mass index			X	
V86	Estrogen receptor status			X	

[1]Generally for use as first listed only but may be used as additional if patient has more than one encounter on one day **or there is more than one reason for the encounter**

[2]These codes may be used as first listed or additional codes

[3]These codes are only for use as additional codes

[4]These codes are primarily for use in the nonacute setting and should be limited to encounters for which no sign or symptom or reason for visit is documented in the record. Their use may be as either a first listed or additional code.

19. Supplemental Classification of External Causes of Injury and Poisoning (E-codes, E800-E999)

Introduction: These guidelines are provided for those who are currently collecting E codes in order that there will be standardization in the process. If your institution plans to begin collecting E codes, these guidelines are to be applied. The use of E codes is supplemental to the application of ICD-9-CM diagnosis codes. E codes are never to be recorded as principal diagnoses (first-listed in non-inpatient setting) and are not required for reporting to CMS.

External causes of injury and poisoning codes (E codes) are intended to provide data for injury research and evaluation of injury prevention strategies. E codes capture how the injury or poisoning happened (cause), the intent (unintentional or accidental; or intentional, such as suicide or assault), and the place where the event occurred.

Some major categories of E codes include:

transport accidents

poisoning and adverse effects of drugs, medicinal substances and biologicals

accidental falls

accidents caused by fire and flames

accidents due to natural and environmental factors

late effects of accidents, assaults or self injury

assaults or purposely inflicted injury

suicide or self inflicted injury

These guidelines apply for the coding and collection of E codes from records in hospitals, outpatient clinics, emergency departments, other ambulatory care settings and provider offices, and nonacute care settings, except when other specific guidelines apply.

a. General E Code Coding Guidelines

1) Used with any code in the range of 001-V84.8

An E code may be used with any code in the range of 001-V84.8, which indicates an injury, poisoning, or adverse effect due to an external cause.

2) Assign the appropriate E code for all initial treatments

Assign the appropriate E code for the initial encounter of an injury, poisoning, or adverse effect of drugs, not for subsequent treatment.

External cause of injury codes (E-codes) may be assigned while the acute fracture codes are still applicable.

See Section I.C.17.b.1 for coding of acute fractures.

3) Use the full range of E codes

Use the full range of E codes to completely describe the cause, the intent and the place of occurrence, if applicable, for all injuries, poisonings, and adverse effects of drugs.

4) Assign as many E codes as necessary

Assign as many E codes as necessary to fully explain each cause. If only one E code can be recorded, assign the E code most related to the principal diagnosis.

5) The selection of the appropriate E code

The selection of the appropriate E code is guided by the Index to External Causes, which is located after the alphabetical index to diseases and by Inclusion and Exclusion notes in the Tabular List.

6) E code can never be a principal diagnosis

An E code can never be a principal (first listed) diagnosis.

7) External cause code(s) with systemic inflammatory response syndrome (SIRS)

An external cause code is not appropriate with a code from subcategory 995.9, unless the patient also has an injury, poisoning, or adverse effect of drugs.

b. Place of Occurrence Guideline

Use an additional code from category E849 to indicate the Place of Occurrence for injuries and poisonings. The Place of Occurrence describes the place where the event occurred and not the patient's activity at the time of the event.

Do not use E849.9 if the place of occurrence is not stated.

c. Adverse Effects of Drugs, Medicinal and Biological Substances Guidelines

1) Do not code directly from the Table of Drugs

Do not code directly from the Table of Drugs and Chemicals. Always refer back to the Tabular List.

2) Use as many codes as necessary to describe

Use as many codes as necessary to describe completely all drugs, medicinal or biological substances.

3) If the same E code would describe the causative agent

If the same E code would describe the causative agent for more than one adverse reaction, assign the code only once.

4) If two or more drugs, medicinal or biological substances

If two or more drugs, medicinal or biological substances are reported, code each individually unless the combination code is listed in the Table of Drugs and Chemicals. In that case, assign the E code for the combination.

5) When a reaction results from the interaction of a drug(s)

When a reaction results from the interaction of a drug(s) and alcohol, use poisoning codes and E codes for both.

6) If the reporting format limits the number of E codes

If the reporting format limits the number of E codes that can be used in reporting clinical data, code the one most related to the principal diagnosis. Include at least one from each category (cause, intent, place) if possible.

If there are different fourth digit codes in the same three digit category, use the code for "Other specified" of that category. If there is no "Other specified" code in that category, use the appropriate "Unspecified" code in that category.

If the codes are in different three digit categories, assign the appropriate E code for other multiple drugs and medicinal substances.

7) Codes from the E930-E949 series

Codes from the E930-E949 series must be used to identify the causative substance for an adverse effect of drug, medicinal and biological substances, correctly prescribed and properly administered. The effect, such as tachycardia, delirium, gastrointestinal hemorrhaging, vomiting, hypokalemia, hepatitis, renal failure, or respiratory failure, is coded and followed by the appropriate code from the E930-E949 series.

d. Multiple Cause E Code Coding Guidelines

If two or more events cause separate injuries, an E code should be assigned for each cause. The first listed E code will be selected in the following order:

E codes for child and adult abuse take priority over all other E codes.

See Section I.C.19.e., Child and Adult abuse guidelines.

E codes for terrorism events take priority over all other E codes except child and adult abuse

E codes for cataclysmic events take priority over all other E codes except child and adult abuse and terrorism.

E codes for transport accidents take priority over all other E codes except cataclysmic events and child and adult abuse and terrorism.

The first-listed E code should correspond to the cause of the most serious diagnosis due to an assault, accident, or self-harm, following the order of hierarchy listed above.

e. Child and Adult Abuse Guideline

1) Intentional injury

When the cause of an injury or neglect is intentional child or adult abuse, the first listed E code should be assigned from categories E960-E968, Homicide and injury purposely inflicted by other persons, (except category E967). An E code from category E967, Child and adult battering and other maltreatment, should be added as an additional code to identify the perpetrator, if known.

2) Accidental intent

In cases of neglect when the intent is determined to be accidental E code E904.0, Abandonment or neglect of infant and helpless person, should be the first listed E code.

f. Unknown or Suspected Intent Guideline

1) If the intent (accident, self-harm, assault) of the cause of an injury or poisoning is unknown

If the intent (accident, self-harm, assault) of the cause of an injury or poisoning is unknown or unspecified, code the intent as undetermined E980-E989.

2) If the intent (accident, self-harm, assault) of the cause of an injury or poisoning is questionable

If the intent (accident, self-harm, assault) of the cause of an injury or poisoning is questionable, probable or suspected, code the intent as undetermined E980-E989.

g. Undetermined Cause

When the intent of an injury or poisoning is known, but the cause is unknown, use codes: E928.9, Unspecified accident, E958.9, Suicide and self-inflicted injury by unspecified means, and E968.9, Assault by unspecified means.

These E codes should rarely be used, as the documentation in the medical record, in both the inpatient outpatient and other settings, should normally provide sufficient detail to determine the cause of the injury.

h. Late Effects of External Cause Guidelines

1) Late effect E codes

Late effect E codes exist for injuries and poisonings but not for adverse effects of drugs, misadventures and surgical complications.

2) Late effect E codes (E929, E959, E969, E977, E989, or E999.1)

A late effect E code (E929, E959, E969, E977, E989, or E999.1) should be used with any report of a late effect or sequela resulting from a previous injury or poisoning (905-909).

3) Late effect E code with a related current injury

A late effect E code should never be used with a related current nature of injury code.

4) Use of late effect E codes for subsequent visits

Use a late effect E code for subsequent visits when a late effect of the initial injury or poisoning is being treated. There is no late effect E code for adverse effects of drugs. Do not use a late effect E code for subsequent visits for follow-up care (e.g., to assess healing, to receive rehabilitative therapy) of the injury or poisoning when no late effect of the injury has been documented.

i. Misadventures and Complications of Care Guidelines

1) Code range E870-E876

Assign a code in the range of E870-E876 if misadventures are stated by the provider.

2) Code range E878-E879

Assign a code in the range of E878-E879 if the provider attributes an abnormal reaction or later complication to a surgical or medical procedure, but does not mention misadventure at the time of the procedure as the cause of the reaction.

j. Terrorism Guidelines

1) Cause of injury identified by the Federal Government (FBI) as terrorism

When the cause of an injury is identified by the Federal Government (FBI) as terrorism, the first-listed E-code should be a code from category E979, Terrorism. The definition of terrorism employed by the FBI is found at the inclusion note at E979. The terrorism E-code is the only E-code that should be assigned. Additional E codes from the assault categories should not be assigned.

2) Cause of an injury is suspected to be the result of terrorism

When the cause of an injury is suspected to be the result of terrorism a code from category E979 should not be assigned. Assign a code in the range of E codes based circumstances on the documentation of intent and mechanism.

3) Code E979.9, Terrorism, secondary effects

Assign code E979.9, Terrorism, secondary effects, for conditions occurring subsequent to the terrorist event. This code should not be assigned for conditions that are due to the initial terrorist act.

4) Statistical tabulation of terrorism codes

For statistical purposes these codes will be tabulated within the category for assault, expanding the current category from E960-E969 to include E979 and E999.1.

SECTION II. SELECTION OF PRINCIPAL DIAGNOSIS

The circumstances of inpatient admission always govern the selection of principal diagnosis. The principal diagnosis is defined in the Uniform Hospital Discharge Data Set (UHDDS) as "that condition established after study to be chiefly responsible for occasioning the admission of the patient to the hospital for care."

The UHDDS definitions are used by hospitals to report inpatient data elements in a standardized manner. These data elements and their definitions can be found in the July 31, 1985, Federal Register (Vol. 50, No, 147), pp. 31038-40.

Since that time the application of the UHDDS definitions has been expanded to include all non-outpatient settings (acute care, short term, long term care and psychiatric hospitals; home health agencies; rehab facilities; nursing homes, etc).

In determining principal diagnosis the coding conventions in the ICD-9-CM, Volumes I and II take precedence over these official coding guidelines.

(See Section I.A., Conventions for the ICD-9-CM)

The importance of consistent, complete documentation in the medical record cannot be overemphasized. Without such documentation the application of all coding guidelines is a difficult, if not impossible, task.

A. Codes for symptoms, signs, and ill-defined conditions

Codes for symptoms, signs, and ill-defined conditions from Chapter 16 are not to be used as principal diagnosis when a related definitive diagnosis has been established.

B. Two or more interrelated conditions, each potentially meeting the definition for principal diagnosis.

When there are two or more interrelated conditions (such as diseases in the same ICD-9-CM chapter or manifestations characteristically associated with a certain disease) potentially meeting the definition of principal diagnosis, either condition may be sequenced first, unless the circumstances of the admission, the therapy provided, the Tabular List, or the Alphabetic Index indicate otherwise.

C. Two or more diagnoses that equally meet the definition for principal diagnosis

In the unusual instance when two or more diagnoses equally meet the criteria for principal diagnosis as determined by the circumstances of admission, diagnostic workup and/or therapy provided, and the Alphabetic Index, Tabular List, or another coding guidelines does not provide sequencing direction, any one of the diagnoses may be sequenced first.

D. Two or more comparative or contrasting conditions.

In those rare instances when two or more contrasting or comparative diagnoses are documented as "either/or" (or similar terminology), they are coded as if the diagnoses were confirmed and the diagnoses are sequenced according to the circumstances of the admission. If no further determination can be made as to which diagnosis should be principal, either diagnosis may be sequenced first.

E. A symptom(s) followed by contrasting/comparative diagnoses

When a symptom(s) is followed by contrasting/comparative diagnoses, the symptom code is sequenced first. All the contrasting/comparative diagnoses should be coded as additional diagnoses.

238   Appendix A   ICD-9-CM Official Guidelines for Coding and Reporting

F. Original treatment plan not carried out

Sequence as the principal diagnosis the condition, which after study occasioned the admission to the hospital, even though treatment may not have been carried out due to unforeseen circumstances.

G. Complications of surgery and other medical care

When the admission is for treatment of a complication resulting from surgery or other medical care, the complication code is sequenced as the principal diagnosis. If the complication is classified to the 996-999 series and the code lacks the necessary specificity in describing the complication, an additional code for the specific complication should be assigned.

H. Uncertain Diagnosis

If the diagnosis documented at the time of discharge is qualified as "probable", "suspected", "likely", "questionable", "possible", or "still to be ruled out", or other similar terms indicating uncertainty, code the condition as if it existed or was established. The bases for these guidelines are the diagnostic workup, arrangements for further workup or observation, and initial therapeutic approach that correspond most closely with the established diagnosis.

Note: This guideline is applicable only to <u>inpatient admissions to</u> short-term, acute, long-term care and psychiatric hospitals.

I. Admission from Observation Unit

1. Admission Following Medical Observation

When a patient is admitted to an observation unit for a medical condition, which either worsens or does not improve, and is subsequently admitted as an inpatient of the same hospital for this same medical condition, the principal diagnosis would be the medical condition which led to the hospital admission.

2. Admission Following Post-Operative Observation

When a patient is admitted to an observation unit to monitor a condition (or complication) that develops following outpatient surgery, and then is subsequently admitted as an inpatient of the same hospital, hospitals should apply the Uniform Hospital Discharge Data Set (UHDDS) definition of principal diagnosis as "that condition established after study to be chiefly responsible for occasioning the admission of the patient to the hospital for care."

J. Admission from Outpatient Surgery

When a patient receives surgery in the hospital's outpatient surgery department and is subsequently admitted for continuing inpatient care at the same hospital, the following guidelines should be followed in selecting the principal diagnosis for the inpatient admission:

• If the reason for the inpatient admission is a complication, assign the complication as the principal diagnosis.

• If no complication, or other condition, is documented as the reason for the inpatient admission, assign the reason for the outpatient surgery as the principal diagnosis.

• If the reason for the inpatient admission is another condition unrelated to the surgery, assign the unrelated condition as the principal diagnosis.

Copyright © 2008, Elsevier Inc. All rights reserved.
CPT only © 2007. Current Procedural Terminology, 2008, Professional Edition, American Medical Association. All rights reserved.

SECTION III. REPORTING ADDITIONAL DIAGNOSES

GENERAL RULES FOR OTHER (ADDITIONAL) DIAGNOSES

For reporting purposes the definition for "other diagnoses" is interpreted as additional conditions that affect patient care in terms of requiring:

clinical evaluation; or

therapeutic treatment; or

diagnostic procedures; or

extended length of hospital stay; or

increased nursing care and/or monitoring.

The UHDDS item #11-b defines Other Diagnoses as "all conditions that coexist at the time of admission, that develop subsequently, or that affect the treatment received and/or the length of stay. Diagnoses that relate to an earlier episode which have no bearing on the current hospital stay are to be excluded." UHDDS definitions apply to inpatients in acute care, short-term, long term care and psychiatric hospital setting. The UHDDS definitions are used by acute care short-term hospitals to report inpatient data elements in a standardized manner. These data elements and their definitions can be found in the July 31, 1985, Federal Register (Vol. 50, No, 147), pp. 31038-40.

Since that time the application of the UHDDS definitions has been expanded to include all non-outpatient settings (acute care, short term, long term care and psychiatric hospitals; home health agencies; rehab facilities; nursing homes, etc).

The following guidelines are to be applied in designating "other diagnoses" when neither the Alphabetic Index nor the Tabular List in ICD-9-CM provide direction. The listing of the diagnoses in the patient record is the responsibility of the attending provider.

A. Previous conditions

If the provider has included a diagnosis in the final diagnostic statement, such as the discharge summary or the face sheet, it should ordinarily be coded. Some providers include in the diagnostic statement resolved conditions or diagnoses and status-post procedures from previous admission that have no bearing on the current stay. Such conditions are not to be reported and are coded only if required by hospital policy.

However, history codes (V10-V19) may be used as secondary codes if the historical condition or family history has an impact on current care or influences treatment.

B. Abnormal findings

Abnormal findings (laboratory, x-ray, pathologic, and other diagnostic results) are not coded and reported unless the provider indicates their clinical significance. If the findings are outside the normal range and the attending provider has ordered other tests to evaluate the condition or prescribed treatment, it is appropriate to ask the provider whether the abnormal finding should be added.

Please note: This differs from the coding practices in the outpatient setting for coding encounters for diagnostic tests that have been interpreted by a provider.

C. Uncertain Diagnosis

If the diagnosis documented at the time of discharge is qualified as "probable", "suspected", "likely", "questionable", "possible", or "still to be ruled out" or other similar terms indicating uncertainty, code the condition as if it existed or was established. The bases for these guidelines are the diagnostic workup, arrangements for further workup or observation, and initial therapeutic approach that correspond most closely with the established diagnosis.

Note: This guideline is applicable only to <u>inpatient admissions to</u> short-term, acute, long-term care and psychiatric hospitals.

SECTION IV. DIAGNOSTIC CODING AND REPORTING GUIDELINES FOR OUTPATIENT SERVICES

These coding guidelines for outpatient diagnoses have been approved for use by hospitals/ providers in coding and reporting hospital-based outpatient services and provider-based office visits.

Information about the use of certain abbreviations, punctuation, symbols, and other conventions used in the ICD-9-CM Tabular List (code numbers and titles), can be found in Section IA of these guidelines, under "Conventions Used in the Tabular List." Information about the correct sequence to use in finding a code is also described in Section I.

The terms encounter and visit are often used interchangeably in describing outpatient service contacts and, therefore, appear together in these guidelines without distinguishing one from the other.

Though the conventions and general guidelines apply to all settings, coding guidelines for outpatient and provider reporting of diagnoses will vary in a number of instances from those for inpatient diagnoses, recognizing that:

The Uniform Hospital Discharge Data Set (UHDDS) definition of principal diagnosis applies only to inpatients in acute, short-term, long-term care and psychiatric hospitals.

Coding guidelines for inconclusive diagnoses (probable, suspected, rule out, etc.) were developed for inpatient reporting and do not apply to outpatients.

A. Selection of first-listed condition

In the outpatient setting, the term first-listed diagnosis is used in lieu of principal diagnosis.

In determining the first-listed diagnosis the coding conventions of ICD-9-CM, as well as the general and disease specific guidelines take precedence over the outpatient guidelines.

Diagnoses often are not established at the time of the initial encounter/ visit. It may take two or more visits before the diagnosis is confirmed.

The most critical rule involves beginning the search for the correct code assignment through the Alphabetic Index. Never begin searching initially in the Tabular List as this will lead to coding errors.

1. Outpatient Surgery

When a patient presents for outpatient surgery, code the reason for the surgery as the first-listed diagnosis (reason for the encounter), even if the surgery is not performed due to a contraindication.

2. Observation Stay

When a patient is admitted for observation for a medical condition, assign a code for the medical condition as the first-listed diagnosis.

When a patient presents for outpatient surgery and develops complications requiring admission to observation, code the reason for the surgery as the first reported diagnosis (reason for the encounter), followed by codes for the complications as secondary diagnoses.

B. Codes from 001.0 through V84.8

The appropriate code or codes from 001.0 through V84.8 must be used to identify diagnoses, symptoms, conditions, problems, complaints, or other reason(s) for the encounter/visit.

C. Accurate reporting of ICD-9-CM diagnosis codes

For accurate reporting of ICD-9-CM diagnosis codes, the documentation should describe the patient's condition, using terminology which includes specific diagnoses as well as symptoms, problems, or reasons for the encounter. There are ICD-9-CM codes to describe all of these.

D. Selection of codes 001.0 through 999.9

The selection of codes 001.0 through 999.9 will frequently be used to describe the reason for the encounter. These codes are from the section of ICD-9-CM for the classification of diseases and injuries (e.g. infectious and parasitic diseases; neoplasms; symptoms, signs, and ill-defined conditions, etc.).

E. Codes that describe symptoms and signs

Codes that describe symptoms and signs, as opposed to diagnoses, are acceptable for reporting purposes when a diagnosis has not been established (confirmed) by the provider. Chapter 16 of ICD-9-CM, Symptoms, Signs, and Ill-defined conditions (codes 780.0-799.9) contain many, but not all codes for symptoms.

F. Encounters for circumstances other than a disease or injury

ICD-9-CM provides codes to deal with encounters for circumstances other than a disease or injury. The Supplementary Classification of factors Influencing Health Status and Contact with Health Services (V01.0- V84.8) is provided to deal with occasions when circumstances other than a disease or injury are recorded as diagnosis or problems. ***See Section I.C. 18 for information on V-codes***

G. Level of Detail in Coding

1.   ICD-9-CM codes with 3, 4, or 5 digits

ICD-9-CM is composed of codes with either 3, 4, or 5 digits. Codes with three digits are included in ICD-9-CM as the heading of a category of codes that may be further subdivided by the use of fourth and/or fifth digits, which provide greater specificity.

2.   Use of full number of digits required for a code

A three-digit code is to be used only if it is not further subdivided. Where fourth-digit subcategories and/or fifth-digit subclassifications are provided, they must be assigned. A code is invalid if it has not been coded to the full number of digits required for that code.

See also discussion under Section I.b.3., General Coding Guidelines, Level of Detail in Coding.

H. ICD-9-CM code for the diagnosis, condition, problem, or other reason for encounter/visit

List first the ICD-9-CM code for the diagnosis, condition, problem, or other reason for encounter/visit shown in the medical record to be chiefly responsible for the services provided. List additional codes that describe any coexisting conditions. In some cases the first-listed diagnosis may be a symptom when a diagnosis has not been established (confirmed) by the physician.

I. Uncertain diagnosis

Do not code diagnoses documented as "probable", "suspected," "questionable," "rule out," or "working diagnosis" or other similar terms indicating uncertainty. Rather, code the condition(s) to the highest degree of certainty for that encounter/visit, such as symptoms, signs, abnormal test results, or other reason for the visit. **Please note:** This differs from the coding practices used by short-term, acute care, long-term care and psychiatric hospitals.

J. Chronic diseases

Chronic diseases treated on an ongoing basis may be coded and reported as many times as the patient receives treatment and care for the condition(s).

K. Code all documented conditions that coexist

Code all documented conditions that coexist at the time of the encounter/visit, and require or affect patient care treatment or management. Do not code conditions that were previously treated and no longer exist. However, history codes (V10-V19) may be used as secondary codes if the historical condition or family history has an impact on current care or influences treatment.

L. Patients receiving diagnostic services only

For patients receiving diagnostic services only during an encounter/visit, sequence first the diagnosis, condition, problem, or other reason for encounter/visit shown in the medical record to be chiefly responsible for the outpatient services provided during the encounter/visit. Codes for other diagnoses (e.g., chronic conditions) may be sequenced as additional diagnoses.

For encounters for routine laboratory/radiology testing in the absence of any signs, symptoms, or associated diagnosis, assign V72.5 and V72.6. If routine testing is performed during the same encounter as a test to evaluate a sign, symptom, or diagnosis, it is appropriate to assign both the V code and the code describing the reason for the non-routine test.

For outpatient encounters for diagnostic tests that have been interpreted by a physician, and the final report is available at the time of coding, code any confirmed or definitive diagnosis(es) documented in the interpretation. Do not code related signs and symptoms as additional diagnoses.

Please note: This differs from the coding practice in the hospital inpatient setting regarding abnormal findings on test results.

M. Patients receiving therapeutic services only

For patients receiving therapeutic services only during an encounter/visit, sequence first the diagnosis, condition, problem, or other reason for encounter/visit shown in the medical record to be chiefly responsible for the outpatient services provided during the encounter/visit. Codes for other diagnoses (e.g., chronic conditions) may be sequenced as additional diagnoses.

The only exception to this rule is that when the primary reason for the admission/encounter is chemotherapy, radiation therapy, or rehabilitation, the appropriate V code for the service is listed first, and the diagnosis or problem for which the service is being performed listed second.

N. Patients receiving preoperative evaluations only

For patients receiving preoperative evaluations only, sequence **first** a code from category V72.8, Other specified examinations, to describe the pre-op consultations. Assign a code for the condition to describe the reason for the surgery as an additional diagnosis. Code also any findings related to the pre-op evaluation.

O. Ambulatory surgery

For ambulatory surgery, code the diagnosis for which the surgery was performed. If the postoperative diagnosis is known to be different from the preoperative diagnosis at the time the diagnosis is confirmed, select the postoperative diagnosis for coding, since it is the most definitive.

P. Routine outpatient prenatal visits

For routine outpatient prenatal visits when no complications are present, codes V22.0, Supervision of normal first pregnancy, or V22.1, Supervision of other normal pregnancy, should be used as the principal diagnosis. These codes should not be used in conjunction with chapter 11 codes.

APPENDIX I

PRESENT ON ADMISSION REPORTING GUIDELINES

Introduction

These guidelines are to be used as a supplement to the *ICD-9-CM Official Guidelines for Coding and Reporting* to facilitate the assignment of the Present on Admission (POA) indicator for each diagnosis and external cause of injury code reported on claim forms (UB-04 and 837 Institutional).

These guidelines are not intended to replace any guidelines in the main body of the *ICD-9-CM Official Guidelines for Coding and Reporting*. The POA guidelines are not intended to provide guidance on when a condition should be coded, but rather, how to apply the POA indicator to the final set of diagnosis codes that have been assigned in accordance with Sections I, II, and III of the official coding guidelines. Subsequent to the assignment of the ICD-9-CM codes, the POA indicator should then be assigned to those conditions that have been coded.

As stated in the Introduction to the ICD-9-CM Official Guidelines for Coding and Reporting, a joint effort between the healthcare provider and the coder is essential to achieve complete and accurate documentation, code assignment, and reporting of diagnoses and procedures. The importance of consistent, complete documentation in the medical record cannot be overemphasized. Medical record documentation from any provider involved in the care and treatment of the patient may be used to support the determination of whether a condition was present on admission or not. In the context of the official coding guidelines, the term "provider" means a physician or any qualified healthcare practitioner who is legally accountable for establishing the patient's diagnosis.

General Reporting Requirements

All claims involving inpatient admissions to general acute care hospitals or other facilities that are subject to a law or regulation mandating collection of present on admission information.

Present on admission is defined as present at the time the order for inpatient admission occurs—conditions that develop during an outpatient encounter, including emergency department, observation, or outpatient surgery, are considered as present on admission.

POA indicator is assigned to principal and secondary diagnoses (as defined in Section II of the Official Guidelines for Coding and Reporting) and the external cause of injury codes.

Issues related to inconsistent, missing, conflicting or unclear documentation must still be resolved by the provider.

If a condition would not be coded and reported based on UHDDS definitions and current official coding guidelines, then the POA indicator would not be reported.

Reporting Options

Y—Yes
N—No
U—Unknown
W—Clinically undetermined
Unreported/Not used—(Exempt from POA reporting)

Reporting Definitions

Y = present at the time of inpatient admission
N = not present at the time of inpatient admission
U = documentation is insufficient to determine if condition is present on admission
W = provider is unable to clinically determine whether condition was present on admission or not

Assigning the POA Indicator

Condition is on the "Exempt from Reporting" list

Leave the "present on admission" field blank if the condition is on the list of ICD-9-CM codes for which this field is not applicable. This is the only circumstance in which the field may be left blank.

POA Explicitly Documented

Assign Y for any condition the provider explicitly documents as being present on admission.

Assign N for any condition the provider explicitly documents as not present at the time of admission.

Conditions diagnosed prior to inpatient admission

Assign "Y" for conditions that were diagnosed prior to admission (example: hypertension, diabetes mellitus, asthma)

Conditions diagnosed during the admission but clearly present before admission

Assign "Y" for conditions diagnosed during the admission that were clearly present but not diagnosed until after admission occurred.

Diagnoses subsequently confirmed after admission are considered present on admission if at the time of admission they are documented as suspected, possible, rule out, differential diagnosis, or constitute an underlying cause of a symptom that is present at the time of admission.

Condition develops during outpatient encounter prior to inpatient admission

Assign Y for any condition that develops during an outpatient encounter prior to a written order for inpatient admission.

Documentation does not indicate whether condition was present on admission

Assign "U" when the medical record documentation is unclear as to whether the condition was present on admission. "U" should not be routinely assigned and used only in very limited circumstances. Coders are encouraged to query the providers when the documentation is unclear.

Documentation states that it cannot be determined whether the condition was or was not present on admission

Assign "W" when the medical record documentation indicates that it cannot be clinically determined whether or not the condition was present on admission.

Chronic condition with acute exacerbation during the admission

If the code is a combination code that identifies both the chronic condition and the acute exacerbation, see POA guidelines pertaining to combination codes.

If the combination code only identifies the chronic condition and not the acute exacerbation (e.g., acute exacerbation of CHF), assign "Y."

Conditions documented as possible, probable, suspected, or rule out at the time of discharge

If the final diagnosis contains a possible, probable, suspected, or rule out diagnosis, and this diagnosis was suspected at the time of inpatient admission, assign "Y."

If the final diagnosis contains a possible, probable, suspected, or rule out diagnosis, and this diagnosis was based on symptoms or clinical findings that were not present on admission, assign "N".

Conditions documented as impending or threatened at the time of discharge

If the final diagnosis contains an impending or threatened diagnosis, and this diagnosis is based on symptoms or clinical findings that were present on admission, assign "Y".

If the final diagnosis contains an impending or threatened diagnosis, and this diagnosis is based on symptoms or clinical findings that were **not** present on admission, assign "N".

Acute and Chronic Conditions

Assign "Y" for acute conditions that are present at time of admission and N for acute conditions that are not present at time of admission.

Assign "Y" for chronic conditions, even though the condition may not be diagnosed until after admission.

If a single code identifies both an acute and chronic condition, see the POA guidelines for combination codes.

Combination Codes

Assign "N" if any part of the combination code was not present on admission (e.g., obstructive chronic bronchitis with acute exacerbation and the exacerbation was not present on admission; gastric ulcer that does not start bleeding until after admission; asthma patient develops status asthmaticus after admission).

Assign "Y" if all parts of the combination code were present on admission (e.g., patient with diabetic nephropathy is admitted with uncontrolled diabetes)

If the final diagnosis includes comparative or contrasting diagnoses, and both were present, or suspected, at the time of admission, assign "Y".

For infection codes that include the causal organism, assign "Y" if the infection (or signs of the infection) was present on admission, even though the culture results may not be known until after admission (e.g., patient is admitted with pneumonia and the provider documents pseudomonas as the causal organism a few days later).

Obstetrical conditions

Whether or not the patient delivers during the current hospitalization does not affect assignment of the POA indicator. The determining factor for POA assignment is whether the pregnancy complication or obstetrical condition described by the code was present at the time of admission or not.

If the pregnancy complication or obstetrical condition was present on admission (e.g., patient admitted in preterm labor), assign "Y".

If the pregnancy complication or obstetrical condition was not present on admission (e.g., 2nd degree laceration during delivery, postpartum hemorrhage that occurred during current hospitalization, fetal distress develops after admission), assign "N".

If the obstetrical code includes more than one diagnosis and any of the diagnoses identified by the code were not present on admission assign "N".

(e.g., Code 642.7, Pre-eclampsia or eclampsia superimposed on pre-existing hypertension).

If the obstetrical code includes information that is not a diagnosis, do not consider that information in the POA determination.

(e.g. Code 652.1x, Breech or other malpresentation successfully converted to cephalic presentation should be reported as present on admission if the fetus was breech on admission but was converted to cephalic presentation after admission (since the conversion to cephalic presentation does not represent a diagnosis, the fact that the conversion occurred after admission has no bearing on the POA determination).

Perinatal conditions

Newborns are not considered to be admitted until after birth. Therefore, any condition present at birth or that developed in utero is considered present at admission and should be assigned "Y". This includes conditions that occur during delivery (e.g., injury during delivery, meconium aspiration, exposure to streptococcus B in the vaginal canal).

Congenital conditions and anomalies

Assign "Y" for congenital conditions and anomalies. Congenital conditions are always considered present on admission.

External cause of injury codes

Assign "Y" for any E code representing an external cause of injury or poisoning that occurred prior to inpatient admission (e.g., patient fell out of bed at home, patient fell out of bed in emergency room prior to admission).

Assign "N" for any E code representing an external cause of injury or poisoning that occurred during inpatient hospitalization (e.g., patient fell out of hospital bed during hospital stay, patient experienced an adverse reaction to a medication administered after inpatient admission).

CATEGORIES AND CODES EXEMPT FROM DIAGNOSIS PRESENT ON ADMISSION REQUIREMENT

Note: "Diagnosis present on admission" for these code categories are exempt because they represent circumstances regarding the healthcare encounter or factors influencing health status that do not represent a current disease or injury or are always present on admission

137-139, Late effects of infectious and parasitic diseases

268.1, Rickets, late effect

326, Late effects of intracranial abscess or pyogenic infection

412, Old myocardial infarction

438, Late effects of cerebrovascular disease

650, Normal delivery

660.7, Failed forceps or vacuum extractor, unspecified

677, Late effect of complication of pregnancy, childbirth, and the puerperium

905-909, Late effects of injuries, poisonings, toxic effects, and other external causes

V02, Carrier or suspected carrier of infectious diseases

V03, Need for prophylactic vaccination and inoculation against bacterial diseases

V04, Need for prophylactic vaccination and inoculation against certain viral diseases

V05, Need for other prophylactic vaccination and inoculation against single diseases

V06, Need for prophylactic vaccination and inoculation against combinations of diseases

V07, Need for isolation and other prophylactic measures

V10, Personal history of malignant neoplasm

V11, Personal history of mental disorder

V12, Personal history of certain other diseases

V13, Personal history of other diseases

V14, Personal history of allergy to medicinal agents

V15, Other personal history presenting hazards to health

V16, Family history of malignant neoplasm

V17, Family history of certain chronic disabling diseases

V18, Family history of certain other specific conditions

V19, Family history of other conditions

V20, Health supervision of infant or child

V21, Constitutional states in development

V22, Normal pregnancy

V23, Supervision of high-risk pregnancy

V24, Postpartum care and examination

V25, Encounter for contraceptive management

V26, Procreative management

V27, Outcome of delivery

V28, Antenatal screening

V29, Observation and evaluation of newborns for suspected condition not found

V30-V39, Liveborn infants according to type of birth

V42, Organ or tissue replaced by transplant

V43, Organ or tissue replaced by other means

V44, Artificial opening status

V45, Other postprocedural states

V46, Other dependence on machines

V49.60-V49.77, Upper and lower limb amputation status

V49.81-V49.84, Other specified conditions influencing health status

V50, Elective surgery for purposes other than remedying health states

V51, Aftercare involving the use of plastic surgery

V52, Fitting and adjustment of prosthetic device and implant

V53, Fitting and adjustment of other device

V54, Other orthopedic aftercare

V55, Attention to artificial openings

V56, Encounter for dialysis and dialysis catheter care

V57, Care involving use of rehabilitation procedures

V58, Encounter for other and unspecified procedures and aftercare

V59, Donors

V60, Housing, household, and economic circumstances

V61, Other family circumstances

V62, Other psychosocial circumstances

V64, Persons encountering health services for specific procedures, not carried out

V65, Other persons seeking consultation

V66, Convalescence and palliative care

V67, Follow-up examination

V68, Encounters for administrative purposes

V69, Problems related to lifestyle

V70, General medical examination

V71, Observation and evaluation for suspected condition not found

V72, Special investigations and examinations

V73, Special screening examination for viral and chlamydial diseases

V74, Special screening examination for bacterial and spirochetal diseases

V75, Special screening examination for other infectious diseases

V76, Special screening for malignant neoplasms

V77, Special screening for endocrine, nutritional, metabolic, and immunity disorders

V78, Special screening for disorders of blood and blood-forming organs

V79, Special screening for mental disorders and developmental handicaps

V80, Special screening for neurological, eye, and ear diseases

V81, Special screening for cardiovascular, respiratory, and genitourinary diseases

V82, Special screening for other conditions

V83, Genetic carrier status

V84, Genetic susceptibility to disease

V85, Body Mass Index

V86, Estrogen receptor status

E800-E807, Railway accidents

E810-E819, Motor vehicle traffic accidents

E820-E825, Motor vehicle nontraffic accidents

E826-E829, Other road vehicle accidents

E830-E838, Water transport accidents

E840-E845, Air and space transport accidents

E846-E848, Vehicle accidents not elsewhere classifiable

E849.0-E849.6, Place of occurrence

E849.8-E849.9, Place of occurrence

E883.1, Accidental fall into well

E883.2, Accidental fall into storm drain or manhole

E884.0, Fall from playground equipment

E884.1, Fall from cliff

E885.0, Fall from (nonmotorized) scooter

E885.1, Fall from roller skates

E885.2, Fall from skateboard

E885.3, Fall from skis

E885.4, Fall from snowboard

E886.0, Fall on same level from collision, pushing, or shoving, by or with other person, In sports

E890.0-E89.9, Conflagration in private dwelling

E893.0, Accident caused by ignition of clothing, from controlled fire in private dwelling

E893.2, Accident caused by ignition of clothing, from controlled fire not in building or structure

E894, Ignition of highly inflammable material

E895, Accident caused by controlled fire in private dwelling

E897, Accident caused by controlled fire not in building or structure

E898.0-E898.1, Accident caused by other specified fire and flames

E917.0, Striking against or struck accidentally by objects or persons, in sports without subsequent fall

E917.1, Striking against or struck accidentally by objects or persons, caused by a crowd, by collective fear or panic without subsequent fall

E917.2, Striking against or struck accidentally by objects or persons, in running water without subsequent fall

E917.5, Striking against or struck accidentally by objects or persons, object in sports with subsequent fall

E917.6, Striking against or struck accidentally by objects or persons, caused by a crowd, by collective fear or panic with subsequent fall

E919.0-E919.1, Accidents caused by machinery

E919.3-E919.9, Accidents caused by machinery

E921.0-E921.9, Accident caused by explosion of pressure vessel

E922.0-E922.9, Accident caused by firearm and air gun missile

E924.1, Caustic and corrosive substances

E926.2, Visible and ultraviolet light sources

E927, Overexertion and strenuous movements

E928.0-E928.8, Other and unspecified environmental and accidental causes

E929.0-E929.9, Late effects of accidental injury

E959, Late effects of self-inflicted injury

E970-E978, Legal intervention

E979, Terrorism

E981.0-E981.8, Poisoning by gases in domestic use, undetermined whether accidentally or purposely inflicted

E982.0-E982.9, Poisoning by other gases, undetermined whether accidentally or purposely inflicted

E985.0-E985.7, Injury by firearms, air guns and explosives, undetermined whether accidentally or purposely inflicted

E987.0, Falling from high place, undetermined whether accidentally or purposely inflicted, residential premises

E987.2, Falling from high place, undetermined whether accidentally or purposely inflicted, natural sites

E989, Late effects of injury, undetermined whether accidentally or purposely inflicted

E990-E999, Injury resulting from operations of war

POA EXAMPLES
General Medical Surgical

1. Patient is admitted for diagnostic work-up for cachexia. The final diagnosis is malignant neoplasm of lung with metastasis.

   Assign "Y" on the POA field for the malignant neoplasm. The malignant neoplasm was clearly present on admission, although it was not diagnosed until after the admission occurred.

2. A patient undergoes outpatient surgery. During the recovery period, the patient develops atrial fibrillation and the patient is subsequently admitted to the hospital as an inpatient.

   Assign "Y" on the POA field for the atrial fibrillation since it developed prior to a written order for inpatient admission.

3. A patient is treated in observation and while in Observation, the patient falls out of bed and breaks a hip. The patient is subsequently admitted as an inpatient to treat the hip fracture.

   Assign "Y" on the POA field for the hip fracture since it developed prior to a written order for inpatient admission.

4. A patient with known congestive heart failure is admitted to the hospital after he develops decompensated congestive heart failure.

   Assign "Y" on the POA field for the congestive heart failure. The ICD-9-CM code identifies the chronic condition and does not specify the acute exacerbation.

5. A patient undergoes inpatient surgery. After surgery, the patient develops fever and is treated aggressively. The physician's final diagnosis documents "possible postoperative infection following surgery."

   Assign "N" on the POA field for the postoperative infection since final diagnoses that contain the terms "possible", "probable", "suspected" or "rule out" and that are based on symptoms or clinical findings that were not present on admission should be reported as "N".

6. A patient with severe cough and difficulty breathing was diagnosed during his hospitalization to have lung cancer.

   Assign "Y" on the POA field for the lung cancer. Even though the cancer was not diagnosed until after admission, it is a chronic condition that was clearly present before the patient's admission.

7. A patient is admitted to the hospital for a coronary artery bypass surgery. Postoperatively he developed a pulmonary embolism.

    Assign "N" on the POA field for the pulmonary embolism. This is an acute condition that was not present on admission.

8. A patient is admitted with a known history of coronary atherosclerosis, status post myocardial infarction five years ago is now admitted for treatment of impending myocardial infarction. The final diagnosis is documented as "impending myocardial infarction."

    Assign "Y" to the impending myocardial infarction because the condition is present on admission.

9. A patient with diabetes mellitus developed uncontrolled diabetes on day 3 of the hospitalization.

    Assign "N" to the diabetes code because the "uncontrolled" component of the code was not present on admission.

10. A patient is admitted with high fever and pneumonia. The patient rapidly deteriorates and becomes septic. The discharge diagnosis lists sepsis and pneumonia. The documentation is unclear as to whether the sepsis was present on admission or developed shortly after admission.

    Query the physician as to whether the sepsis was present on admission, developed shortly after admission, or it cannot be clinically determined as to whether it was present on admission or not.

11. A patient is admitted for repair of an abdominal aneurysm. However, the aneurysm ruptures after hospital admission.

    Assign "N" for the ruptured abdominal aneurysm. Although the aneurysm was present on admission, the "ruptured" component of the code description did not occur until after admission.

12. A patient with viral hepatitis B progresses to hepatic coma after admission.

    Assign "N" for the viral hepatitis B with hepatic coma because part of the code description did not develop until after admission.

13. A patient with a history of varicose veins and ulceration of the left lower extremity strikes the area against the side of his hospital bed during an inpatient hospitalization. It bleeds profusely. The final diagnosis lists varicose veins with ulcer and hemorrhage.

    Assign "Y" for the varicose veins with ulcer. Although the hemorrhage occurred after admission, the code description for varicose veins with ulcer does not mention hemorrhage.

14. The nursing initial assessment upon admission documents the presence of a decubitus ulcer. There is no mention of the decubitus ulcer in the physician documentation until several days after admission.

    Query the physician as to whether the decubitus ulcer was present on admission, or developed after admission. Both diagnosis code assignment and determination of whether a condition was present on admission must be based on provider documentation in the medical record (per the definition of "provider" found at the beginning of these POA guidelines and in the introductory section of the ICD-9-CM Official Guidelines for Coding and Reporting). If it cannot be determined from the provider documentation whether or not a condition was present on admission, the provider should be queried.

Obstetrics

1. A female patient was admitted to the hospital and underwent a normal delivery.

   Leave the "present on admission" (POA) field blank. Code 650, Normal delivery, is on the "exempt from reporting" list.

2. Patient admitted in late pregnancy due to excessive vomiting and dehydration. During admission patient goes into premature labor

   Assign "Y" for the excessive vomiting and the dehydration.

   Assign "N" for the premature labor.

3. Patient admitted in active labor. During the stay, a breast abscess is noted when mother attempted to breast feed. Provider is unable to determine whether the abscess was present on admission

   Assign "W" for the breast abscess.

4. Patient admitted in active labor. After 12 hours of labor it is noted that the infant is in fetal distress and a Cesarean section is performed.

   Assign "N" for the fetal distress.

Newborn

1. A single liveborn infant was delivered in the hospital via Cesarean section. The physician documented fetal bradycardia during labor in the final diagnosis in the newborn record.

   Assign "Y" because the bradycardia developed prior to the newborn admission (birth).

2. A newborn developed diarrhea which was believed to be due to the hospital baby formula.

   Assign "N" because the diarrhea developed after admission.

1995 Guidelines for E/M Services

I. INTRODUCTION

What Is Documentation and Why Is It Important?

Medical record documentation is required to record pertinent facts, findings, and observations about an individual's health history including past and present illnesses, examinations, tests, treatments, and outcomes. The medical record chronologically documents the care of the patient and is an important element contributing to high quality care. The medical record facilitates:

- the ability of the physician and other health care professionals to evaluate and plan the patient's immediate treatment, and to monitor his/her health care over time.

- communication and continuity of care among physicians and other health care professionals involved in the patient's care;

- accurate and timely claims review and payment;

- appropriate utilization review and quality of care evaluations; and

- collection of data that may be useful for research and education.

An appropriately documented medical record can reduce many of the "hassles" associated with claims processing and may serve as a legal document to verify the care provided, if necessary.

What Do Payers Want and Why?

Because payers have a contractual obligation to enrollees, they may require reasonable documentation that services are consistent with the insurance coverage provided. They may request information to validate:

- the site of service;

- the medical necessity and appropriateness of the diagnostic and/or therapeutic services provided; and/or

- that services provided have been accurately reported.

II. GENERAL PRINCIPLES OF MEDICAL RECORD DOCUMENTATION

The principles of documentation listed below are applicable to all types of medical and surgical services in all settings. For Evaluation and Management (E/M) services, the nature and amount of physician work and documentation varies by type of service, place of service and the patient's status. The general principles listed below may be modified to account for these variable circumstances in providing E/M services.

1. The medical record should be complete and legible.

2. The documentation of each patient encounter should include:

   ■ reason for the encounter and relevant history, physical examination findings and prior diagnostic test results;

   ■ assessment, clinical impression or diagnosis;

   ■ plan for care; and

   ■ date and legible identity of the observer.

3. If not documented, the rationale for ordering diagnostic and other ancillary services should be easily inferred.

4. Past and present diagnoses should be accessible to the treating and/or consulting physician.

5. Appropriate health risk factors should be identified.

6. The patient's progress, response to and changes in treatment, and revision of diagnosis should be documented.

7. The CPT and ICD-9-CM codes reported on the health insurance claim form or billing statement should be supported by the documentation in the medical record.

III. DOCUMENTATION OF E/M SERVICES

This publication provides definitions and documentation guidelines for the three *key* components of E/M services and for visits which consist predominately of counseling or coordination of care. The three key components—history, examination, and medical decision making—appear in the descriptors for office and other outpatient services, hospital observation services, hospital inpatient services, consultations, emergency department services, nursing facility services, domiciliary care services, and home services. While some of the text of CPT has been repeated in this publication, the reader should refer to CPT for the complete descriptors for E/M services and instructions for selecting a level of service. **Documentation guidelines are identified by the symbol •*DG*.**

The descriptors for the levels of E/M services recognize seven components which are used in defining the levels of E/M services. These components are:

■ history;

■ examination;

■ medical decision making;

■ counseling;

■ coordination of care;

■ nature of presenting problem; and

■ time.

The first three of these components (i.e., history, examination and medical decision making) are the *key* components in selecting the level of E/M services. An exception to this rule is the case of visits which consist predominantly of counseling or coordination of care; for these services time is the key or controlling factor to qualify for a particular level of E/M service.

For certain groups of patients, the recorded information may vary slightly from that described here. Specifically, the medical records of infants, children, adolescents and pregnant women may have additional or modified information recorded in each history and examination area.

As an example, newborn records may include under history of the present illness (HPI) the details of mother's pregnancy and the infant's status at birth; social history will focus on family structure; family history will focus on congenital anomalies and hereditary disorders in the family. In addition, information on growth and development and/or nutrition will be recorded. Although not specifically defined in these documentation guidelines, these patient group variations on history and examination are appropriate.

A. Documentation of History

The levels of E/M services are based on four types of history (Problem Focused, Expanded Problem Focused, Detailed, and Comprehensive.) Each type of history includes some or all of the following elements:

■ Chief complaint (CC);

■ History of present illness (HPI);

■ Review of systems (ROS); and

■ Past, family and/or social history (PFSH).

The extent of history of present illness, review of systems and past, family and/or social history that is obtained and documented is dependent upon clinical judgement and the nature of the presenting problem(s).

The chart below shows the progression of the elements required for each type of history. To qualify for a given type of history, **all three elements in the table must be met.** (A chief complaint is indicated at all levels.)

History of Present Illness (HPI)	Review of Systems (ROS)	Past, Family, and/or Social History (PFSH)	Type of History
Brief	N/A	N/A	*Problem Focused*
Brief	Problem Pertinent	N/A	*Expanded Problem Focused*
Extended	Extended	Pertinent	*Detailed*
Extended	Complete	Complete	*Comprehensive*

•DG: *The CC, ROS and PFSH may be listed as separate elements of history, or they may be included in the description of the history of the present illness.*

•DG: *A ROS and/or a PFSH obtained during an earlier encounter does not need to be re-recorded if there is evidence that the physician reviewed and updated the previous information. This may occur when a physician updates his or her own record or in an institutional setting or group practice where many physicians use a common record. The review and update may be documented by:*

■ *describing any new ROS and/or PFSH information or noting there has been no change in the information; and*

■ *noting the date and location of the earlier ROS and/or PFSH.*

•DG: The ROS and/or PFSH may be recorded by ancillary staff or on a form completed by the patient. To document that the physician reviewed the information, there must be a notation supplementing or confirming the information recorded by others.

•DG: If the physician is unable to obtain a history from the patient or other source, the record should describe the patient's condition or other circumstance which precludes obtaining a history.

Definitions and specific documentation guidelines for each of the elements of history are listed below.

Chief Complaint (CC)

The CC is a concise statement describing the symptom, problem, condition, diagnosis, physician recommended return, or other factor that is the reason for the encounter.

•DG: The medical record should clearly reflect the chief complaint.

History of Present Illness (HPI)

The HPI is a chronological description of the development of the patient's present illness from the first sign and/or symptom or from the previous encounter to the present. It includes the following elements:

- location,
- quality,
- severity,
- duration,
- timing,
- context,
- modifying factors, and
- associated signs and symptoms.

Brief and **extended** HPIs are distinguished by the amount of detail needed to accurately characterize the clinical problem(s).

A **brief** HPI consists of one to three elements of the HPI.

•DG: The medical record should describe one to three elements of the present illness (HPI).

An **extended** HPI consists of four or more elements of the HPI.

•DG: The medical record should describe four or more elements of the present illness (HPI) or associated comorbidities.

Review of Systems (ROS)

A ROS is an inventory of body systems obtained through a series of questions seeking to identify signs and/or symptoms which the patient may be experiencing or has experienced.

For purposes of ROS, the following systems are recognized:

- Constitutional symptoms (e.g., fever, weight loss)
- Eyes
- Ears, Nose, Mouth, Throat

- Cardiovascular
- Respiratory
- Gastrointestinal
- Genitourinary
- Musculoskeletal
- Integumentary (skin and/or breast)
- Neurological
- Psychiatric
- Endocrine
- Hematologic/Lymphatic
- Allergic/Immunologic

A ***problem pertinent*** ROS inquires about the system directly related to the problem(s) identified in the HPI.

•*DG: The patient's positive responses and pertinent negatives for the system related to the problem should be documented.*

An ***extended*** ROS inquires about the system directly related to the problem(s) identified in the HPI and a limited number of additional systems.

•*DG: The patient's positive responses and pertinent negatives for two to nine systems should be documented.*

A ***complete*** ROS inquires about the system(s) directly related to the problem(s) identified in the HPI plus all additional body systems.

•*DG: At least ten organ systems must be reviewed. Those systems with positive or pertinent negative responses must be individually documented. For the remaining systems, a notation indicating all other systems are negative is permissible. In the absence of such a notation, at least ten systems must be individually documented.*

Past, Family and/or Social History (PFSH)

The PFSH consists of a review of three areas:

- past history (the patient's past experiences with illnesses, operations, injuries and treatments);
- family history (a review of medical events in the patient's family, including diseases which may be hereditary or place the patient at risk); and
- social history (an age appropriate review of past and current activities).

For the categories of subsequent hospital care, follow-up inpatient consultations and subsequent nursing facility care, CPT requires only an "interval" history. It is not necessary to record information about the PFSH.

A ***pertinent*** PFSH is a review of the history area(s) directly related to the problem(s) identified in the HPI.

•*DG: At least one specific item from <u>any</u> of the three history areas must be documented for a pertinent PFSH .*

A ***complete*** PFSH is of a review of two or all three of the PFSH history areas, depending on the category of the E/M service. A review of all three history areas is required for services that by their nature include a comprehensive assessment or reassessment of the patient. A review of two of the three history areas is sufficient for other services.

•*DG: At least one specific item from <u>two</u> of the three history areas must be documented for a complete PFSH for the following categories of E/M services: office or other outpatient services, established patient; emergency department; subsequent nursing facility care; domiciliary care, established patient; and home care, established patient.*

•*DG: At least one specific item from <u>each</u> of the three history areas must be documented for a complete PFSH for the following categories of E/M services: office or other outpatient services, new patient; hospital observation services; hospital inpatient services, initial care; consultations; comprehensive nursing facility assessments; domiciliary care, new patient; and home care, new patient.*

B. Documentation of Examination

The levels of E/M services are based on four types of examination that are defined as follows:

■ *Problem Focused*—a limited examination of the affected body area or organ system.

■ *Expanded Problem Focused*—a limited examination of the affected body area or organ system and other symptomatic or related organ system(s).

■ *Detailed*—an extended examination of the affected body area(s) and other symptomatic or related organ system(s).

■ *Comprehensive*—a general multi-system examination or complete examination of a single organ system.

For purposes of examination, the following *body areas* are recognized:

■ Head, including the face

■ Neck

■ Chest, including breasts and axillae

■ Abdomen

■ Genitalia, groin, buttocks

■ Back, including spine

■ Each extremity

For purposes of examination, the following *organ systems* are recognized:

■ Constitutional (e.g., vital signs, general appearance)

■ Eyes

■ Ears, nose, mouth and throat

■ Cardiovascular

■ Respiratory

■ Gastrointestinal

■ Genitourinary

■ Musculoskeletal

■ Skin

- Neurologic
- Psychiatric
- Hematologic/lymphatic/immunologic

The extent of examinations performed and documented is dependent upon clinical judgement and the nature of the presenting problem(s). They range from limited examinations of single body areas to general multi-system or complete single organ system examinations.

•DG: Specific abnormal and relevant negative findings of the examination of the affected or symptomatic body area(s) or organ system(s) should be documented. A notation of "abnormal" without elaboration is insufficient.

•DG: Abnormal or unexpected findings of the examination of the unaffected or asymptomatic body area(s) or organ system(s) should be described.

•DG: A brief statement or notation indicating "negative" or "normal" is sufficient to document normal findings related to unaffected area(s) or asymptomatic organ system(s).

•DG: The medical record for a general multi-system examination should include findings about 8 or more of the 12 organ systems.

C. Documentation of the Complexity of Medical Decision Making

The levels of E/M services recognize four types of medical decision making (straight-forward, low complexity, moderate complexity and high complexity). Medical decision making refers to the complexity of establishing a diagnosis and/or selecting a management option as measured by:

- the number of possible diagnoses and/or the number of management options that must be considered;
- the amount and/or complexity of medical records, diagnostic tests, and/or other information that must be obtained, reviewed and analyzed; and
- the risk of significant complications, morbidity and/or mortality, as well as comorbidities, associated with the patient's presenting problem(s), the diagnostic procedure(s) and/or the possible management options.

The chart below shows the progression of the elements required for each level of medical decision making. To qualify for a given type of decision making, **two of the three elements in the table must be either met or exceeded.**

Number of Diagnoses or Management Options	Amount and/or Complexity of Data to Be Reviewed	Risk of Complications and/ or Morbidity or Mortality	Type of Decision Making
Minimal	Minimal or None	Minimal	*Straightforward*
Limited	Limited	Low	*Low Complexity*
Multiple	Moderate	Moderate	*Moderate Complexity*
Extensive	Extensive	High	*High Complexity*

Each of the elements of medical decision making is described below.

Number of Diagnoses or Management Options

The number of possible diagnoses and/or the number of management options that must be considered is based on the number and types of problems addressed during the encounter, the complexity of establishing a diagnosis and the management decisions that are made by the physician.

Generally, decision making with respect to a diagnosed problem is easier than that for an identified but undiagnosed problem. The number and type of diagnostic tests employed may be an indicator of the number of possible diagnoses. Problems which are improving or resolving are less complex than those which are worsening or failing to change as expected. The need to seek advice from others is another indicator of complexity of diagnostic or management problems.

•DG: *For each encounter, an assessment, clinical impression, or diagnosis should be documented. It may be explicitly stated or implied in documented decisions regarding management plans and/or further evaluation.*

■ *For a presenting problem with an established diagnosis the record should reflect whether the problem is: a) improved, well controlled, resolving or resolved; or, b) inadequately controlled, worsening, or failing to change as expected.*

■ *For a presenting problem without an established diagnosis, the assessment or clinical impression may be stated in the form of a differential diagnoses or as "possible", "probable", or "rule out" (R/O) diagnoses.*

•DG: *The initiation of, or changes in, treatment should be documented. Treatment includes a wide range of management options including patient instructions, nursing instructions, therapies, and medications.*

•DG: *If referrals are made, consultations requested or advice sought, the record should indicate to whom or where the referral or consultation is made or from whom the advice is requested.*

Amount and/or Complexity of Data to be Reviewed

The amount and complexity of data to be reviewed is based on the types of diagnostic testing ordered or reviewed. A decision to obtain and review old medical records and/or obtain history from sources other than the patient increases the amount and complexity of data to be reviewed.

Discussion of contradictory or unexpected test results with the physician who performed or interpreted the test is an indication of the complexity of data being reviewed. On occasion the physician who ordered a test may personally review the image, tracing or specimen to supplement information from the physician who prepared the test report or interpretation; this is another indication of the complexity of data being reviewed.

•DG: *If a diagnostic service (test or procedure) is ordered, planned, scheduled, or performed at the time of the E/M encounter, the type of service, eg, lab or x-ray, should be documented.*

•DG: *The review of lab, radiology and/or other diagnostic tests should be documented. An entry in a progress note such as "WBC elevated" or "chest x-ray unremarkable" is acceptable. Alternatively, the review may be documented by initialing and dating the report containing the test results.*

•DG: *A decision to obtain old records or decision to obtain additional history from the family, caretaker or other source to supplement that obtained from the patient should be documented.*

•*DG: Relevant finding from the review of old records, and/or the receipt of additional history from the family, caretaker or other source should be documented. If there is no relevant information beyond that already obtained, that fact should be documented. A notation of "Old records reviewed" or "additional history obtained from family" without elaboration is insufficient.*

•*DG: The results of discussion of laboratory, radiology or other diagnostic tests with the physician who performed or interpreted the study should be documented.*

•*DG: The direct visualization and independent interpretation of an image, tracing or specimen previously or subsequently interpreted by another physician should be documented.*

Risk of Significant Complications, Morbidity, and/or Mortality

The risk of significant complications, morbidity, and/or mortality is based on the risks associated with the presenting problem(s), the diagnostic procedure(s), and the possible management options.

•*DG: Comorbidities/underlying diseases or other factors that increase the complexity of medical decision making by increasing the risk of complications, morbidity, and/or mortality should be documented.*

•*DG: If a surgical or invasive diagnostic procedure is ordered, planned or scheduled at the time of the E/M encounter, the type of procedure, eg, laparoscopy, should be documented.*

•*DG: If a surgical or invasive diagnostic procedure is performed at the time of the E/M encounter, the specific procedure should be documented.*

•*DG: The referral for or decision to perform a surgical or invasive diagnostic procedure on an urgent basis should be documented or implied.*

The following table may be used to help determine whether the risk of significant complications, morbidity, and/or mortality is **minimal, low, moderate,** or **high.** Because the determination of risk is complex and not readily quantifiable, the table includes common clinical examples rather than absolute measures of risk. The assessment of risk of the presenting problem(s) is based on the risk related to the disease process anticipated between the present encounter and the next one. The assessment of risk of selecting diagnostic procedures and management options is based on the risk during and immediately following any procedures or treatment. The highest level of risk in any one category (presenting problem(s), diagnostic procedure(s), or management options) determines the overall risk.

TABLE OF RISK

Level of Risk	Presenting Problem(s)	Diagnostic Procedure(s) Ordered	Management Options Selected
Minimal	• One self-limited or minor problem, eg, cold, insect bite, tinea corporis	• Laboratory tests requiring venipuncture • Chest x-rays • EKG/EEG • Urinalysis • Ultrasound, eg, echocardiography • KOH prep	• Rest • Gargles • Elastic bandages • Superficial dressings
Low	• Two or more self-limited or minor problems • One stable chronic illness, eg, well controlled hypertension, non-insulin dependent diabetes, cataract, BPH • Acute uncomplicated illness or injury, eg, cystitis, allergic rhinitis, simple sprain	• Physiologic tests not under stress, eg, pulmonary function tests • Non-cardiovascular imaging studies with contrast, eg, barium enema • Superficial needle biopsies • Clinical laboratory tests requiring arterial puncture • Skin biopsies	• Over-the-counter drugs • Minor surgery with no identified risk factors • Physical therapy • Occupational therapy • IV fluids without additives
Moderate	• One or more chronic illnesses with mild exacerbation, progression, or side effects of treatment • Two or more stable chronic illnesses • Undiagnosed new problem with uncertain prognosis, eg, lump in breast • Acute illness with systemic symptoms, eg, pyelonephritis, pneumonitis, colitis • Acute complicated injury, eg, head injury with brief loss of consciousness	• Physiologic tests under stress, eg, cardiac stress test, fetal contraction stress test • Diagnostic endoscopies with no identified risk factors • Deep needle or incisional biopsy • Cardiovascular imaging studies with contrast and no identified risk factors, eg, arteriogram, cardiac catheterization • Obtain fluid from body cavity, eg, lumbar puncture, thoracentesis, culdocentesis	• Minor surgery with identified risk factors • Elective major surgery (open, percutaneous or endoscopic) with no identified risk factors • Prescription drug management • Therapeutic nuclear medicine • IV fluids with additives • Closed treatment of fracture or dislocation without manipulation
High	• One or more chronic illnesses with severe exacerbation, progression, or side effects of treatment • Acute or chronic illnesses or injuries that pose a threat to life or bodily function, eg, multiple trauma, acute MI, pulmonary embolus, severe respiratory distress, progressive severe rheumatoid arthritis, psychiatric illness with potential threat to self or others, peritonitis, acute renal failure • An abrupt change in neurologic status, eg, seizure, TIA, weakness, sensory loss	• Cardiovascular imaging studies with contrast with identified risk factors • Cardiac electrophysiological tests • Diagnostic endoscopies with identified risk factors • Discography	• Elective major surgery (open, percutaneous or endoscopic) with identified risk factors • Emergency major surgery (open, percutaneous or endoscopic) • Parenteral controlled substances • Drug therapy requiring intensive monitoring for toxicity • Decision not to resuscitate or to de-escalate care because of poor prognosis

D. Documentation of an Encounter Dominated by Counseling or Coordination of Care

In the case where counseling and/or coordination of care dominates (more than 50%) of the physician/patient and/or family encounter (face-to-face time in the office or other outpatient setting or floor/unit time in the hospital or nursing facility), time is considered the key or controlling factor to qualify for a particular level of E/M services.

•*DG: If the physician elects to report the level of service based on counseling and/or coordination of care, the total length of time of the encounter (face-to-face or floor time, as appropriate) should be documented and the record should describe the counseling and/or activities to coordinate care.*

APPENDIX C

1997 Documentation Guidelines for Evaluation and Management Services*

Table of Contents

Introduction	2	[266]
What Is Documentation and Why Is It Important?	2	[266]
What Do Payers Want and Why?	2	[266]
General Principles of Medical Record Documentation	3	[266]
Documentation of E/M Services	4	[267]
Documentation of History	5	[268]
Chief Complaint (CC)	6	[269]
History of Present Illness (HPI)	7	[269]
Review of Systems (ROS)	8	[270]
Past, Family and/or Social History (PFSH)	9	[270]
Documentation of Examination	10	[271]
General Multi-System Examinations	11	[272]
Single Organ System Examinations	12	[273]
Content and Document Requirements	13	[274]
General Multi-System Examination	13	[274]
Cardiovascular Examination	18	[276]
Ears, Nose and Throat Examination	20	[278]
Eye Examination	23	[280]
Genitourinary Examination	25	[281]
Hematologic/Lymphatic/Immunologic Examination	29	[283]
Musculoskeletal Examination	31	[284]
Neurological Examination	34	[286]
Psychiatric Examination	37	[287]
Respiratory Examination	39	[289]
Skin Examination	41	[290]

*Developed jointly by the American Medical Association (AMA) and the Health Care Financing Administration (HCFA) (now Centers for Medicare and Medicaid Services).

Documentation of the Complexity of Medical Decision-Making   43 [292]

   Number of Diagnoses or Management Options   44 [292]

   Amount and/or Complexity of Data to Be Reviewed   45 [293]

   Risk of Significant Complications, Morbidity, and/or Mortality   46 [294]

     Table of Risk   47 [294]

Documentation of an Encounter Dominated by Counseling or Coordination of Care   48 [295]

I. INTRODUCTION

What Is Documentation and Why Is It Important?

Medical record documentation is required to record pertinent facts, findings, and observations about an individual's health history including past and present illnesses, examinations, tests, treatments, and outcomes. The medical record chronologically documents the care of the patient and is an important element contributing to high quality care. The medical record facilitates:

- the ability of the physician and other health care professionals to evaluate and plan the patient's immediate treatment, and to monitor his/her health care over time.

- communication and continuity of care among physicians and other health care professionals involved in the patient's care;

- accurate and timely claims review and payment;

- appropriate utilization review and quality of care evaluations; and

- collection of data that may be useful for research and education.

An appropriately documented medical record can reduce many of the "hassles" associated with claims processing and may serve as a legal document to verify the care provided, if necessary.

What Do Payers Want and Why?

Because payers have a contractual obligation to enrollees, they may require reasonable documentation that services are consistent with the insurance coverage provided. They may request information to validate:

- the site of service;

- the medical necessity and appropriateness of the diagnostic and/or therapeutic services provided; and/or

- that services provided have been accurately reported.

II. GENERAL PRINCIPLES OF MEDICAL RECORD DOCUMENTATION

The principles of documentation listed below are applicable to all types of medical and surgical services in all settings. For Evaluation and Management (E/M) services, the nature and amount of physician work and documentation varies by type of service, place of service and the patient's status. The following list of general principles may be modified to account for these variable circumstances in providing E/M services.

1. The medical record should be complete and legible.

2. The documentation of each patient encounter should include:

   ■ reason for the encounter and relevant history, physical examination findings and prior diagnostic test results;

   ■ assessment, clinical impression or diagnosis;

   ■ plan for care; and

   ■ date and legible identity of the observer.

3. If not documented, the rationale for ordering diagnostic and other ancillary services should be easily inferred.

4. Past and present diagnoses should be accessible to the treating and/or consulting physician.

5. Appropriate health risk factors should be identified.

6. The patient's progress, response to and changes in treatment, and revision of diagnosis should be documented.

7. The CPT and ICD-9-CM codes reported on the health insurance claim form or billing statement should be supported by the documentation in the medical record.

III. DOCUMENTATION OF E/M SERVICES

This publication provides definitions and documentation guidelines for the three key components of E/M services and for visits which consist predominantly of counseling or coordination of care. The three *key* components—history, examination, and medical decision making—appear in the descriptors for office and other outpatient services, hospital observation services, hospital inpatient services, consultations, emergency department services, nursing facility services, domiciliary care services, and home services. While some of the text of CPT has been repeated in this publication, the reader should refer to CPT for the complete descriptors for E/M services and instructions for selecting a level of service. Documentation guidelines are identified by the symbol ■ *DG*.

The descriptors for the levels of E/M services recognize seven components which are used in defining the levels of E/M services. These components are:

■ history;

■ examination;

■ medical decision making;

■ counseling;

■ coordination of care;

■ nature of presenting problem; and

■ time.

The first three of these components (i.e., history, examination and medical decision making) are the key components in selecting the level of E/M services. In the case of visits which consist *predominantly* of counseling or coordination of care, time is the key or controlling factor to qualify for a particular level of E/M service.

Because the level of E/M service is dependent on two or three key components, performance and documentation of one component (e.g., examination) at the highest level does not necessarily mean that the encounter in its entirety qualifies for the highest level of E/M service.

These Documentation Guidelines for E/M services reflect the needs of the typical adult population. For certain groups of patients, the recorded information may vary slightly from that described here. Specifically, the medical records of infants, children, adolescents and pregnant women may have additional or modified information recorded in each history and examination area.

As an example, newborn records may include under history of the present illness (HPI) the details of mother's pregnancy and the infant's status at birth; social history will focus on family structure; family history will focus on congenital anomalies and hereditary disorders in the family. In addition, the content of a pediatric examination will vary with the age and development of the child. Although not specifically defined in these documentation guidelines, these patient group variations on history and examination are appropriate.

A. Documentation of History

The levels of E/M services are based on four types of history (Problem Focused, Expanded Problem Focused, Detailed, and Comprehensive). Each type of history includes some or all of the following elements:

- Chief complaint (CC);

- History of present illness (HPI);

- Review of systems (ROS); and

- Past, family and/or social history (PFSH).

The extent of history of present illness, review of systems and past, family and/or social history that is obtained and documented is dependent upon clinical judgment and the nature of the presenting problem(s).

The chart below shows the progression of the elements required for each type of history. To qualify for a given type of history all three elements in the table must be met. (A chief complaint is indicated at all levels.)

History of Present Illness	Review of Systems (ROS)	Past, Family, and/or Social History	Type of History
Brief	N/A	N/A	Problem Focused
Brief	Problem pertinent	N/A	Expanded Problem Focused
Extended	Extended	Pertinent	Detailed
Extended	Complete	Complete	Comprehensive

- DG: The CC, ROS, and PFSH may be listed as separate elements of history, or they may be included in the description of the history of the present illness.

- DG: A ROS and/or a PFSH obtained during an earlier encounter does not need to be re-recorded if there is evidence that the physician reviewed and updated the previous information. This may occur when a physician updates his or her own record or in an institutional setting or group practice where many physicians use a common record. The review and update may be documented by:

- describing any new ROS and/or PFSH information or noting there has been no change in the information; and

- noting the date and location of the earlier ROS and/or PFSH.

- DG: The ROS and/or PFSH may be recorded by ancillary staff or on a form completed by the patient. To document that the physician reviewed the information, there must be a notation supplementing or confirming the information recorded by others.

- DG: If the physician is unable to obtain a history from the patient or other source, the record should describe the patient's condition or other circumstance which precludes obtaining a history.

Definitions and specific documentation guidelines for each of the elements of history are in the following list.

Chief Complaint (CC)

The CC is a concise statement describing the symptom, problem, condition, diagnosis, physician recommended return, or other factor that is the reason for the encounter, usually stated in the patient's words.

- DG: The medical record should clearly reflect the chief complaint.

History of Present Illness (HPI)

The HPI is a chronological description of the development of the patient's present illness from the first sign and/or symptom or from the previous encounter to the present. It includes the following elements:

- location,

- quality,

- severity,

- duration,

- timing,

- context,

- modifying factors, and

- associated signs and symptoms.

Brief and *extended* HPIs are distinguished by the amount of detail needed to accurately characterize the clinical problem(s).
   A *brief* HPI consists of one to three elements of the HPI.

- DG: The medical record should describe one to three elements of the present illness (HPI).

An *extended* HPI consists of at least four elements of the HPI or the status of at least three chronic or inactive conditions.

- DG: The medical record should describe at least four elements of the present illness (HPI), or the status of at least three chronic or inactive conditions.

Review of Systems (ROS)

A ROS is an inventory of body systems obtained through a series of questions seeking to identify signs and/or symptoms which the patient may be experiencing or has experienced.

For purposes of ROS, the following systems are recognized:

- Constitutional symptoms (e.g., fever, weight loss)
- Eyes
- Ears, Nose, Mouth, Throat
- Cardiovascular
- Respiratory
- Gastrointestinal
- Genitourinary
- Musculoskeletal
- Integumentary (skin and/or breast)
- Neurological
- Psychiatric
- Endocrine
- Hematologic/Lymphatic
- Allergic/Immunologic

A *problem pertinent* ROS inquires about the system directly related to the problem(s) identified in the HPI.

- DG: The patient's positive responses and pertinent negatives for the system related to the problem should be documented.

An *extended* ROS inquires about the system directly related to the problem(s) identified in the HPI and a limited number of additional systems.

- DG: The patient's positive responses and pertinent negatives for two to nine systems should be documented.

A *complete* ROS inquires about the system(s) directly related to the problem(s) identified in the HPI *plus* all additional body systems.

- DG: At least ten organ systems must be reviewed. Those systems with positive or pertinent negative responses must be individually documented. For the remaining systems, a notation indicating all other systems are negative is permissible. In the absence of such a notation, at least ten systems must be individually documented.

Past, Family and/or Social History (PFSH)

The PFSH consists of a review of three areas:

- past history (the patient's past experiences with illnesses, operations, injuries and treatments);
- family history (a review of medical events in the patient's family, including diseases which may be hereditary or place the patient at risk); and
- social history (an age appropriate review of past and current activities).

For certain categories of E/M services that include only an interval history, it is not necessary to record information about the PFSH. Those categories are subsequent hospital care, follow-up inpatient consultations and subsequent nursing facility care.

A *pertinent* PFSH is a review of the history area(s) directly related to the problem(s) identified in the HPI.

- ■ DG: At least one specific item from any of the three history areas must be documented for a pertinent PFSH.

A *complete* PFSH is a review of two or all three of the PFSH history areas, depending on the category of the E/M service. A review of all three history areas is required for services that by their nature include a comprehensive assessment or reassessment of the patient. A review of two of the three history areas is sufficient for other services.

- ■ DG: At least one specific item from two of the three history areas must be documented for a complete PFSH for the following categories of E/M services: office or other outpatient services, established patient; emergency department; domiciliary care, established patient; and home care, established patient.

- ■ DG: At least one specific item from each of the three history areas must be documented for a complete PFSH for the following categories of E/M services: office or other outpatient services, new patient; hospital observation services; hospital inpatient services, initial care; consultations; comprehensive nursing facility assessments; domiciliary care, new patient; and home care, new patient.

B. Documentation of Examination

The levels of E/M services are based on four types of examination:

- ■ *Problem Focused*—a limited examination of the affected body area or organ system.

- ■ *Expanded Problem Focused*—a limited examination of the affected body area or organ system and any other symptomatic or related body area(s) or organ system(s).

- ■ *Detailed*—an extended examination of the affected body area(s) or organ system(s) and any other symptomatic or related body area(s) or organ system(s).

- ■ *Comprehensive*—a general multi-system examination, or complete examination of a single organ system and other symptomatic or related body area(s) or organ system(s).

These types of examinations have been defined for general multi-system and the following single organ systems:

- ■ Cardiovascular
- ■ Ears, Nose, Mouth and Throat
- ■ Eyes
- ■ Genitourinary (Female)
- ■ Genitourinary (Male)
- ■ Hematologic/Lymphatic/Immunologic

- Musculoskeletal

- Neurological

- Psychiatric

- Respiratory

- Skin

A general multi-system examination or a single organ system examination may be performed by any physician regardless of specialty. The type (general multi-system or single organ system) and content of examination are selected by the examining physician and are based upon clinical judgment, the patient's history, and the nature of the presenting problem(s).

The content and documentation requirements for each type and level of examination are summarized following and described in detail in tables beginning on page 571. In the tables, organ systems and body areas recognized by CPT for purposes of describing examinations are shown in the left column. The content, or individual elements, of the examination pertaining to that body area or organ system are identified by bullets (•) in the right column.

Parenthetical examples, "(e.g., . . .)," have been used for clarification and to provide guidance regarding documentation. Documentation for each element must satisfy any numeric requirements (such as "Measurement of *any three of the following seven . . .*") included in the description of the element. Elements with multiple components but with no specific numeric requirement (such as "Examination of *liver* and *spleen*") require documentation of at least one component. It is possible for a given examination to be expanded beyond what is defined here. When that occurs, findings related to the additional systems and/or areas should be documented.

- DG: Specific abnormal and relevant negative findings of the examination of the affected or symptomatic body area(s) or organ system(s) should be documented. A notation of "abnormal" without elaboration is insufficient.

- DG: Abnormal or unexpected findings of the examination of any asymptomatic body area(s) or organ system(s) should be described.

- DG: A brief statement or notation indicating "negative" or "normal" is sufficient to document normal findings related to unaffected area(s) or asymptomatic organ system(s).

General Multi-System Examinations

General multi-system examinations are described in detail beginning on page 571. To qualify for a given level of multi-system examination, the following content and documentation requirements should be met:

- *Problem Focused Examination*—should include performance and documentation of one to five elements identified by a bullet (•) in one or more organ system(s) or body area(s).

- *Expanded Problem Focused Examination*—should include performance and documentation of at least six elements identified by a bullet (•) in one or more organ system(s) or body area(s).

- *Detailed Examination*—should include at least six organ systems or body areas. For each system/area selected, performance and documentation of at least two elements identified by a bullet (•) is expected. Alternatively, a detailed examination may include performance and documentation of at least twelve elements identified by a bullet (•) in two or more organ systems or body areas.

■ *Comprehensive Examination*—should include at least nine organ systems or body areas. For each system/area selected, all elements of the examination identified by a bullet (•) should be performed, unless specific directions limit the content of the examination. For each area/system, documentation of at least two elements identified by a bullet is expected.

Single Organ System Examinations

The single organ system examinations recognized by CPT are described in detail beginning on page 574. Variations among these examinations in the organ systems and body areas identified in the left columns and in the elements of the examinations described in the right columns reflect differing emphases among specialties. To qualify for a given level of single organ system examination, the following content and documentation requirements should be met:

■ *Problem Focused Examination*—should include performance and documentation of one to five elements identified by a bullet (•), whether in a box with a shaded or unshaded border.

■ *Expanded Problem Focused Examination*—should include performance and documentation of at least six elements identified by a bullet (•), whether in a box with a shaded or unshaded border.

■ *Detailed Examination*—examinations other than the eye and psychiatric examinations should include performance and documentation of at least twelve elements identified by a bullet (•), whether in box with a shaded or unshaded border.

■ Eye and psychiatric examinations should include the performance and documentation of at least nine elements identified by a bullet (•), whether in a box with a shaded or unshaded border.

■ *Comprehensive Examination*—should include performance of all elements identified by a bullet (•), whether in a shaded or unshaded box. Documentation of every element in each box with a shaded border and at least one element in each box with an unshaded border is expected.

Content and Document Requirements

GENERAL MULTI-SYSTEM EXAMINATION

System/Body Area	Elements of Examination
Constitutional	• Measurement of any three of the following seven vital signs: 1) sitting or standing blood pressure, 2) supine blood pressure, 3) pulse rate and regularity, 4) respiration, 5) temperature, 6) height, 7) weight (may be measured and recorded by ancillary staff) • General appearance of patient (e.g., development, nutrition, body habitus, deformities, attention to grooming)
Eyes	• Inspection of conjunctivae and lids • Examination of pupils and irises (e.g., reaction to light and accommodation, size and symmetry) • Ophthalmoscopic examination of optic discs (e.g., size, C/D ratio, appearance) and posterior segments (e.g., vessel changes, exudates, hemorrhages)
Ears, Nose, Mouth and Throat	• External inspection of ears and nose (e.g., overall appearance, scars, lesions, masses • Otoscopic examination of external auditory canals and tympanic membranes • Assessment of hearing (e.g., whispered voice, finger rub, tuning fork) • Inspection of nasal mucosa, septum and turbinates • Inspection of lips, teeth and gums • Examination of oropharynx: oral mucosa, salivary glands, hard and soft palates, tongue, tonsils and posterior pharynx
Neck	• Examination of neck (e.g., masses, overall appearance, symmetry, tracheal position, crepitus) • Examination of thyroid (e.g., enlargement, tenderness, mass)
Respiratory	• Assessment of respiratory effort (e.g., intercostal retractions, use of accessory muscles, diaphragmatic movement) • Percussion of chest (e.g., dullness, flatness, hyperresonance) • Palpation of chest (e.g., tactile fremitus) • Auscultation of lungs (e.g., breath sounds, adventitious sounds, rubs)
Cardiovascular	• Palpation of heart (e.g., location, size, thrills) • Auscultation of heart with notation of abnormal sounds and murmurs Examination of: • carotid arteries (e.g., pulse amplitude, bruits) • abdominal aorta (e.g., size, bruits) • femoral arteries (e.g., pulse amplitude, bruits) • pedal pulses (e.g., pulse amplitude) • extremities for edema and/or varicosities
Chest (Breasts)	• Inspection of breasts (e.g., symmetry, nipple discharge) • Palpation of breasts and axillae (e.g., masses or lumps, tenderness)

System/Body Area	Elements of Examination
Gastrointestinal (Abdomen)	• Examination of abdomen with notation of presence of masses or tenderness • Examination of liver and spleen • Examination for presence or absence of hernia • Examination (when indicated) of anus, perineum and rectum, including sphincter tone, presence of hemorrhoids, rectal masses • Obtain stool sample for occult blood test when indicated
Genitourinary	**Male:**
	• Examination of the scrotal contents (e.g., hydrocele, spermatocele, tenderness of cord, testicular mass) • Examination of the penis • Digital rectal examination of prostate gland (e.g., size, symmetry, nodularity, tenderness)
	Female:
	Pelvic examination (with or without specimen collection for smears and cultures), including • Examination of external genitalia (e.g., general appearance, hair distribution, lesions) and vagina (e.g., general appearance, estrogen effect, discharge, lesions, pelvic support, cystocele, rectocele) • Examination of urethra (e.g., masses, tenderness, scarring) • Examination of bladder (e.g., fullness, masses, tenderness) • Cervix (e.g., general appearance, lesions, discharge) • Uterus (e.g., size, contour, position, mobility, tenderness, consistency, descent or support) • Adnexa/parametria (e.g., masses, tenderness, organomegaly, nodularity)
Lymphatic	Palpation of lymph nodes in **two or more areas:** • Neck • Axillae • Groin • Other
Musculoskeletal	• Examination of gait and station • Inspection and/or palpation of digits and nails (e.g., clubbing, cyanosis,) inflammatory conditions, petechiae, ischemia, infections, nodes Examination of joints, bones and muscles of **one or more of the following six areas:** 1) head and neck; 2) spine, ribs and pelvis; 3) right upper extremity; 4) left upper extremity; 5) right lower extremity; and left lower extremity. The examination of a given area includes: • Inspection and/or palpation with notation of presence of any misalignment, asymmetry, crepitation, defects, tenderness, masses, effusions • Assessment of range of motion with notation of any pain, crepitation or contracture • Assessment of stability with notation of any dislocation (luxation), subluxation or laxity • Assessment of muscle strength and tone (e.g., flaccid, cog wheel, spastic) with notation of any atrophy or abnormal movements

System/Body Area	Elements of Examination
Skin	• Inspection of skin and subcutaneous tissue (e.g., rashes, lesions, ulcers) • Palpation of skin and subcutaneous tissue (e.g., induration, subcutaneous nodules, tightening)
Neurologic	• Test cranial nerves with notation of any deficits • Examination of deep tendon reflexes with notation of pathological reflexes (e.g., Babinski) • Examination of sensation (e.g., by touch, pin, vibration, proprioception)
Psychiatric	• Description of patient's judgment and insight Brief assessment of mental status including: • orientation to time, place and person • recent and remote memory • mood and affect (e.g., depression, anxiety, agitation)

Content and Documentation Requirements

LEVEL OF EXAM	PERFORM AND DOCUMENT
Problem Focused	**One to five** elements identified by a bullet.
Expanded Problem Focused	**At least six** elements identified by a bullet.
Detailed	**At least two** elements identified by a bullet **from each of six areas/systems** OR **at least twelve** elements identified by a bullet **in two or more areas/systems.**
Comprehensive	Perform **all elements** identified by a bullet in **at least nine** organ systems or body areas and document **at least two** elements identified by a bullet **from each of nine areas/systems.**

CARDIOVASCULAR EXAMINATION

System/Body Area	Elements of Examination
Constitutional	• Measurement of **any three of the following seven** vital signs: 1) sitting or standing blood pressure, 2) supine blood pressure, 3) pulse rate and regularity, 4) respiration, 5) temperature, 6) height, 7) weight (may be measured and recorded by ancillary staff) • General appearance of patient (e.g., development, nutrition, body habitus, deformities, attention to grooming)
Head and Face	
Eyes	• Inspection of conjunctivae and lids (e.g., xanthelasma)
Ears, Nose, Mouth and Throat	• Inspection of teeth, gums and palate • Inspection of oral mucosa with notation of presence of pallor or cyanosis
Neck	Examination of jugular veins (e.g., distension; a, v or cannon a waves)
	• Examination of thyroid (e.g., enlargement, tenderness, mass)

System/Body Area	Elements of Examination
Respiratory	• Assessment of respiratory effort (e.g., intercostal retractions, use of accessory muscles, diaphragmatic movement) • Auscultation of lungs (e.g., breath sounds, adventitious sounds, rubs)
Cardiovascular	• Palpation of heart (e.g., location, size and forcefulness of the point of maximal impact; thrills; lifts; palpable S3 or S4) • Auscultation of heart including sounds, abnormal sounds and murmurs • Measurement of blood pressure in two or more extremities when indicated (e.g., aortic dissection, coarctation) Examination of: • Carotid arteries (e.g., waveform, pulse amplitude, bruits, apical-carotid delay) • Abdominal aorta (e.g., size, bruits) • Femoral arteries (e.g., pulse amplitude, bruits) • Pedal pulses (e.g., pulse amplitude) • Extremities for peripheral edema and/or varicosities
Chest (Breasts)	
Gastrointestinal (Abdomen)	• Examination of abdomen with notation of presence of masses or tenderness • Examination of liver and spleen • Obtain stool sample for occult blood from patients who are being considered for thrombolytic or anticoagulant therapy
Genitourinary (Abdomen)	
Lymphatic	
Musculoskeletal	• Examination of the back with notation of kyphosis or scoliosis • Examination of gait with notation of ability to undergo exercise testing and/or participation in exercise programs • Assessment of muscle strength and tone (e.g., flaccid, cog wheel, spastic) with notation of any atrophy and abnormal movements
Extremities	• Inspection and palpation of digits and nails (e.g., clubbing, cyanosis, inflammation, petechiae, ischemia, infections, Osler's nodes)
Skin	• Inspection and/or palpation of skin and subcutaneous tissue (e.g., stasis dermatitis, ulcers, scars, xanthomas)
Neurologic/ Psychiatric	Brief assessment of mental status including • Orientation to time, place and person • Mood and affect (e.g., depression, anxiety, agitation)

Content and Documentation Requirements

LEVEL OF EXAM	PERFORM AND DOCUMENT
Problem Focused	**One to five** elements identified by a bullet.
Expanded Problem Focused	**At least six** elements identified by a bullet.
Detailed	**At least twelve** elements identified by a bullet.
Comprehensive	Perform **all** elements identified by a bullet; document every element in each box with a shaded border and at least one element in each box with an unshaded border.

EARS, NOSE AND THROAT EXAMINATION

System/Body Area	Elements of Examination
Constitutional	• Measurement of **any three of the following seven** vital signs: 1) sitting or standing blood pressure, 2) supine blood pressure, 3) pulse rate and regularity, 4) respiration, 5) temperature, 6) height, 7) weight (may be measured and recorded by ancillary staff) • General appearance of patient (e.g., development, nutrition, body habitus, deformities, attention to grooming) • Assessment of ability to communicate (e.g., use of sign language or other communication aids) and quality of voice
Head and Face	• Inspection of head and face (e.g., overall appearance, scars, lesions and masses) • Palpation and/or percussion of face with notation of presence or absence of sinus tenderness • Examination of salivary glands • Assessment of facial strength
Eyes	• Test ocular motility including primary gaze alignment
Ears, Nose, Mouth and Throat	• Otoscopic examination of external auditory canals and tympanic membranes including pneumo-otoscopy with notation of mobility of membranes • Assessment of hearing with tuning forks and clinical speech reception thresholds (e.g., whispered voice, finger rub) • External inspection of ears and nose (e.g., overall appearance, scars, lesions and masses) • Inspection of nasal mucosa, septum and turbinates • Inspection of lips, teeth and gums • Examination of oropharynx: oral mucosa, hard and soft palates, tongue, tonsils and posterior pharynx (e.g., asymmetry, lesions, hydration of mucosal surfaces) • Inspection of pharyngeal walls and pyriform sinuses (e.g., pooling of saliva, asymmetry, lesions) • Examination by mirror of larynx including the condition of the epiglottis, false vocal cords, true vocal cords and mobility of larynx (use of mirror not required in children) • Examination by mirror of nasopharynx including appearance of the mucosa, adenoids, posterior choanae and eustachian tubes (use of mirror not required in children)

System/Body Area	Elements of Examination
Neck	• Examination of neck (e.g., masses, overall appearance, symmetry, tracheal position, crepitus) • Examination of thyroid (e.g., enlargement, tenderness, mass)
Respiratory	• Inspection of chest including symmetry, expansion and/or assessment of respiratory effort (e.g., intercostal retractions, use of accessory muscles, diaphragmatic movement) • Auscultation of lungs (e.g., breath sounds, adventitious sounds, rubs)
Cardiovascular	• Auscultation of heart with notation of abnormal sounds and murmurs • Examination of peripheral vascular system by observation (e.g., swelling, varicosities) and palpation (e.g., pulses, temperature, edema, tenderness)
Chest (Breasts)	
Gastrointestinal (Abdomen)	
Genitourinary	
Lymphatic	• Palpation of lymph nodes in neck, axillae, groin and/or other location
Musculoskeletal	
Extremities	
Skin	
Neurological/ Psychiatric	• Test cranial nerves with notation of any deficits Brief assessment of mental status including • Orientation to time, place and person • Mood and affect (e.g., depression, anxiety, agitation)

Content and Documentation Requirements

LEVEL OF EXAM	PERFORM AND DOCUMENT
Problem Focused	**One to five** elements identified by a bullet.
Expanded Problem Focused	**At least six** elements identified by a bullet.
Detailed	**At least twelve** elements identified by a bullet.
Comprehensive	Perform **all** elements identified by a bullet; document every element in each box with a shaded border and at least one element in each box with an unshaded border.

EYE EXAMINATION

System/Body Area	Elements of Examination
Constitutional	
Head and Face	
Eyes	• Test visual acuity (does not include determination of refractive error) • Gross visual field testing by confrontation • Test ocular motility including primary gaze alignment • Inspection of bulbar and palpebral conjunctivae • Examination of ocular adnexae including lids (e.g., ptosis or lagophthalmos), lacrimal glands, lacrimal drainage, orbits and preauricular lymph nodes • Examination of pupils and irises including shape, direct and consensual reaction (afferent pupil), size (e.g., anisocoria) and morphology • Slit lamp examination of the corneas including epithelium, stroma, endothelium, and tear film • Slit lamp examination of the anterior chambers including depth, cells, and flare • Slit lamp examination of the lenses including clarity, anterior and posterior capsule, cortex, and nucleus • Measurement of intraocular pressures (except in children and patients with trauma or infectious disease) • Ophthalmoscopic examination through dilated pupils (unless contraindicated) of • Optic discs including size, C/D ratio, appearance (e.g., atrophy, cupping, tumor elevation) and nerve fiber layer • Posterior segments including retina and vessels (e.g., exudates and hemorrhages)
Ears, Nose, Mouth and Throat	
Neck	
Respiratory	
Cardiovascular	
Chest (Breasts)	
Gastrointestinal (Abdomen)	
Genitourinary	
Lymphatic	
Musculoskeletal	
Extremities	
Skin	
Neurological/Psychiatric	Brief assessment of mental status including • Orientation to time, place and person • Mood and affect (e.g., depression, anxiety, agitation)

Content and Documentation Requirements

LEVEL OF EXAM	PERFORM AND DOCUMENT
Problem Focused	**One to five** elements identified by a bullet.
Expanded Problem Focused	**At least six** elements identified by a bullet.
Detailed	**At least twelve** elements identified by a bullet.
Comprehensive	Perform **all** elements identified by a bullet; document every element in each box with a shaded border and at least one element in each box with an unshaded border.

GENITOURINARY EXAMINATION

System/Body Area	Elements of Examination
Constitutional	• Measurement of **any three of the following seven** vital signs: 1) sitting or standing blood pressure, 2) supine blood pressure, 3) pulse rate and regularity, 4) respiration, 5) temperature, 6) height, 7) weight (may be measured and recorded by ancillary staff) • General appearance of patient (e.g., development, nutrition, body habitus, deformities, attention to grooming)
Head and Face	
Eyes	
Ears, Nose, Mouth and Throat	
Neck	• Examination of neck (e.g., masses, overall appearance, symmetry, tracheal position, crepitus) • Examination of thyroid (e.g., enlargement, tenderness, mass)
Respiratory	• Assessment of respiratory effort (e.g., intercostal retractions, use of accessory muscles, diaphragmatic movement) • Auscultation of lungs (e.g., breath sounds, adventitious sounds, rubs)
Cardiovascular	• Auscultation of heart with notation of abnormal sounds and murmurs • Examination of peripheral vascular system by observation (e.g., swelling, varicosities) and palpation (e.g., pulses, temperature, edema, tenderness)
Chest (Breasts)	[See genitourinary (female).]
Gastrointestinal (Abdomen)	• Examination of abdomen with notation of presence of masses or tenderness • Examination for presence or absence of hernia • Examination of liver and spleen • Obtain stool sample for occult blood test when indicated

System/Body Area	Elements of Examination
Genitourinary	**Male:**
	• Inspection of anus and perineum Examination (with or without specimen collection for smears and cultures) of genitalia including: • Scrotum (e.g., lesions, cysts, rashes) • Epididymides (e.g., size, symmetry, masses) • Testes (e.g., size, symmetry, masses) • Urethral meatus (e.g., size, location, lesions, discharge) • Penis (e.g., lesions, presence or absence of foreskin, foreskin retractability, plaque, masses, scarring, deformities) Digital rectal examination including: • Prostate gland (e.g., size, symmetry, nodularity, tenderness) • Seminal vesicles (e.g., symmetry, tenderness, masses, enlargement) • Sphincter tone, presence of hemorrhoids, rectal masses **Female:** Includes **at least seven of the following** eleven elements identified by bullets: • Inspection and palpation of breasts (e.g., masses or lumps, tenderness, symmetry, nipple discharge) • Digital rectal examination including sphincter tone, presence of hemorrhoids, rectal masses Pelvic examination (with or without specimen collection for smears and cultures) including: • External genitalia (e.g., general appearance, hair distribution, lesions) • Urethral meatus (e.g., size, location, lesions, prolapse) • Urethra (e.g., masses, tenderness, scarring) • Bladder (e.g., fullness, masses, tenderness) • Vagina (e.g., general appearance, estrogen effect, discharge, lesions, pelvic support, cystocele, rectocele) • Cervix (e.g., general appearance, lesions, discharge) • Uterus (e.g., size, contour, position, mobility, tenderness, consistency, descent or support) • Adnexa/parametria (e.g., masses, tenderness, organomegaly, nodularity) • Anus and perineum
Lymphatic	• Palpation of lymph nodes in neck, axillae, groin and/or other location
Musculoskeletal	
Extremities	
Skin	• Inspection and/or palpation of skin and subcutaneous tissue (e.g., rashes, lesions, ulcers)
Neurological/ Psychiatric	Brief assessment of mental status including • Orientation (e.g., time, place and person) and • Mood and affect (e.g., depression, anxiety, agitation)

Content and Documentation Requirements

LEVEL OF EXAM	PERFORM AND DOCUMENT
Problem Focused	**One to five** elements identified by a bullet.
Expanded Problem Focused	**At least six** elements identified by a bullet.
Detailed	**At least twelve** elements identified by a bullet.
Comprehensive	Perform **all** elements identified by a bullet; document every element in each box with a shaded border and at least one element in each box with an unshaded border.

HEMATOLOGIC/LYMPHATIC/IMMUNOLOGIC EXAMINATION

System/Body Area	Elements of Examination
Constitutional	• Measurement of **any three of the following seven** vital signs: 1) sitting or standing blood pressure, 2) supine blood pressure, 3) pulse rate and regularity, 4) respiration, 5) temperature, 6) height, 7) weight (may be measured and recorded by ancillary staff) • General appearance of patient (e.g., development, nutrition, body habitus, deformities, attention to grooming)
Head and Face	• Palpation and/or percussion of face with notation of presence or absence of sinus tenderness
Eyes	• Inspection of conjunctivae and lids
Ears, Nose, Mouth and Throat	• Otoscopic examination of external auditory canals and tympanic membranes • Inspection of nasal mucosa, septum and turbinates • Inspection of teeth and gums • Examination of oropharynx (e.g., oral mucosa, hard and soft palates, tongue, tonsils, posterior pharynx)
Neck	• Examination of neck (e.g., masses, overall appearance, symmetry, tracheal position, crepitus) • Examination of thyroid (e.g., enlargement, tenderness, mass)
Respiratory	• Assessment of respiratory effort (e.g., intercostal retractions, use of accessory muscles, diaphragmatic movement) • Auscultation of lungs (e.g., breath sounds, adventitious sounds, rubs)
Cardiovascular	• Auscultation of heart with notation of abnormal sounds and murmurs • Examination of peripheral vascular system by observation (e.g., swelling, varicosities) and palpation (e.g., pulses, temperature, edema, tenderness)
Chest (Breasts)	
Gastrointestinal (Abdomen)	• Examination of abdomen with notation of presence of masses or tenderness • Examination of liver and spleen
Genitourinary	
Lymphatic	• Palpation of lymph nodes in neck, axillae, groin, and/or other location
Musculoskeletal	

System/Body Area	Elements of Examination
Extremities	• Inspection and palpation of digits and nails (e.g., clubbing, cyanosis, inflammation, petechiae, ischemia, infections, nodes)
Skin	• Inspection and/or palpation of skin and subcutaneous tissue (e.g., rashes, lesions, ulcers, ecchymoses, bruises)
Neurological/ Psychiatric	Brief assessment of mental status including • Orientation to time, place and person • Mood and affect (e.g., depression, anxiety, agitation)

Content and Documentation Requirements

LEVEL OF EXAM	PERFORM AND DOCUMENT
Problem Focused	**One to five** elements identified by a bullet.
Expanded Problem Focused	**At least six** elements identified by a bullet.
Detailed	**At least twelve** elements identified by a bullet.
Comprehensive	Perform **all** elements identified by a bullet; document every element in each box with a shaded border and at least one element in each box with an unshaded border.

MUSCULOSKELETAL EXAMINATION

System/Body Area	Elements of Examination
Constitutional	• Measurement of **any three of the following seven** vital signs: 1) sitting or standing blood pressure, 2) supine blood pressure, 3) pulse rate and regularity, 4) respiration, 5) temperature, 6) height, 7) weight (may be measured and recorded by ancillary staff) • General appearance of patient (e.g., development, nutrition, body habitus, deformities, attention to grooming)
Head and Face	
Eyes	
Ears, Nose, Mouth and Throat	
Neck	
Respiratory	
Cardiovascular	• Examination of peripheral vascular system by observation (e.g., swelling, varicosities) and palpation (e.g., pulses, temperature, edema, tenderness)
Chest (Breasts)	
Gastrointestinal (Abdomen)	
Genitourinary	
Lymphatic	• Palpation of lymph nodes in neck, axillae, groin and/or other location

System/Body Area	Elements of Examination
Musculoskeletal	• Examination of gait and station Examination of joint(s), bone(s) and muscle(s)/tendon(s) **of four of the following six** areas: 1) head and neck; 2) spine, ribs and pelvis; 3) right upper extremity; 4) left upper extremity; 5) right lower extremity; and 6) left lower extremity. The examination of a given area includes: • Inspection, percussion and/or palpation with notation of any misalignment, asymmetry, crepitation, defects, tenderness, masses or effusions • Assessment of range of motion with notation of any pain (e.g., straight leg raising), crepitation or contracture • Assessment of stability with notation of any dislocation (luxation), subluxation or laxity • Assessment of muscle strength and tone (e.g., flaccid, cog wheel, spastic) with notation of any atrophy or abnormal movements Note: For the comprehensive level of examination, all four of the elements identified by a bullet must be performed and documented for each of four anatomic areas. For the three lower levels of examination, each element is counted separately for each body area. For example, assessing range of motion in two extremities constitutes two elements.
Extremities	[See musculoskeletal and skin.]
Skin	• Inspection and/or palpation of skin and subcutaneous tissue (e.g., scars, rashes, lesions, cafe-au-lait spots, ulcers) **in four of the following six** areas: 1) head and neck; 2) trunk; 3) right upper extremity; 4) left upper extremity; 5) right lower extremity; and 6) left lower extremity. Note: For the comprehensive level, the examination of all four anatomic areas must be performed and documented. For the three lower levels of examination, each body area is counted separately. For example, inspection and/or palpation of the skin and subcutaneous tissue of two extremities constitutes two elements.
Neurological/ Psychiatric	• Test coordination (e.g., finger/nose, heel/ knee/shin, rapid alternating movements in the upper and lower extremities, evaluation of fine motor coordination in young children) • Examination of deep tendon reflexes and/or nerve stretch test with notation of pathological reflexes (e.g., Babinski) • Examination of sensation (e.g., by touch, pin, vibration, proprioception) Brief assessment of mental status including • Orientation to time, place and person • Mood and affect (e.g., depression, anxiety, agitation)

Content and Documentation Requirements

LEVEL OF EXAM	PERFORM AND DOCUMENT
Problem Focused	**One to five** elements identified by a bullet.
Expanded Problem Focused	**At least six** elements identified by a bullet.
Detailed	**At least twelve** elements identified by a bullet.
Comprehensive	Perform **all** elements identified by a bullet; document every element in each box with a shaded border and at least one element in each box with an unshaded border.

NEUROLOGICAL EXAMINATION

System/Body Area	Elements of Examination
Constitutional	• Measurement of **any three of the following seven** vital signs: 1) sitting or standing blood pressure, 2) supine blood pressure, 3) pulse rate and regularity, 4) respiration, 5) temperature, 6) height, 7) weight (may be measured and recorded by ancillary staff) • General appearance of patient (e.g., development, nutrition, body habitus, deformities, attention to grooming)
Head and Face	
Eyes	• Ophthalmoscopic examination of optic discs (e.g., size, C/D ratio, appearance) and posterior segments (e.g., vessel changes, exudates, hemorrhages)
Ears, Nose, Mouth and Throat	
Neck	
Respiratory	
Cardiovascular	• Examination of carotid arteries (e.g., pulse amplitude, bruits) • Auscultation of heart with notation of abnormal sounds and murmurs • Examination of peripheral vascular system by observation (e.g., swelling, varicosities) and palpation (e.g., pulses, temperature, edema, tenderness)
Chest (Breasts)	
Gastrointestinal (Abdomen)	
Genitourinary	
Lymphatic	
Musculoskeletal	• Examination of gait and station Assessment of motor function including: • Muscle strength in upper and lower extremities • Muscle tone in upper and lower extremities (e.g., flaccid, cog wheel, spastic) with notation of any atrophy or abnormal movements (e.g., fasciculation, tardive dyskinesia)
Extremities	[See musculoskeletal.]
Skin	

System/Body Area	Elements of Examination
Neurological	Evaluation of higher integrative functions including: • Orientation to time, place and person • Recent and remote memory • Attention span and concentration • Language (e.g., naming objects, repeating phrases, spontaneous speech) • Fund of knowledge (e.g., awareness of current events, past history, vocabulary) Test the following cranial nerves: • 2nd cranial nerve (e.g., visual acuity, visual fields, fundi) • 3rd, 4th and 6th cranial nerves (e.g., pupils, eye movements) • 5th cranial nerve (e.g., facial sensation, corneal reflexes) • 7th cranial nerve (e.g., facial symmetry, strength) • 8th cranial nerve (e.g., hearing with tuning fork, whispered voice and/or finger rub) • 9th cranial nerve (e.g., spontaneous or reflex palate movement) • 11th cranial nerve (e.g., shoulder shrug strength) • 12th cranial nerve (e.g., tongue protrusion) • Examination of sensation (e.g., by touch, pin, vibration, proprioception) • Examination of deep tendon reflexes in upper and lower extremities with notation of pathological reflexes (e.g., Babinski) • Test coordination (e.g., finger/nose, heel/knee/shin, rapid alternating movements in the upper and lower extremities, evaluation of fine motor coordination in young children)
Psychiatric	

Content and Documentation Requirements

LEVEL OF EXAM	PERFORM AND DOCUMENT
Problem Focused	**One to five** elements identified by a bullet.
Expanded Problem Focused	**At least six** elements identified by a bullet.
Detailed	**At least twelve** elements identified by a bullet.
Comprehensive	Perform **all** elements identified by a bullet; document every element in each box with a shaded border and at least one element in each box with an unshaded border.

PSYCHIATRIC EXAMINATION

System/Body Area	Elements of Examination
Constitutional	• Measurement of **any three of the following seven** vital signs: 1) sitting or standing blood pressure, 2) supine blood pressure, 3) pulse rate and regularity, 4) respiration, 5) temperature, 6) height, 7) weight (may be measured and recorded by ancillary staff) • General appearance of patient (e.g., development, nutrition, body habitus, deformities, attention to grooming)

System/Body Area	Elements of Examination
Head and Face	
Eyes	
Ears, Nose, Mouth and Throat	
Neck	
Respiratory	
Cardiovascular	
Chest (Breasts)	
Gastrointestinal (Abdomen)	
Genitourinary	
Lymphatic	
Musculoskeletal	• Assessment of muscle strength and tone (e.g., flaccid, cog wheel, spastic) with notation of any atrophy and abnormal movements • Examination of gait and station
Extremities	
Skin	
Neurological	
Psychiatric	• Description of speech including: rate; volume; articulation; coherence; and spontaneity with notation of abnormalities (e.g., perseveration, paucity of language) • Description of thought processes including: rate of thoughts; content of thoughts (e.g., logical vs. illogical, tangential); abstract reasoning; and computation • Description of associations (e.g., loose, tangential, circumstantial, intact) • Description of abnormal or psychotic thoughts including: hallucinations; delusions; preoccupation with violence; homicidal or suicidal ideation; and obsessions • Description of the patient's judgment (e.g., concerning everyday activities and social situations) and insight (e.g., concerning psychiatric condition) Complete mental status examination including • Orientation to time, place and person • Recent and remote memory • Attention span and concentration • Language (e.g., naming objects, repeating phrases) • Fund of knowledge (e.g., awareness of current events, past history, vocabulary) • Mood and affect (e.g., depression, anxiety, agitation, hypomania, lability)

Content and Documentation Requirements

LEVEL OF EXAM	PERFORM AND DOCUMENT
Problem Focused	**One to five** elements identified by a bullet.
Expanded Problem Focused	**At least six** elements identified by a bullet.
Detailed	**At least twelve** elements identified by a bullet.
Comprehensive	Perform **all** elements identified by a bullet; document every element in each box with a shaded border and at least one element in each box with an unshaded border.

RESPIRATORY EXAMINATION

System/Body Area	Elements of Examination
Constitutional	• Measurement of **any three of the following seven** vital signs: 1) sitting or standing blood pressure, 2) supine blood pressure, 3) pulse rate and regularity, 4) respiration, 5) temperature, 6) height, 7) weight (may be measured and recorded by ancillary staff) • General appearance of patient (e.g., development, nutrition, body habitus, deformities, attention to grooming)
Head and Face	
Eyes	
Ears, Nose, Mouth and Throat	• Inspection of nasal mucosa, septum and turbinates • Inspection of teeth and gums • Examination of oropharynx (e.g., oral mucosa, hard and soft palates, tongue, tonsils and posterior pharynx)
Neck	• Examination of neck (e.g., masses, overall appearance, symmetry, tracheal position, crepitus) • Examination of thyroid (e.g., enlargement, tenderness, mass) • Examination of jugular veins (e.g., distension; a, v or cannon a waves)
Respiratory	• Inspection of chest with notation of symmetry and expansion • Assessment of respiratory effort (e.g., intercostal retractions, use of accessory muscles, diaphragmatic movement) • Percussion of chest (e.g., dullness, flatness, hyperresonance) • Palpation of chest (e.g., tactile fremitus) • Auscultation of lungs (e.g., breath sounds, adventitious sounds, rubs)
Cardiovascular	• Auscultation of heart including sounds, abnormal sounds and murmurs • Examination of peripheral vascular system by observation (e.g., swelling, varicosities) and palpation (e.g., pulses, temperature, edema, tenderness)
Chest (Breasts)	
Gastrointestinal (Abdomen)	• Examination of abdomen with notation of presence of masses or tenderness • Examination of liver and spleen
Genitourinary	

System/Body Area	Elements of Examination
Lymphatic	• Palpation of lymph nodes in neck, axillae, groin and/or other location
Musculoskeletal	• Assessment of muscle strength and tone (e.g., flaccid, cog wheel, spastic) with notation of any atrophy and abnormal movements • Examination of gait and station
Extremities	• Inspection and palpation of digits and nails (e.g., clubbing, cyanosis, inflammation, petechiae, ischemia, infections, nodes)
Skin	• Inspection and/or palpation of skin and subcutaneous tissue (e.g., rashes, lesions, ulcers)
Neurological/ Psychiatric	Brief assessment of mental status including • Orientation to time, place and person • Mood and affect (e.g., depression, anxiety, agitation)

Content and Documentation Requirements

LEVEL OF EXAM	PERFORM AND DOCUMENT
Problem Focused	**One to five** elements identified by a bullet.
Expanded Problem Focused	**At least six** elements identified by a bullet.
Detailed	**At least twelve** elements identified by a bullet.
Comprehensive	Perform **all** elements identified by a bullet; document every element in each box with a shaded border and at least one element in each box with an unshaded border.

SKIN EXAMINATION

System/Body Area	Elements of Examination
Constitutional	• Measurement of any **three of the following seven** vital signs: 1) sitting or standing blood pressure, 2) supine blood pressure, 3) pulse rate and regularity, 4) respiration, 5) temperature, 6) height, 7) weight (may be measured and recorded by ancillary staff) • General appearance of patient (e.g., development, nutrition, body habitus, deformities, attention to grooming)
Head and Face	
Eyes	• Inspection of conjunctivae and lids
Ears, Nose, Mouth and Throat	• Inspection of lips, teeth and gums • Examination of oropharynx (e.g., oral mucosa, hard and soft palates, tongue, tonsils, posterior pharynx)
Neck	• Examination of thyroid (e.g., enlargement, tenderness, mass)
Respiratory	
Cardiovascular	• Examination of peripheral vascular system by observation (e.g., swelling, varicosities) and palpation (e.g., pulses, temperature, edema, tenderness)
Chest (Breasts)	

System/Body Area	Elements of Examination
Gastrointestinal (Abdomen)	• Examination of liver and spleen • Examination of anus for condyloma and other lesions
Genitourinary	
Lymphatic	• Palpation of lymph nodes in neck, axillae, groin and/or other location
Musculoskeletal	
Extremities	• Inspection and palpation of digits and nails (e.g., clubbing, cyanosis, inflammation, petechiae, ischemia, infections, nodes)
Skin	• Palpation of scalp and inspection of hair of scalp, eyebrows, face, chest, pubic area (when indicated) and extremities • Inspection and/or palpation of skin and subcutaneous tissue (e.g., rashes, lesions, ulcers, susceptibility to and presence of photo damage) in **eight of the following ten** areas • Head, including the face and neck • Chest, including breasts and axillae • Abdomen • Genitalia, groin, buttocks • Back • Right upper extremity • Left upper extremity • Right lower extremity • Left lower extremity *Note:* For the comprehensive level, the examination of at least eight anatomic areas must be performed and documented. For the three lower levels of examination, each body area is counted separately. For example, inspection and/or palpation of the skin and subcutaneous tissue of the right upper extremity and the left upper extremity constitutes two elements. • Inspection of eccrine and apocrine glands of skin and subcutaneous tissue with identification and location of any hyperhidrosis, chromhidroses or bromhidrosis
Neurological/ Psychiatric	Brief assessment of mental status including • Orientation to time, place and person • Mood and affect (e.g., depression, anxiety, agitation)

Content and Documentation Requirements

LEVEL OF EXAM	PERFORM AND DOCUMENT
Problem Focused	**One to five** elements identified by a bullet.
Expanded Problem Focused	**At least six** elements identified by a bullet.
Detailed	**At least twelve** elements identified by a bullet.
Comprehensive	Perform **all** elements identified by a bullet; document every element in each box with a shaded border and at least one element in each box with an unshaded border.

C. Documentation of the Complexity of Medical Decision-Making

The levels of E/M services recognize four types of medical decision-making (straightforward, low complexity, moderate complexity and high complexity). Medical decision-making refers to the complexity of establishing a diagnosis and/or selecting a management option as measured by:

- the number of possible diagnoses and/or the number of management options that must be considered;

- the amount and/or complexity of medical records, diagnostic tests, and/or other information that must be obtained, reviewed and analyzed; and

- the risk of significant complications, morbidity and/or mortality, as well as comorbidities, associated with the patient's presenting problem(s), the diagnostic procedure(s) and/or the possible management options.

The following chart shows the progression of the elements required for each level of medical decision-making. To qualify for a given type of decision-making, **two of the three elements in the table must be either met or exceeded.**

Number of Diagnoses or Management Options	Amount and/or Complexity of Data to Be Reviewed	Risk of Complications and/ or Morbidity or Mortality	Type of Decision Making
Minimal	Minimal or None	Minimal	*Straightforward*
Limited	Limited	Low	*Low Complexity*
Multiple	Moderate	Moderate	*Moderate Complexity*
Extensive	Extensive	High	*High Complexity*

Each of the elements of medical decision-making is described following.

Number of Diagnoses or Management Options

The number of possible diagnoses and/or the number of management options that must be considered is based on the number and types of problems addressed during the encounter, the complexity of establishing a diagnosis and the management decisions that are made by the physician.

Generally, decision-making with respect to a diagnosed problem is easier than that for an identified but undiagnosed problem. The number and type of diagnostic tests employed may be an indicator of the number of possible diagnoses. Problems which are improving or resolving are less complex than those which are worsening or failing to change as expected. The need to seek advice from others is another indicator of complexity of diagnostic or management problems.

- DG: For each encounter, an assessment, clinical impression, or diagnosis should be documented. It may be explicitly stated or implied in documented decisions regarding management plans and/or further evaluation.

- For a presenting problem with an established diagnosis the record should reflect whether the problem is: a) improved, well controlled, resolving or resolved; or, b) inadequately controlled, worsening, or failing to change as expected.

- For a presenting problem without an established diagnosis, the assessment or clinical impression may be stated in the form of differential diagnoses or as a "possible," "probable," or "rule out" (R/O) diagnosis.

- DG: The initiation of, or changes in, treatment should be documented. Treatment includes a wide range of management options including patient instructions, nursing instructions, therapies, and medications.

- DG: If referrals are made, consultations requested or advice sought, the record should indicate to whom or where the referral or consultation is made or from whom the advice is requested.

Amount and/or Complexity of Data to Be Reviewed

The amount and complexity of data to be reviewed is based on the types of diagnostic testing ordered or reviewed. A decision to obtain and review old medical records and/or obtain history from sources other than the patient increases the amount and complexity of data to be reviewed.

Discussion of contradictory or unexpected test results with the physician who performed or interpreted the test is an indication of the complexity of data being reviewed. On occasion the physician who ordered a test may personally review the image, tracing or specimen to supplement information from the physician who prepared the test report or interpretation; this is another indication of the complexity of data being reviewed.

- DG: If a diagnostic service (test or procedure) is ordered, planned, scheduled, or performed at the time of the E/M encounter, the type of service, eg, lab or x-ray, should be documented.

- DG: The review of lab, radiology and/or other diagnostic tests should be documented. A simple notation such as "WBC elevated" or "chest x-ray unremarkable" is acceptable. Alternatively, the review may be documented by initialing and dating the report containing the test results.

- DG: A decision to obtain old records or decision to obtain additional history from the family, caretaker or other source to supplement that obtained from the patient should be documented.

- DG: Relevant findings from the review of old records, and/or the receipt of additional history from the family, caretaker or other source to supplement that obtained from the patient should be documented. If there is no relevant information beyond that already obtained, that fact should be documented. A notation of "Old records reviewed" or "additional history obtained from family" without elaboration is insufficient.

- DG: The results of discussion of laboratory, radiology or other diagnostic tests with the physician who performed or interpreted the study should be documented.

- DG: The direct visualization and independent interpretation of an image, tracing or specimen previously or subsequently interpreted by another physician should be documented.

Risk of Significant Complications, Morbidity, and/or Mortality

The risk of significant complications, morbidity, and/or mortality is based on the risks associated with the presenting problem(s), the diagnostic procedure(s), and the possible management options.

- ■ DG: Comorbidities/underlying diseases or other factors that increase the complexity of medical decision making by increasing the risk of complications, morbidity, and/or mortality should be documented.

- ■ DG: If a surgical or invasive diagnostic procedure is ordered, planned or scheduled at the time of the E/M encounter, the type of procedure, e.g., laparoscopy, should be documented.

- ■ DG: If a surgical or invasive diagnostic procedure is performed at the time of the E/M encounter, the specific procedure should be documented.

- ■ DG: The referral for or decision to perform a surgical or invasive diagnostic procedure on an urgent basis should be documented or implied.

The following table may be used to help determine whether the risk of significant complications, morbidity, and/or mortality is *minimal, low, moderate,* or *high*. Because the determination of risk is complex and not readily quantifiable, the table includes common clinical examples rather than absolute measures of risk. The assessment of risk of the presenting problem(s) is based on the risk related to the disease process anticipated between the present encounter and the next one. The assessment of risk of selecting diagnostic procedures and management options is based on the risk during and immediately following any procedures or treatment. **The highest level of risk in any one category (presenting problem(s), diagnostic procedure(s), or management options) determines the overall risk.**

TABLE OF RISK

Level of Risk	Presenting Problem(s)	Diagnostic Procedure(s) Ordered	Management Options Selected
Minimal	• One self-limited or minor problem, eg, cold, insect bite, tinea corporis	• Laboratory tests requiring venipuncture • Chest x-rays • EKG/EEG • Urinalysis • Ultrasound, eg, echocardiography • KOH prep	• Rest • Gargles • Elastic bandages • Superficial dressings
Low	• Two or more self-limited or minor problems • One stable chronic illness, eg, well controlled hypertension, non-insulin dependent diabetes, cataract, BPH • Acute uncomplicated illness or injury, eg, cystitis, allergic rhinitis, simple sprain	• Physiologic tests not under stress, eg, pulmonary function tests • Non-cardiovascular imaging studies with contrast, eg, barium enema • Superficial needle biopsies • Clinical laboratory tests requiring arterial puncture • Skin biopsies	• Over-the-counter drugs • Minor surgery with no identified risk factors • Physical therapy • Occupational therapy • IV fluids without additives

Level of Risk	Presenting Problem(s)	Diagnostic Procedure(s) Ordered	Management Options Selected
Moderate	• One or more chronic illnesses with mild exacerbation, progression, or side effects of treatment • Two or more stable chronic illnesses • Undiagnosed new problem with uncertain prognosis, eg, lump in breast • Acute illness with systemic symptoms, eg, pyelonephritis, pneumonitis, colitis • Acute complicated injury, eg, head injury with brief loss of consciousness	• Physiologic tests under stress, eg, cardiac stress test, fetal contraction stress test • Diagnostic endoscopies with no identified risk factors • Deep needle or incisional biopsy • Cardiovascular imaging studies with contrast and no identified risk factors, eg, arteriogram, cardiac catheterization • Obtain fluid from body cavity, eg, lumbar puncture, thoracentesis, culdocentesis	• Minor surgery with identified risk factors • Elective major surgery (open, percutaneous or endoscopic) with no identified risk factors • Prescription drug management • Therapeutic nuclear medicine • IV fluids with additives • Closed treatment of fracture or dislocation without manipulation
High	• One or more chronic illnesses with severe exacerbation, progression, or side effects of treatment • Acute or chronic illnesses or injuries that pose a threat to life or bodily function, eg, multiple trauma, acute MI, pulmonary embolus, severe respiratory distress, progressive severe rheumatoid arthritis, psychiatric illness with potential threat to self or others, peritonitis, acute renal failure • An abrupt change in neurologic status, eg, seizure, TIA, weakness, sensory loss	• Cardiovascular imaging studies with contrast with identified risk factors • Cardiac electrophysiological tests • Diagnostic endoscopies with identified risk factors • Discography	• Elective major surgery (open, percutaneous or endoscopic) with identified risk factors • Emergency major surgery (open, percutaneous or endoscopic) • Parenteral controlled substances • Drug therapy requiring intensive monitoring for toxicity • Decision not to resuscitate or to de-escalate care because of poor prognosis

D. Documentation of an Encounter Dominated by Counseling or Coordination of Care

In the case where counseling and/or coordination of care dominates (more than 50%) of the physician/patient and/or family encounter (face-to-face time in the office or other or outpatient setting, floor/unit time in the hospital or nursing facility), time is considered the key or controlling factor to qualify for a particular level of E/M services.

■ DG: If the physician elects to report the level of service based on counseling and/or coordination of care, the total length of time of the encounter (face-to-face or floor time, as appropriate) should be documented and the record should describe the counseling and/or activities to coordinate care.

E/M Audit Form

HISTORY ELEMENTS				Documented
HISTORY OF PRESENT ILLNESS (HPI)				
1. Location (site on body)				
2. Quality (characteristic: throbbing, sharp)				
3. Severity (1/10 or how intense)				
4. Duration (how long for problem or episode)				
5. Timing (when it occurs)				
6. Context (under what circumstances does it occur)				
7. Modifying factors (what makes it better or worse)				
8. Associated signs and symptoms (what else is happening when it occurs)				
			TOTAL	4
			LEVEL	4
REVIEW OF SYSTEMS (ROS)				Documented
1. Constitutional (e.g., weight loss, fever)				
2. Ophthalmologic (eyes)				
3. Otolaryngologic (ears, nose, mouth, throat)				
4. Cardiovascular				
5. Respiratory				
6. Gastrointestinal				
7. Genitourinary				
8. Musculoskeletal				
9. Integumentary (skin and/or breasts)				
10. Neurologic				
11. Psychiatric				
12. Endocrine				
13. Hematologic/Lymphatic				
14. Allergic/Immunologic				
			TOTAL	
			LEVEL	
PAST, FAMILY, AND/OR SOCIAL HISTORY (PFSH)				Documented
1. Past illness, operations, injuries, treatments, and current medications				
2. Family medical history for heredity and risk				
3. Social activities, both past and present				
			TOTAL	
			LEVEL	

History Level	1	2	3	4
	Problem Focused	Expanded Problem Focused	Detailed	Comprehensive
HPI	Brief 1-3	Brief 1-3	Extended 4+	Extended 4+
ROS	None	Problem Pertinent	Extended 2-9	Complete 10+
PFSH	None	None	Pertinent 1	Complete 2-3
			HISTORY LEVEL	3

EXAMINATION ELEMENTS	Documented
CONSTITUTIONAL	
1. Blood pressure, sitting	
2. Blood pressure, lying	
3. Pulse	
4. Respirations	
5. Temperature	
6. Height	
7. Weight	
8. General appearance	
NUMBER	
BODY AREAS (BA)	Documented
1. Head (including face)	
2. Neck	
3. Chest (including breasts and axillae)	
4. Abdomen	
5. Genitalia, groin, buttocks	
6. Back (including spine)	
7. Each extremity	
NUMBER	
ORGAN SYSTEMS (OS)	Documented
1. Ophthalmologic (eyes)	
2. Otolaryngologic (ears, nose, mouth, throat)	
3. Cardiovascular	
4. Respiratory	
5. Gastrointestinal	
6. Genitourinary	
7. Musculoskeletal	
8. Integumentary	
9. Neurologic	
10. Psychiatric	
11. Hematologic/Lymphatic/Immunologic	
NUMBER	
TOTAL BA/OS	

Exam Level	1	2	3	4
	Problem Focused	Expanded Problem Focused	Detailed	Comprehensive
	Limited to affected BA/OS	Limited to affected BA/OS & other related OSs	Extended of affected BA & other related OSs	General multi-system or complete single OS
# of OS or BA	1	2-7 limited	2-7 extended	8+
			EXAMINATION LEVEL	

MDM ELEMENTS	Documented
# OF DIAGNOSIS/MANAGEMENT OPTIONS	
1. Minimal	
2. Limited	
3. Multiple	
4. Extensive	
LEVEL	
AMOUNT OR COMPLEXITY OF DATA TO REVIEW	Documented
1. Minimal/None	
2. Limited	
3. Moderate	
4. Extensive	
LEVEL	
RISK OF COMPLICATION OR DEATH IF NOT TREATED	Documented
1. Minimal	
2. Low	
3. Moderate	
4. High	
LEVEL	

MDM*	1	2	3	4
	Straightforward	Low	Moderate	High
Number of DX or management options	Minimal	Limited	Multiple	Extensive
Amount or complexity of data	Minimal/None	Limited	Moderate	Extensive
Risks	Minimal	Low	Moderate	High
			MDM LEVEL	4

*To qualify for a given type of MDM complexity, 2 of 3 elements in the table must be met or exceeded.

History:
Examination:
MDM:

Number of Key Components:

Code:

HISTORY ELEMENTS	Documented
HISTORY OF PRESENT ILLNESS (HPI)	
1. Location (site on body)	
2. Quality (characteristic: throbbing, sharp)	
3. Severity (1/10 or how intense)	
4. Duration (how long for problem or episode)	
5. Timing (when it occurs)	
6. Context (under what circumstances does it occur)	
7. Modifying factors (what makes it better or worse)	
8. Associated signs and symptoms (what else is happening when it occurs)	
TOTAL	4
LEVEL	4

REVIEW OF SYSTEMS (ROS)	Documented
1. Constitutional (e.g., weight loss, fever)	
2. Ophthalmologic (eyes)	
3. Otolaryngologic (ears, nose, mouth, throat)	
4. Cardiovascular	
5. Respiratory	
6. Gastrointestinal	
7. Genitourinary	
8. Musculoskeletal	
9. Integumentary (skin and/or breasts)	
10. Neurologic	
11. Psychiatric	
12. Endocrine	
13. Hematologic/Lymphatic	
14. Allergic/Immunologic	
TOTAL	
LEVEL	

PAST, FAMILY, AND/OR SOCIAL HISTORY (PFSH)	Documented
1. Past illness, operations, injuries, treatments, and current medications	
2. Family medical history for heredity and risk	
3. Social activities, both past and present	
TOTAL	
LEVEL	

History Level	1 Problem Focused	2 Expanded Problem Focused	3 Detailed	4 Comprehensive
HPI	Brief 1-3	Brief 1-3	Extended 4+	Extended 4+
ROS	None	Problem Pertinent	Extended 2-9	Complete 10+
PFSH	None	None	Pertinent 1	Complete 2-3
			HISTORY LEVEL	3

EXAMINATION ELEMENTS	Documented
CONSTITUTIONAL	
1. Blood pressure, sitting	
2. Blood pressure, lying	
3. Pulse	
4. Respirations	
5. Temperature	
6. Height	
7. Weight	
8. General appearance	
NUMBER	

BODY AREAS (BA)	Documented
1. Head (including face)	
2. Neck	
3. Chest (including breasts and axillae)	
4. Abdomen	
5. Genitalia, groin, buttocks	
6. Back (including spine)	
7. Each extremity	
NUMBER	

ORGAN SYSTEMS (OS)	Documented
1. Ophthalmologic (eyes)	
2. Otolaryngologic (ears, nose, mouth, throat)	
3. Cardiovascular	
4. Respiratory	
5. Gastrointestinal	
6. Genitourinary	
7. Musculoskeletal	
8. Integumentary	
9. Neurologic	
10. Psychiatric	
11. Hematologic/Lymphatic/Immunologic	
NUMBER	
TOTAL BA/OS	

Exam Level	1 Problem Focused	2 Expanded Problem Focused	3 Detailed	4 Comprehensive
	Limited to affected BA/OS	Limited to affected BA/OS & other related OSs	Extended of affected BA & other related OSs	General multi-system or complete single OS
# of OS or BA	1	2-7 limited	2-7 extended	8+
			EXAMINATION LEVEL	

MDM ELEMENTS	Documented
# OF DIAGNOSIS/MANAGEMENT OPTIONS	
1. Minimal	
2. Limited	
3. Multiple	
4. Extensive	
LEVEL	
AMOUNT OR COMPLEXITY OF DATA TO REVIEW	Documented
1. Minimal/None	
2. Limited	
3. Moderate	
4. Extensive	
LEVEL	
RISK OF COMPLICATION OR DEATH IF NOT TREATED	Documented
1. Minimal	
2. Low	
3. Moderate	
4. High	
LEVEL	

MDM*	1 Straightforward	2 Low	3 Moderate	4 High
Number of DX or management options	Minimal	Limited	Multiple	Extensive
Amount or complexity of data	Minimal/None	Limited	Moderate	Extensive
Risks	Minimal	Low	Moderate	High
			MDM LEVEL	4

*To qualify for a given type of MDM complexity, 2 of 3 elements in the table must be met or exceeded.

History:
Examination:
MDM:

Number of Key Components:

Code:

HISTORY ELEMENTS	Documented
HISTORY OF PRESENT ILLNESS (HPI)	
1. Location (site on body)	
2. Quality (characteristic: throbbing, sharp)	
3. Severity (1/10 or how intense)	
4. Duration (how long for problem or episode)	
5. Timing (when it occurs)	
6. Context (under what circumstances does it occur)	
7. Modifying factors (what makes it better or worse)	
8. Associated signs and symptoms (what else is happening when it occurs)	
TOTAL	4
LEVEL	4

REVIEW OF SYSTEMS (ROS)	Documented
1. Constitutional (e.g., weight loss, fever)	
2. Ophthalmologic (eyes)	
3. Otolaryngologic (ears, nose, mouth, throat)	
4. Cardiovascular	
5. Respiratory	
6. Gastrointestinal	
7. Genitourinary	
8. Musculoskeletal	
9. Integumentary (skin and/or breasts)	
10. Neurologic	
11. Psychiatric	
12. Endocrine	
13. Hematologic/Lymphatic	
14. Allergic/Immunologic	
TOTAL	
LEVEL	

PAST, FAMILY, AND/OR SOCIAL HISTORY (PFSH)	Documented
1. Past illness, operations, injuries, treatments, and current medications	
2. Family medical history for heredity and risk	
3. Social activities, both past and present	
TOTAL	
LEVEL	

History Level	1	2	3	4
	Problem Focused	Expanded Problem Focused	Detailed	Comprehensive
HPI	Brief 1-3	Brief 1-3	Extended 4+	Extended 4+
ROS	None	Problem Pertinent	Extended 2-9	Complete 10+
PFSH	None	None	Pertinent 1	Complete 2-3
			HISTORY LEVEL	3

EXAMINATION ELEMENTS	Documented
CONSTITUTIONAL	
1. Blood pressure, sitting	
2. Blood pressure, lying	
3. Pulse	
4. Respirations	
5. Temperature	
6. Height	
7. Weight	
8. General appearance	
NUMBER	

BODY AREAS (BA)	Documented
1. Head (including face)	
2. Neck	
3. Chest (including breasts and axillae)	
4. Abdomen	
5. Genitalia, groin, buttocks	
6. Back (including spine)	
7. Each extremity	
NUMBER	

ORGAN SYSTEMS (OS)	Documented
1. Ophthalmologic (eyes)	
2. Otolaryngologic (ears, nose, mouth, throat)	
3. Cardiovascular	
4. Respiratory	
5. Gastrointestinal	
6. Genitourinary	
7. Musculoskeletal	
8. Integumentary	
9. Neurologic	
10. Psychiatric	
11. Hematologic/Lymphatic/Immunologic	
NUMBER	
TOTAL BA/OS	

Exam Level	1	2	3	4
	Problem Focused	Expanded Problem Focused	Detailed	Comprehensive
	Limited to affected BA/OS	Limited to affected BA/OS & other related OSs	Extended of affected BA & other related OSs	General multi-system or complete single OS
# of OS or BA	1	2-7 limited	2-7 extended	8+
			EXAMINATION LEVEL	

MDM ELEMENTS	Documented
# OF DIAGNOSIS/MANAGEMENT OPTIONS	
1. Minimal	
2. Limited	
3. Multiple	
4. Extensive	
LEVEL	

AMOUNT OR COMPLEXITY OF DATA TO REVIEW	Documented
1. Minimal/None	
2. Limited	
3. Moderate	
4. Extensive	
LEVEL	

RISK OF COMPLICATION OR DEATH IF NOT TREATED	Documented
1. Minimal	
2. Low	
3. Moderate	
4. High	
LEVEL	

MDM*	1	2	3	4
	Straightforward	Low	Moderate	High
Number of DX or management options	Minimal	Limited	Multiple	Extensive
Amount or complexity of data	Minimal/None	Limited	Moderate	Extensive
Risks	Minimal	Low	Moderate	High
			MDM LEVEL	4

*To qualify for a given type of MDM complexity, 2 of 3 elements in the table must be met or exceeded.

History:
Examination:
MDM:

Number of Key Components:

Code:

HISTORY ELEMENTS	Documented
HISTORY OF PRESENT ILLNESS (HPI)	
1. Location (site on body)	
2. Quality (characteristic: throbbing, sharp)	
3. Severity (1/10 or how intense)	
4. Duration (how long for problem or episode)	
5. Timing (when it occurs)	
6. Context (under what circumstances does it occur)	
7. Modifying factors (what makes it better or worse)	
8. Associated signs and symptoms (what else is happening when it occurs)	
TOTAL	4
LEVEL	4

REVIEW OF SYSTEMS (ROS)	Documented
1. Constitutional (e.g., weight loss, fever)	
2. Ophthalmologic (eyes)	
3. Otolaryngologic (ears, nose, mouth, throat)	
4. Cardiovascular	
5. Respiratory	
6. Gastrointestinal	
7. Genitourinary	
8. Musculoskeletal	
9. Integumentary (skin and/or breasts)	
10. Neurologic	
11. Psychiatric	
12. Endocrine	
13. Hematologic/Lymphatic	
14. Allergic/Immunologic	
TOTAL	
LEVEL	

PAST, FAMILY, AND/OR SOCIAL HISTORY (PFSH)	Documented
1. Past illness, operations, injuries, treatments, and current medications	
2. Family medical history for heredity and risk	
3. Social activities, both past and present	
TOTAL	
LEVEL	

History Level	1	2	3	4
	Problem Focused	Expanded Problem Focused	Detailed	Comprehensive
HPI	Brief 1-3	Brief 1-3	Extended 4+	Extended 4+
ROS	None	Problem Pertinent	Extended 2-9	Complete 10+
PFSH	None	None	Pertinent 1	Complete 2-3
HISTORY LEVEL				3

EXAMINATION ELEMENTS	Documented
CONSTITUTIONAL	
1. Blood pressure, sitting	
2. Blood pressure, lying	
3. Pulse	
4. Respirations	
5. Temperature	
6. Height	
7. Weight	
8. General appearance	
NUMBER	

BODY AREAS (BA)	Documented
1. Head (including face)	
2. Neck	
3. Chest (including breasts and axillae)	
4. Abdomen	
5. Genitalia, groin, buttocks	
6. Back (including spine)	
7. Each extremity	
NUMBER	

ORGAN SYSTEMS (OS)	Documented
1. Ophthalmologic (eyes)	
2. Otolaryngologic (ears, nose, mouth, throat)	
3. Cardiovascular	
4. Respiratory	
5. Gastrointestinal	
6. Genitourinary	
7. Musculoskeletal	
8. Integumentary	
9. Neurologic	
10. Psychiatric	
11. Hematologic/Lymphatic/Immunologic	
NUMBER	
TOTAL BA/OS	

Exam Level	1	2	3	4
	Problem Focused	Expanded Problem Focused	Detailed	Comprehensive
	Limited to affected BA/OS	Limited to affected BA/OS & other related OSs	Extended of affected BA & other related OSs	General multi-system or complete single OS
# of OS or BA	1	2-7 limited	2-7 extended	8+
EXAMINATION LEVEL				

MDM ELEMENTS	Documented
# OF DIAGNOSIS/MANAGEMENT OPTIONS	
1. Minimal	
2. Limited	
3. Multiple	
4. Extensive	
LEVEL	
AMOUNT OR COMPLEXITY OF DATA TO REVIEW	Documented
1. Minimal/None	
2. Limited	
3. Moderate	
4. Extensive	
LEVEL	
RISK OF COMPLICATION OR DEATH IF NOT TREATED	Documented
1. Minimal	
2. Low	
3. Moderate	
4. High	
LEVEL	

MDM*	1	2	3	4
	Straightforward	Low	Moderate	High
Number of DX or management options	Minimal	Limited	Multiple	Extensive
Amount or complexity of data	Minimal/None	Limited	Moderate	Extensive
Risks	Minimal	Low	Moderate	High
MDM LEVEL				4

*To qualify for a given type of MDM complexity, 2 of 3 elements in the table must be met or exceeded.

History:
Examination:
MDM:

Number of Key Components:

Code:

HISTORY ELEMENTS	Documented
HISTORY OF PRESENT ILLNESS (HPI)	
1. Location (site on body)	
2. Quality (characteristic: throbbing, sharp)	
3. Severity (1/10 or how intense)	
4. Duration (how long for problem or episode)	
5. Timing (when it occurs)	
6. Context (under what circumstances does it occur)	
7. Modifying factors (what makes it better or worse)	
8. Associated signs and symptoms (what else is happening when it occurs)	
TOTAL	4
LEVEL	4

REVIEW OF SYSTEMS (ROS)	Documented
1. Constitutional (e.g., weight loss, fever)	
2. Ophthalmologic (eyes)	
3. Otolaryngologic (ears, nose, mouth, throat)	
4. Cardiovascular	
5. Respiratory	
6. Gastrointestinal	
7. Genitourinary	
8. Musculoskeletal	
9. Integumentary (skin and/or breasts)	
10. Neurologic	
11. Psychiatric	
12. Endocrine	
13. Hematologic/Lymphatic	
14. Allergic/Immunologic	
TOTAL	
LEVEL	

PAST, FAMILY, AND/OR SOCIAL HISTORY (PFSH)	Documented
1. Past illness, operations, injuries, treatments, and current medications	
2. Family medical history for heredity and risk	
3. Social activities, both past and present	
TOTAL	
LEVEL	

History Level	1	2	3	4
	Problem Focused	Expanded Problem Focused	Detailed	Comprehensive
HPI	Brief 1-3	Brief 1-3	Extended 4+	Extended 4+
ROS	None	Problem Pertinent	Extended 2-9	Complete 10+
PFSH	None	None	Pertinent 1	Complete 2-3
HISTORY LEVEL				3

EXAMINATION ELEMENTS	Documented
CONSTITUTIONAL	
1. Blood pressure, sitting	
2. Blood pressure, lying	
3. Pulse	
4. Respirations	
5. Temperature	
6. Height	
7. Weight	
8. General appearance	
NUMBER	

BODY AREAS (BA)	Documented
1. Head (including face)	
2. Neck	
3. Chest (including breasts and axillae)	
4. Abdomen	
5. Genitalia, groin, buttocks	
6. Back (including spine)	
7. Each extremity	
NUMBER	

ORGAN SYSTEMS (OS)	Documented
1. Ophthalmologic (eyes)	
2. Otolaryngologic (ears, nose, mouth, throat)	
3. Cardiovascular	
4. Respiratory	
5. Gastrointestinal	
6. Genitourinary	
7. Musculoskeletal	
8. Integumentary	
9. Neurologic	
10. Psychiatric	
11. Hematologic/Lymphatic/Immunologic	
NUMBER	
TOTAL BA/OS	

Exam Level	1	2	3	4
	Problem Focused	Expanded Problem Focused	Detailed	Comprehensive
	Limited to affected BA/OS	Limited to affected BA/OS & other related OSs	Extended of affected BA & other related OSs	General multi-system or complete single OS
# of OS or BA	1	2-7 limited	2-7 extended	8+
EXAMINATION LEVEL				

MDM ELEMENTS	Documented
# OF DIAGNOSIS/MANAGEMENT OPTIONS	
1. Minimal	
2. Limited	
3. Multiple	
4. Extensive	
LEVEL	

AMOUNT OR COMPLEXITY OF DATA TO REVIEW	Documented
1. Minimal/None	
2. Limited	
3. Moderate	
4. Extensive	
LEVEL	

RISK OF COMPLICATION OR DEATH IF NOT TREATED	Documented
1. Minimal	
2. Low	
3. Moderate	
4. High	
LEVEL	

MDM*	1	2	3	4
	Straightforward	Low	Moderate	High
Number of DX or management options	Minimal	Limited	Multiple	Extensive
Amount or complexity of data	Minimal/None	Limited	Moderate	Extensive
Risks	Minimal	Low	Moderate	High
MDM LEVEL				4

*To qualify for a given type of MDM complexity, 2 of 3 elements in the table must be met or exceeded.

History:
Examination:
MDM:

Number of Key Components:

Code:

HISTORY ELEMENTS				Documented
HISTORY OF PRESENT ILLNESS (HPI)				
1. Location (site on body)				
2. Quality (characteristic: throbbing, sharp)				
3. Severity (1/10 or how intense)				
4. Duration (how long for problem or episode)				
5. Timing (when it occurs)				
6. Context (under what circumstances does it occur)				
7. Modifying factors (what makes it better or worse)				
8. Associated signs and symptoms (what else is happening when it occurs)				
			TOTAL	4
			LEVEL	4

REVIEW OF SYSTEMS (ROS)				Documented
1. Constitutional (e.g., weight loss, fever)				
2. Ophthalmologic (eyes)				
3. Otolaryngologic (ears, nose, mouth, throat)				
4. Cardiovascular				
5. Respiratory				
6. Gastrointestinal				
7. Genitourinary				
8. Musculoskeletal				
9. Integumentary (skin and/or breasts)				
10. Neurologic				
11. Psychiatric				
12. Endocrine				
13. Hematologic/Lymphatic				
14. Allergic/Immunologic				
			TOTAL	
			LEVEL	

PAST, FAMILY, AND/OR SOCIAL HISTORY (PFSH)				Documented
1. Past illness, operations, injuries, treatments, and current medications				
2. Family medical history for heredity and risk				
3. Social activities, both past and present				
			TOTAL	
			LEVEL	

History Level	1	2	3	4
	Problem Focused	Expanded Problem Focused	Detailed	Comprehensive
HPI	Brief 1-3	Brief 1-3	Extended 4+	Extended 4+
ROS	None	Problem Pertinent	Extended 2-9	Complete 10+
PFSH	None	None	Pertinent 1	Complete 2-3
			HISTORY LEVEL	3

EXAMINATION ELEMENTS	Documented
CONSTITUTIONAL	
1. Blood pressure, sitting	
2. Blood pressure, lying	
3. Pulse	
4. Respirations	
5. Temperature	
6. Height	
7. Weight	
8. General appearance	
NUMBER	

BODY AREAS (BA)	Documented
1. Head (including face)	
2. Neck	
3. Chest (including breasts and axillae)	
4. Abdomen	
5. Genitalia, groin, buttocks	
6. Back (including spine)	
7. Each extremity	
NUMBER	

ORGAN SYSTEMS (OS)	Documented
1. Ophthalmologic (eyes)	
2. Otolaryngologic (ears, nose, mouth, throat)	
3. Cardiovascular	
4. Respiratory	
5. Gastrointestinal	
6. Genitourinary	
7. Musculoskeletal	
8. Integumentary	
9. Neurologic	
10. Psychiatric	
11. Hematologic/Lymphatic/Immunologic	
NUMBER	
TOTAL BA/OS	

Exam Level	1	2	3	4
	Problem Focused	Expanded Problem Focused	Detailed	Comprehensive
	Limited to affected BA/OS	Limited to affected BA/OS & other related OSs	Extended of affected BA & other related OSs	General multi-system or complete single OS
# of OS or BA	1	2-7 limited	2-7 extended	8+
			EXAMINATION LEVEL	

MDM ELEMENTS				Documented
# OF DIAGNOSIS/MANAGEMENT OPTIONS				
1. Minimal				
2. Limited				
3. Multiple				
4. Extensive				
			LEVEL	
AMOUNT OR COMPLEXITY OF DATA TO REVIEW				Documented
1. Minimal/None				
2. Limited				
3. Moderate				
4. Extensive				
			LEVEL	
RISK OF COMPLICATION OR DEATH IF NOT TREATED				Documented
1. Minimal				
2. Low				
3. Moderate				
4. High				
			LEVEL	

MDM*	1	2	3	4
	Straightforward	Low	Moderate	High
Number of DX or management options	Minimal	Limited	Multiple	Extensive
Amount or complexity of data	Minimal/None	Limited	Moderate	Extensive
Risks	Minimal	Low	Moderate	High
			MDM LEVEL	4

*To qualify for a given type of MDM complexity, 2 of 3 elements in the table must be met or exceeded.

History:
Examination:
MDM:

Number of Key Components:

Code:

Abbreviations

ABG	arterial blood gases
ACLS	Advanced Cardiac Life Support
AIC	amino-imidazole carboxamide, anti-inflammatory corticoid
ALT	alanine transaminase (formerly SGPT)
ARDS	acute or adult respiratory distress syndrome
AST	aspartate amino-transferase (formerly SGOT)
ATN	acute tubular necrosis
AV	arteriovenous
b.i.d.	twice a day
BOOP	bronchiolitis obliterans organizing pneumonia
BSO	bilateral salpingo-oophorectomy
BUN	blood urea nitrogen
CABG	coronary artery bypass graft
CBC	complete blood count
CEA	carcinoembryonic antigen
CHF	congestive heart failure
CK	creatine kinase
COPD	chronic obstructive pulmonary disease
CPK	creatine phosphokinase
CT	computed tomography
CVA	cardiovascular accident
D	deciliter
D5	dextrose 5% water
ENT	ear, nose, throat
EOMs	extraocular movements
FI	forced inspiration
GERD	gastroesophageal reflux
GI	gastrointestinal
GU	genitourinary
h	hour
H_2	histamine-2
H&H	hematocrit and hemoglobin, also stated HH
HEENT	head, ears, eyes, nose, throat
Hs	at bedtime
I&O	intake and output
IM	intramuscular
INR	International Normalized Ratio
IV	intravenous
JP	jugular process, jugular pulse
JVD	jugular vein distention

LMP	last menstrual period
MAP	mean aortic pressure, mean arterial pressure
MB	methylene blue, mesio-buccal
MDM	medical decision making
mEq	milliequivalent
mg	milligram
MI	myocardial infarction
mL	milliliter
mm	millimeter
neb	nebula, a spray
NG	nasogastric, nitroglycerin
n.p.o	nothing by mouth
O_2	oxygen
OBT	occult blood test
OP	outpatient
OPC	outpatient clinic
OPD	outpatient department
OPS	outpatient surgery
OPV	oral poliovirus vaccine
OR	operating room
OTC	over-the-counter
OURQ	outer upper-right quadrant
OV	office visit
PCO_2	partial pressure of carbon dioxide
PEEP	positive end expiration pressure
pH	potential of hydrogen
p.o.	by mouth
p.r.n.	as needed
PT	prothrombin time
PTH	parathyroid hormone, post-transfusional hepatitis
q	every
q.2wk	every 2 weeks
q.3h	every 3 hours
q.4h	every 4 hours
q.4wk	every 4 weeks
q.a.m.	every morning
q.d.	every day
q.d.s.	four times a day
q.h.	every hour
q.h.s.	each bedtime
q.i.d.	four times a day
q.m.	every morning
q.o.d.	every other day
q.os.	as needed
q.p.m.	every afternoon or every evening
q.q.h.	every fourth hour
q.s.	quantity sufficient
qq.	each, every
qq.h	every hour
QRS	Q-wave R-wave S-wave
RLQ	right lower quadrant
s	sans (without), sigma (sign, mark), semis (half)
S1	first heart sound
S2	second heart sound
S3	third heart sound

S4	fourth heart sound
SBE	subacute bacterial endocarditis
SIMV	synchronized intermittent mandatory ventilation
T_4	thyroxine
TMJ	temporomandibular joint
URI	upper respiratory infection

APPENDIX F

Further Text Resources

ANATOMY AND PHYSIOLOGY

Book Title	Author	Imprint	Publication Date	ISBN-13
The Anatomy and Physiology Learning System, 3rd Edition	Applegate	Saunders	2006	978-1-4160-2586-3
Gray's Anatomy for Students	Drake, Vogl, Mitchell	Churchill Livingstone	2005	978-0-443-06612-2
Anthony's Textbook of Anatomy and Physiology, 18th edition	Thibodeau, Patton	Mosby	2006	978-0-323-03982-6

CODING

Book Title	Author	Imprint	Publication Date	ISBN-13
Step-by-Step Medical Coding, 2008 Edition	Buck	Saunders	2008	978-1-4160-4567-0
Saunders 2008 ICD-9-CM, Volumes 1 & 2 (Professional Edition)	Buck	Saunders	2008	978-1-4160-4414-7
Saunders 2008 ICD-9-CM, Volumes 1, 2, & 3 (Professional Edition)	Buck	Saunders	2008	978-1-4160-4413-0
Saunders 2008 HCPCS Level II	Buck	Saunders	2008	978-1-4160-4892-3
The Next Step, Advanced Medical Coding, 2008 edition	Buck	Saunders	2008	978-1-4160-4042-2
The Extra Step: Facility-Based Coding Practice	Buck	Saunders	2006	978-1-4160-3450-6
The Extra Step: Physician-Based Coding Practice	Buck	Saunders	2006	978-1-4160-3451-3
CPC Coding Exam Review 2008: The Certification Step	Buck	Saunders	2008	978-1-4160-3711-8
CCS Coding Exam Review 2008: The Certification Step	Buck	Saunders	2008	978-1-4160-3683-8
CCS-P Coding Exam Review 2008: The Certification Step	Buck	Saunders	2008	978-1-4160-3692-0
CPC-H Coding Exam Review 2008: The Certification Step	Buck	Saunders	2008	978-1-4160-3721-7

PATHOPHYSIOLOGY

Book Title	Author	Imprint	Publication Date	ISBN-13
Pathology for the Health Professions, 3rd Edition	Damjanov	Saunders	2006	978-1-4160-0031-0
Essentials of Human Diseases and Conditions, 4th Edition	Frazier, Drzymkowski	Saunders	2008	978-1-4160-4714-8
Pathophysiology for the Health Related Professions, 3rd Edition	Gould	Saunders	2006	978-1-4160-0210-9
The Human Body in Health and Illness, 3rd Edition	Herlihy	Saunders	2007	978-1-4160-2885-7
The Human Body in Health and Disease, 4th Edition	Thibodeau, Patton	Mosby	2005	978-0-323-03162-2

MEDICAL TERMINOLOGY

Book Title	Author	Imprint	Publication Date	ISBN-13
The Language of Medicine, 8th Edition	Chabner	Saunders	2007	978-1-4160-3492-6
Dictionary of Medical Acronyms & Abbreviations, 5th edition	Jablonski	Hanley & Belfus	2005	978-1-560-53632-1
Exploring Medical Language, 7th Edition	LaFleur, Brooks	Mosby	2008	978-0-323-04950-4
Building a Medical Vocabulary (with Spanish Translations), 6th Edition	Leonard	Saunders	2005	978-0-7216-0464-0
Quick & Easy Medical Terminology, 5th Edition	Leonard	Saunders	2007	978-1-4160-2494-1
Mastering Healthcare Terminology, 2nd Edition	Shiland	Mosby	2006	978-0-323-03572-9
Dorland's Illustrated Medical Dictionary, 31st Edition		Saunders	2007	978-1-4160-2364-7

INTRODUCTION TO COMPUTER

Book Title	Author	Imprint	Publication Date	ISBN-13
Computerized Medical Office Procedures: A Worktext 2nd Edition	Larsen	Saunders	2008	978-1-4160-4834-3

BASICS OF WRITING/MEDICAL TRANSCRIPTION

Book Title	Author	Imprint	Publication Date	ISBN-13
Medical Transcription Guide: Do's and Don'ts, 3rd edition	Diehl	Saunders	2005	978-0-7216-0684-2
Diehl & Fordney's Medical Transcribing: Techniques and Procedures, 6th Edition	Diehl	Saunders	2007	978-1-4160-2347-0

COMPREHENSION BUILDING/STUDY SKILLS

Book Title	Author	Imprint	Publication Date	ISBN-13
Career Development for Health Professionals: Success in School and on the Job 2nd edition	Haroun	Saunders	2006	978-0-7216-0609-5

BASIC MATH

Book Title	Author	Imprint	Publication Date	ISBN-13
Basic Mathematics for the Health-Related Professions	Doucette	Saunders	2000	978-0-7216-7938-9
Using Maths in Health Sciences	Gunn	Churchill Livingstone	2001	978-0-443-07074-7

MEDICAL BILLING/INSURANCE

Book Title	Author	Imprint	Publication Date	ISBN-13
Health Insurance Today A Practical Approach	Buck	Saunders	2007	978-1-4160-0054-9
Medical Insurance Made Easy: Understanding the Claim Cycle, 2nd Edition	Brown	Saunders	2006	978-0-7216-0556-2
Quick Guide to HIPAA for the Physician's Office	Burton	Saunders	2004	978-0-7216-3935-2
Insurance Handbook for the Medical Office, 10th Edition	Fordney	Saunders	2008	978-1-4160-3666-1

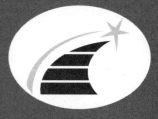

Trust **Carol J. Buck** and **Elsevier** for the resources you need at *each step* of your coding career!

Track your progress toward complete coding success!

Step 1: Learn

Step-by-Step Medical Coding 2008 Edition • ISBN: 978-1-4160-4567-0
Workbook for Step-by-Step Medical Coding 2008 Edition • ISBN: 978-1-4160-4568-7
Medical Coding Online for Step-by-Step Medical Coding 2008 • ISBN: 978-1-4160-5539-6
Virtual Medical Office for Step-by-Step Medical Coding 2008 Edition • ISBN: 978-1-4160-3040-9

Step 2: Practice

The Next Step, Advanced Medical Coding: A Worktext 2008 Edition • ISBN: 978-1-4160-4042-2
Advanced Medical Coding Online for the Next Step: Medical Coding 2008 Edition • ISBN: 978-1-4160-5542-6

Step 3: Certify

CCS Coding Exam Review 2008: The Certification Step • ISBN: 978-1-4160-3683-8
CCS-P Coding Exam Review 2008: The Certification Step • ISBN: 978-1-4160-3692-0
CPC Coding Exam Review 2008: The Certification Step • ISBN: 978-1-4160-3711-8
CPC-H Coding Exam Review 2008: The Certification Step • ISBN: 978-1-4160-3721-7
The Extra Step: Facility-Based Coding Practice • ISBN: 978-1-4160-3450-6
The Extra Step: Physician-Based Coding Practice • ISBN: 978-1-4160-3451-3

Step 4: Specialize

Evaluation and Management Step: An Auditing Tool • ISBN: 978-1-4160-3596-1

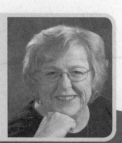

Coding References

Saunders 2008 ICD-9-CM, Volumes 1 and 2, Professional Edition • ISBN: 978-1-4160-4414-7
Saunders 2008 ICD-9-CM, Volumes 1, 2, and 3, Professional Edition • ISBN: 978-1-4160-4413-0
Saunders 2008 ICD-9-CM, Volumes 1 and 2, Standard Edition • ISBN: 978-1-4160-4416-1
Saunders 2008 ICD-9-CM, Volumes 1, 2, and 3, Standard Edition • ISBN: 978-1-4160-4415-4
Saunders 2008 HCPCS Level II • ISBN: 978-1-4160-4892-3

Get the next resource on your list today!

- Order securely at **www.elsevierhealth.com**
- Call toll-free **1-800-545-2522**
- Visit your local bookstore

ELSEVIER